HEALTH AT THE CROSSROADS

TRANSPORT POLICY AND URBAN HEALTH

London School of Hygiene & Tropical Medicine
Fifth Annual Public Health Forum

HEALTH AT THE CROSSROADS

TRANSPORT POLICY AND URBAN HEALTH

Edited by
Tony Fletcher and Anthony J. McMichael

Series Editor
Barbara M. Judge

*London School of Hygiene
& Tropical Medicine, London, UK*

JOHN WILEY & SONS

Chichester · New York · Brisbane · Toronto · Singapore

Other Wiley Editorial Offices

John Wiley & Sons, Inc., 605 Third Avenue,
New York, NY 10158-0012, USA

Jacaranda Wiley Ltd, 33 Park Road, Milton,
Queensland 4064, Australia

John Wiley & Sons (Canada) Ltd, 22 Worcester Road,
Rexdale, Ontario M9W 1LI, Canada

John Wiley & Sons (Asia) Pte Ltd, 2 Clementi Loop #02-01,
Jin Xing Distripark, Singapore 129809

Library of Congress Cataloging-in-Publication Data

London School of Hygiene and Tropical Medicine Public Health Forum
(5th : 1995 : London, England)
   Health at the crossroads : transport policy and urban health /
edited by Tony Fletcher and Anthony J. McMichael.
      p.   cm.
   "London School of Hygience & Tropical Medicine Fifth Annual
Public Health Forum."
   Forum held in April 1995, London.
   Includes bibliographical references and index.
   ISBN 0-471-96272-4 (hbk : alk. paper)
   1. Urban transportation policy—Health aspects—Congresses.
   2. Urban transportation—Health aspects—Congresses.
   I. Fletcher, Tony.   II. McMichael, Anthony, J.   III. Title.
   RA615.L66 1995
   614—dc20   96–4969
                                                        CIP

British Library Cataloguing in Publication Data

A catalogue record for this book is available from the British Library

ISBN 0-471-96272-4

Typeset in 10/12pt Times from the author's disks by Vision Typesetting, Manchester
Printed and bound in Great Britain by Biddles Ltd, Guildford and King's Lynn
This book is printed on acid-free paper responsibly manufactured from sustainable forestation, for which at least two trees are planted for each one used for paper production.

Contents

Contributors

Ross Anderson, Department of Public Health Sciences, St George's Hospital Medical School, Cranmer Terrace, London SW17 0RE, UK.

John R. Ashton, Director of Public Health, North West Regional Health Authority, 930–932 Birchwood Boulevard, Millennium Park, Warrington WA3 7QN, UK.

Philip H. Bly, Research Director, Transport Research Laboratory, Old Wokingham Road, Crowthorne, Berkshire RG45 6AU, UK.

Ekkehard Brühning, Bundesanstahlt für Straβenwesen, Postfach 100150, 51401 Bergisch Gladbach 1, Germany.

Bert Brunekreef, Department of Epidemiology & Public Health, Agricultural University of Wageningen, PO Box 238, NL-6700 AE Wageningen, Netherlands.

Jørgen Bunde, Head of Traffic Planning, City Engineer's Office, Århus Council, Stansingeniørens kontor, Orla Lehmanns Alle 3, Postboks 539, 8100 Århus C, Denmark.

Kenneth J. Button, Professor of Applied Economics and Transport, Centre for Research in European Economics and Finance, Economics Department, University of Loughborough, Loughborough, LE11 3TU, UK.

Jake Ferguson, Drugs Services, 112 Hampstead Road, London NW1 2LT, UK.

Tony Fletcher, Environmental Epidemiology Unit, London School of Hygiene & Tropical Medicine, Keppel Street, London WC1E 7HT, UK.

David Gee, WBMG Environmental Communications, 28 Broomwood Road, London SW11 6HT, UK.

Gregory Goldstein, Urban Environmental Health Programme, World Health Organization, CH-1211 Geneva 27, Switzerland.

Philip B. Goodwin, ESRC Transport Studies Unit, University of Oxford, 11 Bevington Road, Oxford OX2 6NB, UK.

Daniel S. Greenbaum, President, Health Effects Institute, 141 Portland Street, Cambridge, MA 02139, USA.

Carmen Hass-Klau, Transport Consultant, Environment and Transport Planning, Stanford House, 9 South Road, Brighton BN1 6SB, UK.

Mayer Hillman, Senior Fellow Emeritus, Policy Studies Institute, 100 Park Village East, London NW1 3SR, UK.

Godfrey D. Jacobs, Programme Director–Overseas, Transport Research Laboratory, Old Wokingham Road, Crowthorne, Berkshire RG45 6AU, UK.

Klea Katsouyanni, University of Athens Medical School, Dept of Hygiene & Epidemiology, 75 Mikras Asias Street, 115 27 Goudi, Athens, Greece.

Jeffrey R. Kenworthy, Lecturer in Urban Environments, Institute for Science & Technology Policy, Murdoch University, Perth, Western Australia 6150, Australia.

Mark McCarthy, Director of Public Health, Camden and Islington Health Authority, 110 Hampstead Road, London NW1 2LJ, UK.

Anthony J. McMichael, Head, Epidemiology Unit, London School of Hygiene & Tropical Medicine, Keppel Street, London WC1E 7HT, UK.

Dinesh Mohan, Head, Centre for Biomedical Engineering, Indian Institute of Technology, New Delhi 110016, India.

René Neuenschwander, ECOPLAN, Seidenweg 63, CH-3012 Bern, Switzerland.

Isabelle Romieu, Pan American Center of Human Ecology and Health, Pan American Health Organization, Apartado 37-473, 06696 Mexico D.F., Mexico.

Joel Schwartz, Department of Environmental Health, Harvard School of Public Health, 665 Huntington Avenue, Boston, 02115 MA, USA.

Jens Steensberg, Public Health Medical Officer, Embedslægeinstitutionen Frederiksborg AMT, Kongens Vænge 4, 3400 Hillerød, Denmark.

Stefan Suter, ECOPLAN, Seidenweg 63, CH-3012 Bern, Switzerland.

Anthony R. Taig, Business Development Director, Utilities & Infrastructure AEA Technology Consultancy Services, Thomson House, Risley, Warrington WA3 6AT, UK.

Geetam Tiwari, Applied Systems Research Programme, Indian Institute of Technology, New Delhi 110016, India.

Felix Walter, ECOPLAN, Seidenweg 63, CH-3012 Bern, Switzerland.

John Whitelegg, Ecologica Limited, 713 Cameron House, White Cross, Lancaster LA1 4XQ, UK.

Foreword

By the
Rt Hon. the Baroness Chalker of Wallasey,
Minister for Overseas Development

The Overseas Development Administration (ODA) is delighted to be associated with the London School's Annual Public Health Forum, and subsequently this publication, on a topic which is of increasing concern to people of many disciplines in both developed and developing countries.

There are three main areas where transport policy impacts on urban health and all are covered in the forum papers. The first is the effect of vehicle exhausts on air pollution and the consequent effect on human health. The second is the effect of traffic management and congestion on personal injury accidents and the third is related to health benefits arising from encouraging the use of non-motorized transport.

In the 1950s less than one third of the world's population lived in urban areas, but by the year 2000 it is forecast that this proportion will rise to over 50%. Over two thirds of the world's urban population will be living in cities of the developing world that already have great difficulty in feeding, housing, providing medical services and transporting the millions who live there.

In many cities, but especially in the developing world, the rapid increase in population, coupled with limited finance for investment in urban services, has produced severe transport and environmental problems.

By the year 2000 it is expected that 23 cities worldwide will have populations over 10 million. As cities grow, travel distances increase, and so the demand for motorised travel continues to rise. With public transport struggling to keep pace, motor vehicle ownership keeps on rising, leading to congested city streets and a host of other environmental problems. This brings with it an increasing economic and environmental cost that is often paid by those least able to afford it.

Health is affected by pollution. There is a close link between the lead content of petrol and average blood lead levels. Emissions of fine particles in vehicle exhaust have been associated with increases in deaths from respiratory illness and heart disease. Emissions from motor vehicles contribute to wind borne acid deposition, and other pollutants affect the ozone layer.

In the developing world, continuing increases in traffic will cancel out improvements in vehicle emissions. Good traffic-management measures are needed to ease congestion and the air quality problems that it brings.

Independent studies by both the World Health Organization and the ODA have estimated that about 500 000 people worldwide lose their lives each year as a result of road accidents and over 15 million suffer injuries. The majority of these, about 70%, occur in low- or middle-income countries.

While the road-accident situation is slowly improving in high-income countries, for most developing countries accidents are increasing. In Thailand, for example, more years of potential life are lost through road accidents than from tuberculosis and malaria combined. In Mexico, accidents as a cause of death rose from 4% in 1955 to 11% in 1980, with traffic accidents predominating.

ODA-funded research has shown that road accidents annually cost any nation, whether developing or developed, about 1% of its gross national product (GNP). Collectively, this suggests that the global annual cost of road accidents is approximately $230 US billion; and 60% of these accidents occur in urban areas.

In developing countries, there are major challenges associated with the development of efficient cities. The benefits are very high, since most of a country's GNP is generated in urban areas, but the cost of pollution and accidents is also very steep.

A truly effective framework for decision-making in this field will only be achieved when researchers can put values on all the costs and benefits. This is not easy. However, people will only be convinced of the need for painful measures if they are presented with sound economic and scientific arguments.

Good interdisciplinary research is vital if we are to produce solutions to these problems. The Annual Public Health Forum and this publication are an important part of that process.

In conclusion, you may wish to know that recently ODA has formed a new 'Urban Development Focus Group' from its specialist advisers in many disciplines. The issue of Transport Policy and Urban Health is one of the subject areas which will be kept under constant review by that group.

Preface

This volume comprises papers presented at the Fifth Annual Public Health Forum held in April 1995 at the London School of Hygiene & Tropical Medicine, entitled *Health at the Crossroads: Transport Policy and Urban Health*. This notion of 'Health at the Crossroads' was chosen to imply not only that a choice needs to be made about what level of health impacts is tolerated, but also that health concerns are now helping to influence policy, a trend we are seeking to reinforce. There is an increasing awareness that human health and well-being is in a complex way affected by transport arrangements, with arguably the disbenefits outweighing the benefits, especially for certain vulnerable subgroups. Public health professionals need to appreciate better these complex inter-relationships. The Forum and this book come at a time when it appears that concerns about health impacts are starting to filter through more substantially to policy-makers, and influencing their choices. If there was one over-riding objective in organizing the Forum it was to try and place more firmly on the map the place of health impacts in the policy-making arena. This volume contributes to that process.

The Public Health Forum, the fifth in the series organized by the School, brought together over 200 people interested in the dialogue between transport policy-makers, members of local and national government, non-governmental organizations, and public health professionals. They discussed important questions, including: Can we better understand the positive and negative consequences of transport planning decisions on public health? Can we feed that understanding back into the policy process? Taking the enormous diversity of experience what can we learn from experiments in urban transport policy already undertaken?

This Forum would not have been viable without the generous support of our sponsors who contributed directly to the Forum and to the travel costs of overseas participants. We are especially grateful to the UK Overseas Development Administration who contributed in both respects, and to the Health Education Authority, who have funded this publication. Other sponsors include the Commission of the European Communities, the Health Effects Institute, The Wellcome Trust and the British Council.

We are grateful to the Forum Executive Committee, and to the following individuals who were particularly helpful in the development of the programme: Professor Charles Normand, Dr Carolyn Stephens, Dr Philip Goodwin and Ms Lynn Sloman.

Alice Dickens, the Conference Organizer, once again demonstrated her expertise and hard work in the organization and smooth running of the Forum. We are also indebted to her for her contribution to the production of this book.

Tony Fletcher
Anthony J. McMichael
Barbara M. Judge

1
Introduction

Tony Fletcher and Anthony J. McMichael

London School of Hygiene & Tropical Medicine, UK

The world's cities are growing in size nearly everywhere. As a result, urban transport systems and patterns of population mobility are evolving restlessly and rapidly. In particular, car ownership and travel have increased spectacularly over the past half-century, creating new freedoms, new opportunities—and new social and public health problems.

At one level, car-dominated city traffic looks to be a clear-cut, discrete, public health problem. Technical and engineering solutions could therefore be sought. However, at another level, it is a manifestation of what many people now recognize as a wider malaise of modern cities, and as a part of the general overloading of the world's ecological systems as human populations consume more materials, more energy, more space, and generate more effluent. Most of us prefer the former, narrower-visioned, view, as part of an unquestioned expectation that private motorized transport is essential to our foreseeable future. Yet it is becoming clear that the issue is more complex, the need to re-think city life and form is becoming more urgent, and in any case, the range of adverse public health impacts of prevailing patterns of urban transport is greater than is usually thought.

So, how has this urban transport situation arisen? The reasons for the burgeoning move from non-motorized, and latterly from public motorized, transport to private cars are many. They include: gains in average personal wealth; an increase in leisure time; the seductive imagery of advertising; the techno-industrial culture of road-building; deterioration in public transport facilities; greater mobility of women outside the home; a growth in the proportion of elderly retired persons likely to prefer the convenience and safety of the private car; and, in Western countries, the superseding of the urbanization phase of city development by the ('edge city') decentralization of place-of-residence, work and shopping.

Assessing the overall public health burden attributable to urban transport is a kaleidoscopic task. While much of the public concern in developed countries is

Health at the Crossroads: Transport Policy and Urban Health.
Edited by Tony Fletcher and Anthony J. McMichael © 1997 John Wiley & Sons Ltd

focused on the effects of exhaust emissions on respiratory health (especially childhood asthma), and much of the concern in developing countries is over the escalating rate of physical injury and death, there are four broad categories of health hazard from car traffic. Exhaust emissions cause a range of toxic effects: respiratory disorders, exacerbated heart disease, lead-impaired child intellectual development, and, via fine particulates, increased deaths. Emissions also contribute to acid rain and to the global 'greenhouse' accumulation of carbon dioxide, each of which have wide-ranging consequences for health. Fatal and non-fatal injuries affect pedestrians, cyclists and car-users—and the hazards to children tend to be much greater in poorer areas of cities in both rich and poor countries. Meanwhile, the chronic, traffic-related effects of fragmented neighbourhoods, intrusive noise and restricted exercise impair various other aspects of health.

The benefits of freedom and comfort conferred by private car use are clear. But we live in an increasingly car-dominated society in which the debits, assessed comprehensively, have come to outweigh the credits. Not surprisingly, tourists in Europe find car-restricted cities—such as Amsterdam, Bremen, Copenhagen and Delft—to be havens of safety and sanity compared to cities elsewhere. London, Athens, Los Angeles, Taipei and Bangkok have become symbols of traffic blight. The Los Angeles car debacle has prompted Californian law-makers to require a phased move away from combustion-engine cars to electric cars. Part of notoriously air-polluted downtown Athens, in 1995, went car-free; residents and retailers liked the results—despite their initial misgivings about adverse effects on convenience and commerce.

We must re-think the role and form of city living and, therefore, of urban transport. As is argued by various contributors to this book, the documented detrimental effects of urban transport upon our health, safety and quality of life makes the need for change overwhelming. It is not just that motor vehicles have transformed the physical urban environment and the quality of its air; they also contribute increasingly to global pressures on the world's atmosphere and future climate and to the declining sustainability of expanding cities.

The phrase 'sustainability of cities' needs critical consideration. Human settlements, by their nature, make demands on the surrounding land, air, water, food and other natural resources. The more consumption-based is the lifestyle of citizens, the wider is the environmental area and the greater is the supply of resources needed to sustain that settlement. Settlements that consume no more than can be replaced, whether by natural or managed processes, could continue indefinitely. They are therefore 'sustainable'.

In modern culture, however, with its physical and electronic interconnections between populations around the world, the sustainability equation is no longer based on fixed localized relationships. Furthermore, the dynamic balance between input, consumption and effluent is influenced by changes in human aspirations and technology. Nevertheless, there is a recurring and escalating problem: the typical modern urban population attains an *apparent* sustainability by dint of inputs of materials and energy from distant, often vulnerable, sources. (Consider the well-known example of US imports of beef produced in the erstwhile rainforest regions of Central America. Likewise, the world's urban car fleet requires massive inputs of materials, oil and industrial energy, the winning of which entails diverse stresses upon distant environments.) Such environmental damage or depletion beyond the urban horizon can only mean that, in fact, the 'sustainability' of the privileged urban population is illusory.

As urbanization and its wider-ranging environmental impacts become global, we must re-define 'sustainability' within a closed-system context. The global aggregate ('bottom line') equation must be balanced for the world *in toto*. Indeed, in an equitable world, each large city would achieve a balanced lifestyle with zero-sum impact within and beyond its regional environment. The management of urban transport everywhere, with its potential impacts on resources, environment and health, will be a crucial part of this global sustainability.

As national governments are (somewhat begrudgingly) recognizing, there is a particular and urgent need to curb greenhouse gas emissions. This must include reducing carbon dioxide emissions from motorized transport. In developed countries, cars contribute around one-quarter of all such emissions at a national level. Internal combustion engines in cars and trucks, and the fossil fuel burning power-plants that supply electricity to rail-borne transport, are a central part of our modern dependence on this source of stored (non-renewable) energy. In view of the acknowledged serious potential consequences for human health and well-being of a greenhouse-warming world over the coming century or two, we would have our priorities wrong if we worried only about the immediate health impacts of toxic exhaust emissions, physical injury and social–environmental disruption.

Yet there is a morally and politically difficult international issue lurking here. Today's 'developed' countries were yesterday's 'developing' countries, and, in making the transition, they have incurred substantial ecological debts: they have emitted most of the currently accumulated greenhouse gases, done most of the damage to the ozone layer, and exerted much of the pressure on the world's forests, farmlands and fisheries. The rich countries may now forswear the profligate use of fossil fuels, but what concession is to be made to those developing countries (China, India, Indonesia, and other smaller developing countries) whose level of *per capita* usage is still a long way behind? This has become one of the main sticking points in recent international climate-change negotiations.

Meanwhile, reverting to a more familiar problem, the public policy dilemma over patterns of urban transport is increasing in developing countries. In many of their large cities, air quality is poor and the risk of physical injury in heterogeneous and poorly controlled traffic is high. Yet, the surge of car ownership appears unstoppable, as developing countries accumulate wealth, modernize, and become fully paid-up members of today's much-vaunted free-market world economy.

Contradictions emerge. While public investment in roads and highways is encouraged via international loans, international agencies urge a multipronged approach to road safety, including the expansion of public transport. So, economic and social values appear to come into conflict.

Shifts in the approach taken by economists may reduce this apparent conflict, as new brands of economics emerge which do not merely take the endless expansion of 'Gross National Product' as an unquestioned goal. An economics which attempts to cost the 'externalities' of transport, such as the values assigned to resource depletion, adverse health effects and long-term environmental impacts, will more fully reflect the overall costs of road transport. An awareness of these external costs appear to be filtering through to policy makers. Doubts clearly remain whether price mechanisms, even with the extra costs forced in, can deliver the improved environment that many yearn for, especially for targets such as environmental equity and the preservation of the long-term sustainability of human health. Visionary large scale planning that reduces car dependence or unnnecessary road freight at a national and international level is necessary.

The case studies presented in this book well illustrate the beneficial and deleterious impacts of government actions and inactions in the transport policy arena. At a local level, popular pressure for improved quality of urban living, reinforced by concerns raised by Agenda 21, are leading to many imaginative initiatives. Networks such as that organized in the framework of the WHO *Health Cities* programme or the Car Free Cities Networks, among many others, lead to a publicizing and sharing of experience. We see a convergence of interest between those concerned with public health, the environment and engineering—perhaps enough to overcome the barriers of language in these often separated sectors. This volume is a contribution to that multi-disciplinary effort to improve our environment, health, life expectancy and quality of life.

SECTION 1

POLLUTION AND HEALTH

2
Introduction

Tony Fletcher and Anthony J. McMichael

London School of Hygiene & Tropical Medicine, UK

Around the world, cars are displacing industry as the major source of urban air pollution. As the profile of inhaled air pollutants changes, epidemiologists have striven to differentiate and quantify the impacts upon health. This has not been easy: the exposures are complex; they impinge on whole communities; the measurement of cumulative personal exposure is always difficult; and confounding factors (especially smoking and occupation) lie in ambush for the unwary.

This section examines the nature of these health hazards and the attendant problems for science and society. McMichael reviews the rise of urban transport as a source of health hazards, and the limitations of prevailing research designs. He queries the reliance on time-series analyses and (for the study of mortality) the meaning of their measures of short-term 'effect'. He emphasizes the need to consolidate disparate research findings into quantitative estimates of population-level risk, to help policy-makers make decisions. Gee explores the many types of uncertainty to be dealt with: the intrinsic uncertainty of all science; the uncertainties in constructing dose–response relationships from multiple studies and disciplines; and the philosophical uncertainties about whether to act sceptically (thus allowing profligate exposure) or prudently. He argues for prudence, and that proof-of-causation at the level of the 'balance of probabilities' is appropriate.

Katsouyanni describes the types of research question addressed in air pollution epidemiology, and then systematically classifies and explains the types of study designs used. The different roles and attributes of population-level ('ecological') and individual-level ('analytic') studies are discussed critically. Much of the recent sophistication in research methods, especially in such matters as exposure assessment and the handling of interactive effects, has been driven by the need to study exposures lower than those of earlier decades.

Schwartz takes two major contemporary air pollutants—particulates and ozone—and reviews the rapidly expanding health effects literature on each. Particulates are of special interest because of recent evidence, from US studies, of

Health at the Crossroads: Transport Policy and Urban Health.
Edited by Tony Fletcher and Anthony J. McMichael © 1997 John Wiley & Sons Ltd

substantial risks of death (especially from heart and lung disease) at levels often encountered in today's cities. He concentrates on the short-term impacts on daily deaths and hospital admissions of acute increases in exposure to each of these two pollutants. Anderson, reviewing further some of these same issues, examines the following: the uses and limitations of time-series analyses; how better to deal with complex mixed exposures; and the need to consider the underlying biology. He points out that UK asthma rates have increased in recent decades while levels of SO_2 and total particulates have declined. Maybe, he suggests, certain particulate fractions contribute to exacerbating (but not causing) asthma, along with modern car-associated photochemical oxidant pollutants (such as ozone).

Turning to policy-setting, Romieu reviews the rationale for air quality guidelines and standards. The former are indicative; helpful for defining targets. The latter should be enforceable, directed at specified sources. She explores the contribution of science to their development, and the interface with quantitative risk assessment (QRA). By summarizing population-wide risks, QRA informs the setting of 'standards' that would attain socially acceptable levels of risk. Romieu also considers the use of these several criteria to monitor population exposure and changes in health risk. Brunekreef then notes that, while guidelines propose 'safe' exposures, standards usually entail compromise borne of cost–benefit analysis and technical limitations. Guidelines are never based on full knowledge; 'safeness' entails knowing how to define adverse effect; and a somewhat arbitrary margin-of-safety is needed to protect susceptible subgroups. Brunekreef also reminds us that certain limitations of air pollution epidemiology (and hence the reliance on experimental exposure-chamber studies or high-exposure occupational studies) limit the confidence with which guidelines and standards can be proposed.

3
Transport and health: assessing the risks

Anthony J. McMichael

London School of Hygiene & Tropical Medicine, UK

When we cross a busy road, we reflexly assess the *personal* risk involved. In contrast, public health research addresses health risks at the *population* level. There are several senses in which 'risk' is used. They are: as a *probability* measure by statisticians and gamblers; as an *impact* measure of 'damage' to health (i.e. product of probability times severity); and to reflect, in the lay mind, the *acceptability* of that impact, as influenced, for example, by differences in the familiarity and controllability of the perceived risks.

Assessing the risk to population health from an environmental health hazard requires quantitative information from epidemiological research. Boundaries must also be defined, since 'risk' can be conceived of either in a local or in a more all-embracing context. We typically ignore the 'externalized' environmental and health costs of urban transport, such as those associated with extracting and transporting oil, mining metals, manufacturing vehicles and building roads. Some of those externalized, and substantial, risks may accrue remotely (McMichael *et al.*, 1994).

This chapter examines some of the epidemiological evidence of health risks in relation to transport patterns, the associated research difficulties, and how research results can be used to predict the aggregate health risk in other (perhaps distant) populations. The chapter focuses on health hazards from cars, which dominate the world's urban transport—as evidenced by the following statistics. Since 1950, the worldwide number of private cars has increased from around 50 million to 500 million. Cars produce 40–80% of various major air pollutants (Holman, 1994) and around 20% of two major heat-trapping gases (carbon dioxide and chlorofluorocarbons) (OECD, 1994). Roads, highways, garages and

Health at the Crossroads: Transport Policy and Urban Health.
Edited by Tony Fletcher and Anthony J. McMichael © 1997 John Wiley & Sons Ltd

parking lots now occupy about 10% of all arable space in the USA (Renner, 1988). In the UK, as population has increased by 15% since mid-century so car travel has increased tenfold (Great Britain Department of Transport, 1993). Meanwhile, bus travel in the UK has halved, train travel has remained constant, and bicycle travel has declined fivefold.

In the UK, the Department of Transport forecasts that, by 2025, there will be at least a doubling in national traffic (Great Britain Department of Transport, 1989)—although the Great Britain Royal Commission on Environmental Pollution (1994) deemed such an increase environmentally unmanageable. The OECD anticipates that: 'policies for urban land use and travel in operation in all OECD countries will lead to increased use of cars and trucks. The same is true of Central Europe, South-East Asia and other developing countries. In all of them, the trend is towards urban dispersal, growing car travel and increasing road-goods distribution' (OECD, 1994).

Clearly, there are strong commercial, economic, political and cultural determinants of urban transport patterns. In that robust company, if the assessment of transport-related health risks is to influence transport policy it is essential that:

1. Good studies are done on the health impacts of urban transport.
2. Researchers, policy-makers and interest groups learn how to deal with the uncertainties that surround all science (including epidemiological research, done in an unavoidably noisy real-world).
3. The research results are synthesized, for application to assessing the wider risk to public health.
4. The results of such health risk assessments, and their limitations, are conveyed clearly to participants in the risk management process.

Adverse health impacts of urban transport: an overview

Motor vehicle air pollution

Various health hazards arise from transport-related air pollution. The main hazards, from the exhausts of cars, lorries and buses, arise from particulates and from nitrogen dioxide, volatile organics and their photochemical progeny (principally ozone). The traffic-associated brown-yellow photochemical smog occurs primarily in summer, in temperate climates, when anticyclonic conditions enhance the photochemical activation of becalmed air pollutants. They occur frequently in large traffic-filled cities, such as Los Angeles, Taipei, Mexico City, Athens and Milan. In winter, nitrogen dioxide-rich smogs can occur (as in London in December 1991 and 1994). While such pollutants predominate in many Western cities, more diverse air pollution (characterized by sulphur dioxide, particulates and acid aerosols) from a mix of industry, power-generation, cars and heavy vehicles, afflicts cities such as Mexico City, São Paulo, Bangkok,

Seoul, Shanghai and Jakarta. These various pollutants have adverse effects upon the respiratory and cardiovascular systems.

Photochemical oxidants and acid aerosols also adversely affect crops and waterways—which may then affect food and water supplies. Some transport-related air pollutants (especially CO_2) also affect the heat-trapping properties of the lower atmosphere, and may thus contribute to global climate change (Great Britain Royal Commission on Environmental Pollution, 1994), which may have a range of longer-term and wide-ranging adverse impacts on human health (Last, 1993; McMichael, 1993). These risks are much less easy to identify and quantify than those due to direct-acting toxicological effects. Further, they entail forecasts of more distant future risks to population health.

Road trauma

Motor vehicle crashes account for an increasing global burden of injury and death, particularly in developing countries and in Central-Eastern Europe. Yearly, road traffic crashes (including with pedestrians) cause around 850 000 deaths (Murray and Lopez, 1994; World Bank, 1993). Young people (especially males) and the elderly are particularly vulnerable, as are pedestrians and—especially in developing countries—drivers of non-motorized vehicles. The World Bank estimates that road trauma accounts for over 2% of the estimated total global burden of impaired health (World Bank, 1993).

In the UK, transport currently causes almost 40% of 'accidental' deaths; mostly from road crashes. Even so, mortality from road crashes in developed countries has generally declined markedly in recent decades. In the UK, for example, deaths have halved in the past thirty years, and injuries have declined by one-third (Great Britain Royal Commission on Environmental Pollution, 1994). Meanwhile, road fatalities and injuries in developing countries are rising rapidly with urbanization and growth in traffic (World Bank, 1993; PAHO, 1994).

The roads are particularly risky for cyclists, who share the roads with fast-moving, momentum-rich, motor vehicles. In the UK, the death rate per unit distance travelled is approximately ten times higher for bicyclists than for car travellers (OECD, 1994). This rate is two to three times higher than for cyclists in the Netherlands, Sweden or Denmark, presumably because the higher prevalence of cyclists makes them less likely to be overlooked by motorists—on a road layout that is more cyclist-friendly anyway (Transport 2000, 1992; Great Britain Royal Commission on Environmental Pollution, 1994).

Noise

Noise causes annoyance and stress, disturbs sleep, and may marginally affect blood pressure (World Health Organization, 1980; Rylander, 1992). In Roman times, nocturnal noise from iron wheels on paved roads was regulated. In mediaeval Europe, horse riding and carriages were forbidden at night in certain cities on behalf of the sleeping citizenry. Today, the problem is much greater. Noise confronts us from industry, transport, amusement centres, and over the back-fence.

Transport is the most pervasive source of noise in the UK daily environment (Great Britain Royal Commission on Environmental Pollution, 1994). Objective surveys of types of noise impinging on houses show that road transport noise is much more prevalent than aircraft or railway noise. Surveys of people's perceptions show that road traffic is the major source of nuisance noise, followed by aircraft and, rather less, by railways. Epidemiological studies have shown that noise disturbs sleep patterns and, consequently, mood, functioning, and symptoms (headaches, fatigue, etc.). One study, comparing people living in quiet and noisy residential areas, found clear differences in sleep disturbance and in impairments of healthy functioning (Ohrstrom, 1989). Peak noise, above 45 dB(A), appears to cause most of the problem, suggesting that large proportions of urban populations are regularly disturbed while asleep. The OECD describes noise levels above 55 dB(A) as undesirable, and, thus, almost half of the urban population in countries of the European Union is adversely affected by road traffic noise (OECD, 1994).

Disruption of social relations and neighbourhoods

The needs of the automobile now dominate city landscapes throughout the developed world. Two-thirds of inner Los Angeles is devoted to roads and parking lots. Residential communities are surgically divided by roads and freeways. The proportion of UK primary school children walking to school has declined by a precipitous tenfold since 1970 (Hillman and Adams, 1992). Corner stores and neighbourhood shops, once within easy walking or cycling distance, have been widely superseded by soulless peri-suburban shopping centres. Peter Newman, an Australian urban-environmental scientist, observes that: 'The standard approach to [building] roads has been to see them as a conduit for traffic where little was allowed to get in the way of a smooth flow ... This is reductionist engineering that forces cities into a mould of concrete and bitumen, denying the importance of streets as meeting places, recreation areas, flora and fauna havens and the aesthetic glue that holds the city together'(Newman, 1992).

Air pollution: some research challenges

As urban settlements have grown, so has the public health problem of air pollution. Coal-burning was long the major source of air pollution in Europe. In 1661, the squire-diarist, Dr John Evelyn, attributed many of London's 'pulmonic distempers, coughs and importunate rheumatisms' to its filthy air and smoky fogs (Evelyn, 1661). Today, urban air pollution has become a worldwide health hazard, as industrialization and car ownership continue to spread.

The starting point for health risk assessment is the epidemiological estimation of risk in selected study populations. However, epidemiologists must heed four cautions:

1. Vehicle emissions almost always coexist with those of industry, power generation, and domestic activities. Hence it is difficult to study the effects of specific air pollutants.
2. Coincident exposures may interact. (For example, particulates and gaseous air pollutants may interact, since acidic gases are adsorbed to respirable particulates and can thus lodge within the lung.)
3. Although low-level exposures may not noticeably increase death rates, they may cause many other less easily documented non-fatal health disorders.
4. Most environmental hazards act 'directly' by toxicological, physical or infective mechanisms. However, pollutants may have serious *indirect* impacts on health. Consider, for example, fossil fuel combustion:
   - local pollutants cause respiratory disorders via toxicity;
   - acid rain has some regional effects, including those mediated by aerosol exposure and the acidification of waterways and topsoils; and
   - CO_2 emissions amplify the greenhouse effect. Consequent (anticipated) changes in global climate could have various adverse effects on human population health. Road traffic accounts for around one-quarter of Britain's greenhouse gas emissions (OECD, 1994).

To characterize some of the difficulties in aetiological research and in risk assessment, several examples are referred to briefly below: photochemical smog, carbon monoxide, particulates, airborne carcinogens and lead.

The range of adverse health effects of air pollutants

Air pollutants have various acute and longer-term adverse health effects. Short-term exposures can impair lung function, cause mucosal inflammation, increase tissue sensitivity to repeated exposure, and cause respiratory symptoms. Although the effects of short-term exposure are often reversible, repetition can damage tissues. The acute effects of short-term exposures have typically been studied in small groups of experimental subjects, or in locally enrolled panel studies, or by population-level time-series analysis of fluctuations in health events and exposure. In the latter two non-experimental types of study, it is often difficult to distinguish between the effects of coexistent pollutants.

Long-term or repeated exposure to air pollutants can cause chronic bronchitis, emphysema and lung fibrosis. These are best studied by community-based epidemiological studies that follow, over time, representative groups of exposed individuals. This type of study, in school-age children, has found that respiratory disorders and impaired lung function increase when particulates or SO_2 levels exceed around 100 μg/cubic metre (Romieu et al., 1990; Ware et al., 1986).

Long-term follow-up studies of adults have shown increased risks of death from exposure to these same pollutants (Dockery *et al.*, 1993; Ostro, 1993; Seaton *et al.*, 1995).

Photochemical smog: ozone and nitrogen dioxide

Photochemical smog (a variable mixture of ozone, NO_2 acid sulphate aerosol and other reactive gases) appears to cause various respiratory disorders. However, few good epidemiological studies have been able to yield specific evidence about the health effects of photochemical smog *per se*. In those Latin American cities most affected by complex photochemical air pollution, with a combined population of over 80 million, more than two million children may, in consequence, develop chronic cough each year, over 100 000 elderly may develop chronic bronchitis, and over 20 000 people may die because of air pollution (Romieu *et al.*, 1990). These, however, are very coarse-grained risk assessments.

Epidemiologists conventionally prefer to elucidate the health effects of individual constituent pollutants. This, while conforming to classical reductionism, may actually miss some of the real-world point. Nevertheless, what do we know about the effects of the two-man constituents of photochemical smog?

Ozone. Last century, Victorian Britons promenaded along the jetties of Brighton, believing that the ozone-laden sea air was doing them good. Today we treat this atmospheric gas more warily. Ozone is highly reactive; it can oxidize target molecules directly, and can create 'free radicals' that damage cell membranes. It has various acute effects upon the respiratory tract.

Ozone reacts rapidly with respiratory tissues, impeding lung functioning and causing structural or functional damage to cells (Tilton, 1989; Romieu, 1992). It affects the lungs at concentrations approximating current exposure standards in developed countries (0.1 ppm). In experimental studies, ozone concentrations of around 0.1–0.2 ppm impair lung functioning. Controlled chamber studies of ozone exposure in volunteer children demonstrate an exposure–response relationship between the effective dose of ozone and a symptom score (Avol *et al.*, 1987). The score comprised various respiratory and non-respiratory symptoms. A similar exposure–response relationship comes from controlled studies of effective ozone dose and change in FEV_1 (Romieu, 1992). However, these observations come from single-factor experiments and may not well describe how ozone behaves in the complex real world.

Ozone and other air pollutants may interact. In asthmatic children previously exposed to low concentrations of ozone, subsequent exposure to sulphur dioxide impairs lung functioning at concentrations that would otherwise have no effect (Koenig *et al.*, 1990). Ozone increases bronchial reactivity in asthmatics (Molfino *et al.*, 1991). The occurrence of these potentiating effects means that the various modelled estimates of exposure–response relationships for ozone and its respiratory effects (e.g. those of Ostro (1994)) can only be approximations, since the effect depends on levels of other pollutants.

The effects of long-term exposure to ozone are uncertain. Animal studies indicate progressive, persistent, inflammatory damage to respiratory epithelium (Tepper *et al.*, 1987). Epidemiological studies of US children repeatedly or chronically exposed to ambient ozone at concentrations at around 0.1 ppm show impaired lung function. However, these studies have had difficulty excluding coexistent effects of other air pollutants, and, in adults, occupational exposures and smoking (Romieu, 1992).

Nitrogen dioxide. The other dominant component of photochemical smog is nitrogen dioxide. Nitrogen dioxide is less biologically reactive than ozone and its effects are more delayed. It appears to impair deep lung function and to cause chest discomfort during deep breathing. Controlled studies of the effect of short-term exposure upon volunteer subjects, at around 500–2000 $\mu g/m^3$, show modest lung function changes in healthy individuals and evidence of greater responsiveness in asthmatics (Romieu, 1992).

Longer-term ambient exposure appears to increase respiratory symptoms and impaired lung functioning—although it is difficult to discount the effects of ambient co-pollutants. Hence, most of the epidemiologically-derived risk estimates have relied on studies of higher-level, simpler, indoor exposure, especially of children at home and at school. These studies indicate an increase in respiratory infection associated with high and persistent exposures. A meta-analysis of 11 such studies yielded an estimate of a 20% increase in respiratory infection occurrence for an increase in NO_2 exposure of 30 $\mu g/m^3$ (Romieu, 1992). However, to estimate the risks from outdoor exposures requires assuming that the risk function observed at higher exposures can reasonably be extrapolated to lower (ambient) exposures.

Carbon monoxide

Carbon monoxide (CO) is a colourless, odourless gas (which may account for the relatively little attention it has received as an air pollutant). Its concentrations are typically much higher in urban than in rural environments. Most urban CO comes from motor vehicle emissions, especially where vehicles lack catalytic converters and adequate maintenance. The in-vehicle concentrations of CO are much higher than those occurring at ambient monitoring sites (Peterson and Sabersky, 1975; Chan, 1991), and are positively correlated with traffic density and the slowness of traffic flow (Flachsbart and Brown, 1985; Flachsbart *et al.*, 1987; Koushki *et al.*, 1992). The exposure is several times higher for commuters in automobiles than in buses and light rail (Fernandez-Bremauntz, 1992).

CO in the blood competes with haemoglobin to bind with oxygen; by forming carboxyhaemoglobin (COHb) it lowers the oxygen-carrying capacity of blood.

Tissues sensitive to reduced oxygenation, such as the brain and heart, are thus jeopardized. However, ambient urban environmental exposures, particularly in non-smoking commuters, are unlikely to achieve the approximately 5% COHb that is associated with manifest adverse cardiovascular effects—except in situations of prolonged peak exposures to heavy traffic.

Epidemiological data specific to CO, especially at ambient environmental levels, are elusive. Controlled experiments of the effects of CO exposure on human subjects and toxicological experiments in animals have therefore been important. The main adverse health effect of CO is upon the cardiovascular system. As for many of the health effects of photochemical smog, there are few quantitative data; the epidemiological literature provides little exposure–response information about the relationship of CO exposure to the main health endpoints (Ostro, 1994). Without such empirical risk estimates, the quantitative assessment of the risk in other exposed populations is not possible.

Consistent clinical–experimental evidence shows that CO exposure induces exercise-induced angina in persons with pre-existing cardiovascular disease (CVD) (Anderson et al., 1973; Allred et al., 1989; Adams et al., 1988; Kleinman et al., 1989). The onset-to-angina time is reduced at 50–100 ppm CO and the duration of angina increases (Allred et al., 1991; Weir and Fabiano, 1982). Exposures at these levels therefore constrain the activity of persons with ischaemic heart disease. However, empirical epidemiological evidence of increased risks of actual cardiovascular disease events remains elusive. The evidence has either been positive but non-specific, as in cigarette smokers and traffic-tunnel workers (Stern et al., 1988), or inconclusive, as in foundry workers (Weir and Fabiano, 1982). CO exposure at 50–100 ppm also reduces exercise performance, measured as maximal oxygen uptake (Weir and Fabiano, 1982; Grant et al., 1993). This effect may marginally reduce the capacity for sustained work.

Air pollution and health: methodological issues in estimating risks

Ambient air pollution illustrates well the research challenge posed by a predominantly 'ecological' (that is, community-wide) exposure. The estimation of health risks due to air pollution typically relies on studies at the population level because it is difficult to make discriminating measures of exposure at the individual level. The three types of ecologically based study design are: cross-sectional correlation study, time-series analysis, and quasi-cohort follow-up study (in which individuals' exposure levels are deduced from some community-based measurement of exposure).

The *acute* health effects can be studied in a single population by time-series analysis of the correlation between short-term fluctuations in pollutant concentrations and health outcomes. It may also be possible to examine the cross-sectional correlation of location-specific mean pollutant levels and some index of acute health events (e.g. hospital admissions for asthma). Time-series analysis avoids the problem of inter-population confounding (e.g. due to variations in smoking prevalence or other unknown/unmeasured factors) that afflict cross-sectional ecological correlations. For this reason, and because of the often ready availability of historical single-city data sets, research into air pollution and health (especially mortality) has recently been dominated by time-series analyses.

In contrast, the study of *long-term* health effects (e.g. the incidence of chronic obstructive lung disease or death) usually requires comparison *between* populations or groups, exposed at different levels. Cross-sectional geographic correlation studies may illuminate these longer-term relationships, so long as current exposure levels are representative of past levels. However, much better are cohort-type studies in which detailed information (age, smoking, occupation, etc.) is obtained from sets of healthy individuals, exposed at different levels, and who are then followed up over time. The relationship between the three different study designs is illustrated in Figure 3.1.

Studies of acute effects and those of long-term effects address substantially different aetiological questions. This difference is best illustrated by the studies of mortality. The causation of life-shortening chronic disease by long-term exposure to air pollution entails a different biological process from the precipitation, by short-term severe exposure, of death in susceptible persons. Whereas the former influences the population's mean level of health (that is, disease prevalence), the latter refers more to the intra-population timing and distribution of individual deaths. Thus, long-term exposure of a population to air pollution may cause an

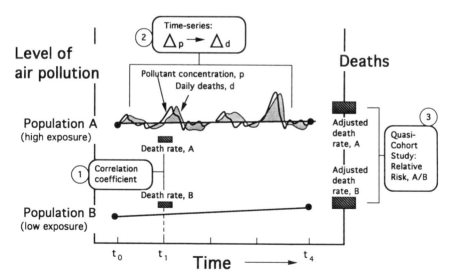

Figure 3.1 Approaches to estimating the mortality impact of air pollution. Diagrammatic representation of the three major, contrasting, study designs: cross-sectional correlation (ecological) studies, time-series studies, and cohort studies

increase in the prevalence of chronic respiratory disease and asthma and in mortality from cardiopulmonary diseases, while short-term fluctuations in air pollution may cause extra deaths among susceptible subgroups (e.g. those with pre-existing heart disease, or the elderly and frail), temporary increases in respiratory symptoms, and exacerbations of asthma in susceptible persons.

Perhaps this issue can be clarified by analogy. Around Europe, the *per capita* consumption of alcohol is positively correlated with mortality from liver cirrhosis. The underlying pathogenesis of cirrhosis takes decades. However, within one population (say France), the daily death rate from acute alcohol poisoning (plus accidental and violent deaths) is correlated with occasions of excessive drinking, such as holidays and football finals. The magnitude of that latter (time-series) correlation has little to do with the strength of the underlying longitudinal relationship between long-term consumption and the incidence of (eventually fatal) cirrhosis.

This distinction is well illustrated by reference to recent follow-up studies of mortality in persons with long-term exposure to particulates. The numerous time-series analyses of the correlation between daily fluctuations in fine particulate air pollution and mortality show that, for an increase in particulate concentration of 10 μg/m^3, there is an approximately 1% increase in daily deaths (Ostro, 1994). By contrast, two large cohort-based follow-up studies in the USA indicate that lifelong exposure to an extra 10 μg/m^3 of fine particulates entails a several-fold larger increase in mortality rates (Ostro, 1993; Pope *et al.*, 1995). The relationship between these two estimates of excess mortality risk per 10 μg/m^3 is still unclear—but clearly they address substantially different health-impact processes. Nevertheless, there has been some uncritical use of the first (acute) risk estimate to assess overall (including longer-term) population health risks (Ostro, 1994).

Further, many of the deaths from acute pollution episodes probably occur in susceptible people who would have died soon anyway. This short-term forward-displacement of deaths has been referred to (perhaps a little callously) as 'harvesting'. Recent research in Erfurt, East Germany, indicates that harvesting occurs for mortality from exposure to particulates but not SO$_2$ (Spix *et al.*, 1993). This idea is conceptually straightforward for mortality. But how much of the non-fatal health impact of short-term pollutant fluctuations is genuinely 'extra' (i.e. would not otherwise have occurred)? Most episode-associated visits to GPs are presumably 'extra'. Probably many hospital admissions are also 'extra'.

Quantitative risk assessment

Role and function

In 1994, *New Scientist* estimated that around 10000 deaths per year in the UK are due to particulates in urban air (Brown, 1994). This figure was based on the above-mentioned average impact of particulate-pollution episodes, as estimated from time-series analyses: i.e. a 10 μg/m^3 increase in particulate concentration causes a 1% increase in daily deaths. By knowing the average particulate levels in UK cities, and the annual total number of deaths in those cities, it was possible to calculate (predict) the number of particulates-induced deaths. For example, for London, with a particulate level of 29 $\mu g/m^3$ and approximately 66 000 deaths annually, the calculated excess number of deaths is (66 000 × 2.9%) = approximately 1900 deaths. The aggregate national urban total is 10 000 excess deaths. So, if half of the fine particulates comes from transport sources, then around 5000 of those deaths are attributable to transport emissions.

It is clear that such calculations entail simplified arithmetic, such as the assumption of an underlying exposure–response log-linearity. Further, acute mortality risks relating to brief exposure fluctuations have been used to predict risks from prolonged exposure to average levels of pollution. Nevertheless, the exercise is a modest illustration of quantitative risk assessment (QRA).

QRA has evolved, particularly within the modern North American regulatory environment, to assist the rational social management of public health risks. It strives for a data-based and objective estimation of the aggregate health risk posed to a specific population by some exposure factor. The role of QRA within the overall framework of risk assessment-and-management is shown in Figure 3.2.

Environmental epidemiological research typically estimates, from empirical data, the increased health risk associated with a specific exposure. Some studies, with detailed exposure data, allow definition of the exposure–response relationship. The subsequent application of these research-based risk estimates to predict the *aggregate* risk to a target population due to its known/estimated profile of exposure to that same factor is the essence of the QRA process (summarized in Table 3.1).

QRA, as a prediction of the exposure-induced additional health risk within the target population, entails a calculation similar to the epidemiologist's conventional population attributable risk (PAR). However, where the PAR refers a study-specific risk estimate back to its source population—and is thus strictly an exercise in *estimation*—QRA applies the literature-derived risk estimates to *predict* health impact in some new, perhaps distant, target population.

The derivation of the exposure–response relationship is often limited by a lack of prior epidemiological data pertaining to the lower exposure levels within the actual ambient environmental range. Further, there are often difficulties in extrapolating risks from the data-rich high-dose region to the data-poor low-dose region, or in extrapolating from experimental animals to humans. All such extrapolations introduce additional uncertainties and complexities into the QRA process.

Cancer risk assessment illustrates well these scientific difficulties. Typically, there is a need to extrapolate health risks via either of the following two excursions: (1) high human dose → low human dose; or (2) high animal dose → low animal dose → low human dose. The pitfalls in such extrapolation are well-known. Romieu (1992) cites a revealing example: model-based extrapolations of the

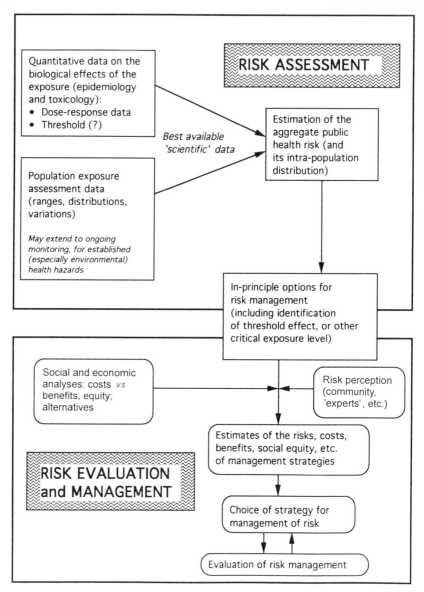

Figure 3.2 Assessing and managing public risks: the role of epidemiological research and quantitative risk assessment as input to policy-making

leukaemia risk from lifetime exposure to ambient airborne benzene at $1 \, \mu g/m^3$ show a 100-fold variation. Nevertheless, molecular biochemical and biological techniques are emerging that should reinforce QRA procedures and thus improve the prediction of cancer risk (IARC, in press).

Table 3.1 Quantitative risk assessment: four-point approach

1. Qualitative question: Is exposure X a hazard for health-outcome Y?
2. Determine X–Y exposure–response relationship (from epidemiological data and by extrapolation, as necessary, from cognate data)
3. Estimate profile of exposure to X of target population
4. 'Multiply' items 2 and 3 to estimate aggregate impact on population health

QRA example 1: Air pollution and lung cancer

Lung cancer is, numerically, only of minor concern in relation to traffic emissions. Some emissions (polycyclic aromatic hydrocarbons, benzene, and formaldehyde) may cause cancer. The topic, at least, affords insights into the possibilities for QRA.

The first experimental evidence that urban air pollutants could cause cancer came from animal bioassay studies (of mouse skin) in the 1940s (Leiter and Shear, 1942). Studies of human populations exposed to ambient air pollution, however, have provided little clear evidence of increased cancer risk. Perhaps at these low ambient concentrations any increased risk is too small for ready detection. Cancer risks are evident at much higher levels of exposure to some of the same pollutants. For example, diesel exhaust is associated with increased lung cancer risks in railway workers (Garshick *et al.*, 1988).

There is, nevertheless, some empirical epidemiological evidence of lung cancer risks in populations exposed to urban air pollution. Risks appear to be increased by around 10% by long-term exposure (Tomatis, 1990). A case-control study in heavily polluted Cracow, Poland, which assessed personal (residential) exposure to urban air pollution, occupational carcinogens and cigarette smoking, estimated that 4% of lung cancers in men and 10% in women were attributable to air pollution (Jedrychowski *et al.*, 1990).

The alternative approach entails the QRA-based aggregation of predicted risks for each constituent pollutant. From the published literature on each pollutant, the exposure–response relationship is estimated over the range of ambient environmental exposures. (This often entails back-extrapolation from observations in occupationally exposed humans or in experimental animals exposed at higher levels.) By combining each such estimate with information about the target population's exposure profile, pollutant-specific population health risks are predicted, and then summed. For example, the US Environmental Protection Agency estimated the number of cancers attributable to a real-world mix of 90 air pollutants (US Environmental Protection Agency, 1990). By aggregating pollutant-specific estimates, the Agency estimated an annual excess of 1700–2700 cases of cancer (mostly lung cancer) in the USA; that is, 10 cancer cases per million persons per year. Motor vehicle emissions would account for around 60% of these excess cancers.

QRA Example 2: Health impact of air lead exposure

Ostro has recently reviewed the health effects of various major air pollutants, including airborne lead (Ostro, 1994). For each pollutant and health outcome he has derived the average exposure–response relationship from the published literature. The aggregate excess burden of a specified health outcome within a population exposed to an increment of a particular air pollutant is given by:

$$dH_i = b_i * Pop_i * dA \qquad (1)$$

where: $\quad dH_i$ = change in aggregate risk of health effect i
$\qquad\qquad b_i$ = slope of exposure–response graph
$\qquad\qquad Pop_i$ = exposed population, at risk of health effect i
$\qquad\qquad dA$ = change in concentration of air pollutant, A

For example, to estimate the attributable loss of IQ points in an urban population of 40 000 young children exposed to an (avoidable) excess of 4 $\mu g/m^3$ of lead in air, the equation becomes:

$$dIQ = 0.975* 40\,000* 4 = 156\,000 \text{ IQ points} \qquad (2)$$

The b_i coefficient is (0.975) the air-lead equivalent of the average coefficient for blood-lead (PbB) concentration (i.e. 0.25 IQ points per 1 $\mu g/dl$ PbB), which measure of exposure has been used in nearly all epidemiological studies.

In populations with heterogeneous exposure, the aggregate health impact is predicted by summing the estimates given by the equation (1) for each of the differently exposed sub-populations. For example, if there were an adjoining rest-of-population 60 000 young children with an avoidable exposure of 3 $\mu g/m^3$ of lead in air, then their 'excess' IQ loss would (by equation (2)) be 175 500 IQ points.

Hence, the total 'excess' IQ loss in the combined population of 100 000 young children would be (156 000 + 175 500) = 331 500 IQ points. The average individual IQ loss would be 3.3 IQ points; and this would be greater in some residential areas than in others. This simplified example illustrates the process of population health risk assessment in relation to air pollution.

Conclusions

The quantitative assessment of health risk is a difficult, imperfect, exercise. But must we, in our dealings with policy-makers and general community, banish or hide the complexities and uncertainties? Of course not. Rather, we must all learn to accommodate and communicate the inherent uncertainties of population health risk assessment.

Quantitative risk assessment has manifest strengths and weaknesses (Romieu, 1992). The strengths are:

- It assists risk evaluation and priority-setting.
- It yields readily understood summary measures.
- It can be used for cost assessments, to evaluate control strategies.

The weaknesses are:

- Risk estimates are population-specific, and so extrapolation to other populations is risky.
- The mathematical derivation of the exposure–response function often entails debatable assumptions.
- A reductionist approach to risk estimation ignores potentially important interactive effects between coexistent exposures.
- The attribution of risk to a specific constituent factor within a complex exposure may be erroneous. The effects of coexistent exposures may be difficult to disentangle.

Technicalities aside, transport emissions clearly have many adverse health effects. As better and larger epidemiological studies are reported, as meta-analyses are done, as the complementarity and coherence of laboratory, clinical and epidemiological research becomes better understood, and as exposure–response estimation is enhanced by biological measures in toxicology and epidemiology, so our capacity to quantify these health risks improves. Meanwhile, if we consider the many adverse health impacts of car-dominated urban transport systems, and if we could reduce them to a bottom-line estimate of public health impact, then doubtless we would confirm the widespread, growing, view that this is not a healthy way for an urban society to live.

References

Adams KF, Koch G, Chattergee B et al., (1988) Acute elevation of blood carboxyhemoglobin to 6% impairs exercise performance and aggravates symptoms in patients with ischaemic heart disease. *Journal of American College of Cardiology, 12*, 900–909

Allred EN, Bleecker ER, Chaitman BR et al. (1989) Short-term effects of carbon monoxide exposure on the exercise performance of subjects with coronary artery disease. *New England Journal of Medicine, 321*, 1426–1432

Allred EN, Bleecker ER, Chaitman BR et al. (1991) Effects of carbon monoxide on myocardial ischaemia. *Environmental Health Perspectives, 91*, 89–132

Anderson EW, Andelman RJ, Strauch JM et al. (1973) Effects of low-level carbon monoxide exposure on onset and duration of angina pectoris. *Annals of Internal Medicine, 79*, 46–50

Avol EL, Linn WS, Shamoo DA et al. (1987) Short-term respiratory effects of photochemical oxidant exposure in exercising children *Journal of the Air Pollution Control Association, 37*, 158–162

Brown W (1994) Dying from too much dust. *New Scientist, 141*, 12–13

Chan C (1991) Driver exposure to volatile organic compounds, CO, ozone, and NO_2 under different driving conditions. *Environmental Science and Technology, 25*, 964–972

Dockery DW, Pope CA, Xu X, et al. (1993) An association between air pollution and mortality in six US cities. *New England Journal of Medicine, 329,* 1753–1759

Evelyn J (1661) *The Inconvenience of the Air and Smoke of London Dissipated, London 1661.* London 1661 (cited in Dubos R (1965) *Man Adapting.* Yale: Yale University Press)

Fernandez-Bremauntz A (1992) *Commuters' Exposure to Carbon Monoxide in the Metropolitan Area of Mexico City.* Centre for Environmental Technology, Imperial College of Science, Technology & Medicine, London. (PhD Thesis)

Flachsbart P, Brown D (1985) *Surveys of Personal Exposure to Vehicle Exhaust in Honolulu Microenvironments.* Department of Urban & Regional Planning, University of Hawaii at Manoa, Hawaii

Flachsbart PG, Mack GA, Howes JE, Rodes CE (1987) Carbon monoxide exposures of Washington commuters. *Journal of the Air Pollution Control Association, 37,* 135–142

Garshick E, Schenker MB, Munoz A *et al.,* (1988) A retrospective cohort study of lung cancer and diesel exhaust exposure in railroad workers. *American Review of Respiratory Disease, 137,* 820–825

Grant L, Raub JA, Graham JA *et al.,* (1993) Health effects of motor vehicle-related criteria air pollutants. In Manuell R, Callan P, Bentley K *et al.,* (eds) *International Workshop on Human Health and Environmental Effects of Motor Vehicle Fuels and Their Exhaust Emissions.* International Programme on Chemical Safety, 101–173, Geneva

Great Britain Department of Transport (1989) *National Road Traffic Forecasts (Great Britain),* 1989. HMSO, London

Great Britain Department of Transport (1993) *Transport Statistics of Great Britain,* 1993. HMSO, London

Great Britain Royal Commission on Environmental Pollution (1994) *Eighteenth Report. Transport and the Environment.* HMSO, London

Hillman M, Adams J (1992) Safer driving—safer for whom? In *Conference Report Eurosafe 1992,* Association of London Borough Road Safety Officers, London

Holman C (1994) How much does road traffic contribute to air pollution? In Read C (ed) *How Vehicle Pollution Affects Our Health.* Ashden Trust, London

IARC (1996) *The Quantitative Estimation and Prediction of Cancer Risk.* International Agency for Research on Cancer, Lyon (in press)

Jedrychowski W, Becher H, Wahrendorf J, Basa-Cierpalek Z (1990) A case-control study of lung cancer with special reference to the effect of air pollution in Poland. *Journal of Epidemiology and Community Health, 44,* 114–120

Kleinman MT, Davidson DM, Vandagriff RB *et al.* (1989) Effects of short-term exposure to carbon monoxide in subjects with coronary artery disease. *Archives of Environmental Health, 44,* 361–369

Koenig JQ, Covert DS, Hanley QS *et al.* (1990) Prior exposure to ozone potentiates subsequent response to sulphur dioxide in adolescent asthmatic subjects. *American Review of Respiratory Disease, 141,* 377–380

Koushki PA, al-Dhowalia KH, Niaizi SA (1992) Vehicle occupant exposure to carbon monoxide. *Journal of the Air and Waste Management Association, 42,* 1603–1608

Last JM (1993) Global change: ozone depletion, global warming and public health. *Annual Review of Public Health, 14,* 115–136

Leiter J, Shear MJ (1942) Production of tumors in mice with tars from city air dusts. *Journal of the National Cancer Institute, 3,* 167–174

McMichael AJ (1993) Global environmental change and human population health: A conceptual and scientific challenge for epidemiology. *International Journal of Epidemiology, 22,* 1–8

McMichael AJ, Martens WJM (1995) Assessing health impacts of global environmental change: grappling with scenarios, predictive models, and uncertainty. *Ecosystem Health, 1,* 15–25

McMichael AJ, Woodward AJ, van Leeuwen RE (1994) The impact of energy use in industrialised countries upon global population health. *Medicine and Global Survival, 1*, 23–32

Molfino NA, Wright SC, Katz I *et al.* (1991) Effect of low concentrations of ozone on inhaled allergen responses in asthmatic subjects. *Lancet, 338*, 199–203

Murray CJL, Lopez AD (eds) (1994) *Global Comparative Assessments in the Health Sector.* World Health Organization, Geneva, p. 53

Newman PWG (1992) *Sustainable cities: International and Australian progress.* (Unpublished paper presented at EcoCity Conference, Adelaide, April 1992.)

OECD (1994) *The State of the Environment.* OECD, Paris

Ohrstrom E (1989) Sleep disturbance, psychosocial and medical symptoms—a pilot survey among persons exposed to high levels of road traffic noise. *Journal of Sound Vibration, 133*, 117–128

Ostro BD (1993) The association of air pollution and mortality: examining the case for inference. *Archives of Environmental Health, 48*, 336–342

Ostro B (1994) *Estimating the Health Effects of Air Pollutants.* Policy Research Working Paper 1301. World Bank, Washington, DC

PAHO (1994) Motor Vehicle Traffic Accidents. *Epidemiological Bulletin, 15*, 7–8

Peterson G, Sabersky R (1975) Measurement of pollutants inside an automobile. *Journal of the Air Pollution Control Association, 25*, 1028–1032

Pope CA, Thun MJ, Namboodiri MM *et al.* (1995) Particulate air pollution as a predictor of mortality in a prospective study of US adults. *American Journal of Respiratory Critical Care Medicine, 151*, 669–674

Renner M (1988) *Rethinking the Role of the Automobile.* Worldwatch Institute, Washington DC

Romieu I (1992) Epidemiological studies of the health effects of air pollution due to motor vehicles. In Mage DT, Zali O (eds) *Motor Vehicle Air Pollution. Public Health Impact and Control Measures.* World Health Organization, Geneva

Romieu I Weitzenfeld H, Finkelman J (1990) Urban air pollution in Latin America and the Caribbean: health perspectives. *World Health Statistics Quarterly, 43*, 153–167

Rylander R (1992) Effects on humans of environmental noise, particularly from road traffic. In Mage DT, Zali O (eds) *Motor Vehicle Air Pollution. Public Health Impact and Control Measures.* World Health Organization, Geneva

Seaton A, MacNee W, Donaldson K, Godden D (1995) Particulate air pollution and acute health effects. *Lancet, 345*, 176–178

Spix C, Heinrich J, Dockery D *et al.* (1993) Air pollution and daily mortality in Erfurt, East Germany, 1980–1989. *Environmental Health Perspectives, 101*, 518–526

Stern F, Halperin WE, Hornung RW *et al.* (1988) Heart disease mortality among bridge and tunnel officers exposed to carbon monoxide. *American Journal of Epidemiology, 128, 1276–1288*

Tepper JS, Costa DL, Weber MF *et al.* (1987) Functional and organic changes in rats: a model of ozone adaptation. *American Review of Respiratory Disease, 135*, A283

Tilton BE (1989) Health effects of tropospheric ozone. *Environmental Science and Technology, 23*, 254–263

Tomatis L (1990) Air pollution and cancer: an old and new problem. In Tomatis L (ed) *Air Pollution and Human Cancer.* Springer-Verlag, Berlin.

Transport 2000 (1992) *Travelling Cleaner: Dutch and British Transport Policy Compared.* Transport 2000, London

US Environmental Protection Agency (1990) *Cancer Risk from Outdoor Exposure to Air Toxics.* Final Report, US EPA, Research Triangle Park, North Carolina

Ware JH, Ferris BG, Dockery DW *et al.* (1986) Effects of ambient sulfur oxides and suspended particles on respiratory health of preadolescent children. *American Review of Respiratory Disease, 133,* 834–842

Weir FW, Fabiano VL (1982) Re-evaluation of the role of carbon monoxide in production or aggravation of cardiovascular disease processes. *Journal of Occupational Medicine, 24,* 519–525

World Bank (1993) *World Development Report 1993: Investing in Health.* Oxford University Press, Oxford

World Health Organization (1980) *Noise* (Environmental Health Criteria, 12). World Health Organization, Geneva

4
Approaches to scientific uncertainty

David Gee

WBMG Environmental Communications, London, UK

Introduction

I am not a scientist, and I am very uncertain. If I were a scientist, I would probably be even more uncertain. But perhaps because I am not a scientist I am certain that 'uncertainty' will continue to be one certain feature of debates about health hazards for years to come. As both scientists and citizens therefore we need to agree on ways of dealing with uncertainty.

This chapter looks at the main sources of uncertainty in dose/response models; identifies some useful lessons from the history of other controversial health hazards; examines the 'profligacy' and the 'precautionary' approaches to dealing with uncertainty; and concludes with some recommendations for action on traffic fumes.

Sources of scientific uncertainty

Scientific uncertainties abound, due to data deficiencies, ignorance of processes and pathways in both humans and nature, and to the elements of 'surprise' that nature always holds out to us. Who would have guessed that the 'inert' chlorofluorocarbons (CFCs) would turn out to be dangerous in the ozone layer some 25 kilometres above our heads?

Table 4.1 lists some of the main uncertainties surrounding the basic hazard equation of 'Exposure + Toxicity = Harm'. Most toxicity relates to single substances, and the toxicity of mixtures is largely unknown, yet there are some 15 000 substances in traffic fumes (Swedish Environmental Protection Agency, 1994). Exposure variation is also large and unknown, and personal monitoring has shown that some indoor exposures to NO_2 for example, such as at skating rinks, are high in comparison to urban air pollution.

Health at the Crossroads: Transport Policy and Urban Health.
Edited by Tony Fletcher and Anthony J. McMichael © 1997 John Wiley & Sons Ltd

Table 4.1 Sources of uncertainty in the dose/response relationships for occupational/environmental hazards

Exposure +	Toxicity =	Harm
Emissions:	*Host:*	*Predicted from:*
• Single substances	• Adult	• Structural analogies
• Mixtures (e.g. c. 15k in traffic fumes)	• Children	• Plant/animals
• Carriers (e.g. gases on particles)	• Infants	• Cell changes (e.g. 'rad equivalent dose')
	• Embryo	• Additive/multiplicative models
	• Genetics	
	• Immune state	*Actual:*
Exposures:	• Sensitized	• Changes in cells/functions
• Work		• Increased susceptibility to other harm
• Home	*Response:*	• Reversible/irreversible
• Leisure (e.g. skating rinks)	• Pathways	• Acute
• Urban	• Clearance mechanisms	• Chronic
• Rural	• Immune/defence reactions	• Severity
	• Thresholds	• Duration
Monitoring:	• Latency	• Evaluation
• Background	• Interactions with other exposures	• 'Surprises'
• Personal	• Co-factors	
• Chemical (DNA adducts)	• Additive	
• Target organ/s dose	• Synergistic	
• Duration		
• Concentration		
• Peaks		
• Cumulative		
• Timing (age, season)		

More specialized monitoring of 'biological markers' for exposure, such as DNA adducts (Figure 4.1), which provide a measure of cancer potential, probably get nearer actual target organ doses than conventional background or personal monitoring, but these also show considerable variability in exposure, depending on the location, timing and pattern of exposure (Figure 4.2). The significance of 'peak' and 'cumulative' exposures is also uncertain, as is the variation in response amongst individuals caused by different genetic make-up, age and immune state. Whilst much of this individual variability is easily identifiable (e.g. albinism), some is not, such as a person's ability to detoxify a particular active metabolite intermediate. Whilst many variations in individual susceptibility seem to confer only minor increases in say, cancer risk (Finkel, 1987), some are more significant, such as carcinogenic metabolism (e.g. a 10-fold difference between individuals has been observed for benzo(a)pyrene metabolism, Petruzzelli *et al.*, 1988); DNA adduct formation (inter-individual and inter-tissue variations within an individual, of 10–150 times have been observed; Harris, 1989); DNA repair rates (e.g. a 40 times difference for one kind of repair activity, D'Ambrosio *et al.*, 1987), synergistic effect (e.g. asbestos and smoking); and age, with children and the elderly being particularly sensitive to harmful agents. (US National Research Council, 1993). Similar variations are likely for some of the reactions involved in exposure to traffic fumes.

The existence of 'thresholds' are particularly difficult to deal with, especially when both the 'critical' dose, and how near we are (or nature is) to that dose are both unknown. As O'Riordan and Cameron (1994) point out in their recent work on 'the precautionary principle' 'the usual scientific approaches, dependent on observation, verification, falsification and replication, coupled to prediction by reference to statistical interference, hypothesis testing and modelling may not be sufficient to instil confidence' when confronted by possible threshold effects. Defence mechanisms and natural resilience are impressive but 'homo stupidus' can overwhelm them with sometimes catastrophic results.

Finally, the uncertainties involved in predicting and evaluating harm are also substantial, and further research can often expand the number of questions that remain unanswered, rather than serving to reduce them. In the meantime, whilst there needs to be ever more sophistication and qualification in risk assessment, with 'uncertainty analysis guidelines' being developed for each step in risk assessment (US National Research Council, 1994), the unknowable complexity of dose/response models in the context of large-scale exposures of the public calls for a robust method of dealing with uncertainty.

However, before examining the two basic approaches to uncertainty that have been developed, let us look at the history of some relevant and contentious health hazards which may provide some useful lessons that we can apply to current issues like transport fumes and health.

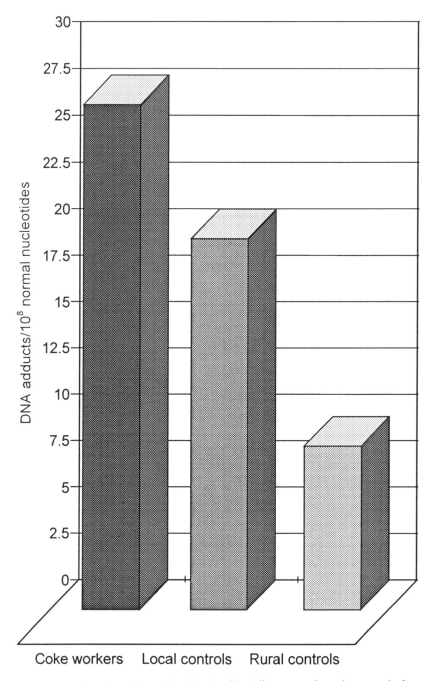

Figure 4.1   Adduct levels in white blood cells. Adjustments have been made for age, smoking and occupational exposure in the control groups. Source: Swedish Environmental Protection Agency (1994)

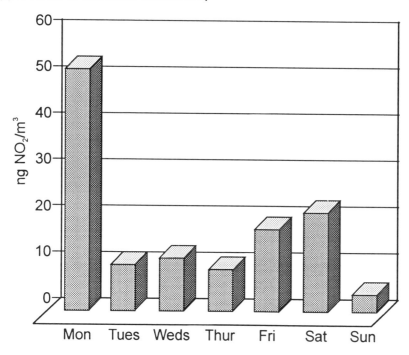

Figure 4.2   An example of how exposure to nitrogen dioxide varies on a day-to-day basis for urban children, depending on the activites they are involved in. On Monday this child went skating for 2 hours at an indoor rink. On Saturday she spent 3 hours in the town centre, 2 hours indoors and 1 hour out of doors. Sunday was spent at home. Source: Swedish Environmental Protection Agency (1994)

Dealing with uncertainty: lessons from the history of some harmful substances

Many substances that are today considered harmful were once treated as harmless. If we look at the history of how scientific uncertainty has been dealt with in the past, and how we move from 'unknown' to 'known' causes of ill health then we may be able to better manage the process of dealing with the uncertainties currently surrounding the debate about traffic fumes and health. It is particularly helpful to look at the ways in which experience in the occupational health field can help us identify and deal with risks in the public health field. We will look at asbestos, diesel fumes, benzene and occupational asthma. These substances and diseases have been chosen because they illustrate much about the *process* of dealing with health hazards and scientific uncertainty, and because the lessons we can draw are relevant to the issue of traffic fumes and health. (In other respects, these examples are quite different. For example, asbestos certainly does not cause asthma: and there is no known connection between asthma and cancer.)

Asbestos

Asbestos used to be called the 'magic' mineral before it was recognized as a deadly substance, now being responsible for about 3000 deaths a year in the UK (GB Health and Safety Commission, 1993). Table 4.2 summarizes the history of asbestos as it moved from the harmless substance of the 1890s to the recognized killer of the 1990s. An astute observation by a lady factory inspector in 1898 concluded: 'The evil effects of asbestos dust have also attracted my attention. A microscopic inspection clearly revealed the sharp, glass-like, jagged nature of particles and . . . the effects have been found to be injurious, as might have been expected' (ARCI, 1898).

Her fears were confirmed 30 years later. A government-funded study in 1929 which found that one-third of asbestos workers had asbestosis, a form of pneumoconiosis. By 1955, a study of workers by Sir Richard Doll (1955) showed that asbestos also caused lung cancer, and by 1964 other cancers, including the most deadly, mesothelioma, were added to the list of 'evil effects of asbestos dust'. However, because of the economic and political power of the asbestos industry, who did not want to accept (or at least publicly admit to) the mounting evidence of its danger, poorly controlled asbestos use expanded right up until the 1980s, by which time it had killed thousands of people, and condemned thousands of others to die in the next 20–30 years as a result of their past exposure. The costs of failing to control asbestos early enough are not just health costs—dealing with compensation and asbestos in buildings is costing billions of pounds and was partly responsible for the bankruptcy of some Lloyds insurance underwriters.

Table 4.2 Asbestos: from unknown to known causes of death

Exposed group	Asbestosis	Lung cancer	Mesothelioma cancer
Occupational:			
Workers	(1898–1929)	1955	1960s
Mates	1964	1964	1964
Environmental:			
Relatives	1960s	?	1960s
Public	?	?	1980s

There are now 3000 asbestos induced deaths a year, including lung cancers (GB Health and Safety Commission, 1993).
Asbestos also causes other cancers, e.g. cancer of the larynx.

What are the relevant lessons for health hazard control that we can learn from the history of smoking and asbestos?

1. The experience of victims and other common sense observations often predate confirmation by experts, sometimes by several decades.

2. Vested interests, such as those who have an economic stake in the substance, will resist the evidence until it is overwhelming.
3. 'If you don't look, and look properly, you don't find' in other words, evidence of harm can exist, but unless it is looked for by focused and comprehensive studies of people at risk, it will not be seen properly. (The statement that 'there is no evidence of harm' usually means 'we have not yet done the relevant studies'.)
4. Evidence of harm at high levels of exposure is easier to get, but as scientific investigations get more sophisticated, they usually uncover evidence of harm at much lower levels of exposure.
5. Diseases that have long-term (i.e. over two or three decades) and irreversible effects are particularly difficult to deal with because:

   (a) evidence of disease in humans comes too late to save both those victims whose ill health provides the evidence, and those who are exposed before the substance is controlled; there is a 'pipeline' effect of future damage that is unavoidable once exposure takes place; and
   (b) the conditions of exposure to the substances will have usually changed (e.g. cleaner asbestos factories, low tar cigarettes) by the time conclusive evidence of harm is finally assembled, and this allows those who wish to defend the substance to say that it is no longer harmful at current levels of exposure; and this point cannot be 'proven' one way or the other for another 20–30 years.
6. Asbestos and the chemicals in cigarette smoke act together to produce more lung cancer than either exposure does separately (Table 4.3). This 'synergistic' response increases risks by multiples of the separate risks from each exposure, rather than by additions, giving very high risks of lung cancer to those who both smoke and breathe in asbestos dust.
7. Exposures in children are particularly damaging because they are often more sensitive to chemicals and dusts; they have many more years in which to both express, and suffer from, disease initiated in childhood; and they usually derive no off-setting benefit from exposures to the substances, unlike workers or smokers.

Table 4.3   Asbestos, smoking and synergy

Exposure	Relative risk of lung cancer
Non-exposed	1
Asbestos only	5 ×
Smoking only	10 ×
Asbestos and smoking	50 ×

A synergistic effect multiplies rather than adds the risks from each separate harmful agent.
Source: Hammond *et al.* (1979).

Diesel fumes

Since at least 1955 it has been recognized that some of the gases—the polycyclic aromatic hydrocarbons (PAHs)—produced during the combustion of diesel fumes cause cancer in rats; that most of the particulates in diesel fumes have got PAHs stuck to them, and that most of the particulates are small enough to penetrate deep into the lungs where they deposit their cancer-causing load. In addition, tests for the cancer-causing potential of substances, such as mutagenicity tests, had also shown that diesel fumes were potentially carcinogenic. Unfortunately, the studies of diesel fumes and cancer, in both workers and animals, had produced mixed results by the early 1980s—some found a weak link between lung cancer and exposure to diesel fumes (a 'positive' result), and some did not (a 'negative' result). When the overall evidence was assessed by expert committees in 1981 their conclusion was that 'excess cancer of the lung ... has not been convincingly demonstrated.' (US National Research Council, 1982). UK experts took the same view: diesel fumes were not carcinogenic.

However, most of the studies did not allow for enough time for exposure to the fumes, or time for the cancers to appear properly. The workers were also exposed to tobacco smoke and asbestos, both causes of lung cancer, and it was difficult to separate their effects from those of diesel fumes. However, bigger and better studies of workers were reported in 1987, and the US government department charged with assessing workers' health risks concluded that: 'a potential occupational carcinogenic hazard exists in human exposure to diesel exhaust' (US National Institute for Occupational Safety and Health, 1988). Two years later, the world authority on cancer concluded that diesel engine exhaust was 'probably carcinogenic to humans' (International Agency for Research on Cancer, 1989). The earlier conclusion had turned out to be what scientists call a 'false negative'. Workers had been unnecessarily exposed to high levels of diesel fumes during the long process of deciding that the fumes were dangerous.

If workers who work in confined spaces with diesel fumes, such as truck, rail and mining workers, are at risk from cancer, what about the public? Their exposure will be much less, being in the open air, and most of the exposure to traffic fumes will come from the much less carcinogenic petrol fuel. But diesels contribute most of the particulates which provide the 'carriers' for the carcinogenic PAHs. And studies of filling station workers, whose exposure is mid-way between indoor rail, truck and mining workers, and the public, also show evidence of cancer from their work. Given this evidence, and that there is no *threshold* effect (i.e. no known safe level of exposure) for a carcinogen like diesel fumes, then it is very probable that the public is also at some risk of cancer from diesel fumes. This is now the current expert view:

As vehicle pollution is a major source of PAHs in urban areas, an increase in emissions in particulates that can carry PAHs into the lungs, particularly from diesel vehicles, is likely to increase lung cancer risk. However the magnitude of the risk is difficult to estimate at present. (Phillips, 1994).

It is likely that the higher lung cancer rate in urban areas is due in part to traffic fumes, as well as to domestic coal burning, industrial pollution and smoking, causing possibly several thousand extra cancer deaths a year.

Recent studies in the USA have shown that particulates also seem to cause increased deaths from other respiratory diseases, and from heart disease, in addition to extra lung cancers. The Six Cities study, for example, has shown almost 40% extra heart and lung disease deaths in cities with exposure to fine particulates (less than 10 microns in size—those that are 2.5 microns seem particularly dangerous), compared to cities with less pollution. (Pope *et al.*, 1992; Schwartz, 1994; Schwartz and Dockery, 1992). The pattern of disease and particulate pollution is similar to that which caused the extra 4000 deaths in the London 'smog' of December 1952, and which led to the Clean Air Act of 1954. In all these studies, the detailed composition of the particulates seemed not to be important for the association with respiratory ill health—the effect was similar whether the particulate came from coal, a steel mill, or cars. And it was the particulate, not the sulphur dioxide, that was having the main effect. The level of exposure was much lower than in London in 1952 (ten times lower in Philadelphia, for example), so the level of disease was proportionately lower, but with a similar pattern i.e. increased heart and lung disease, particularly in the elderly, and with increased contributions of respiratory conditions to heart disease deaths. None of the dozen studies found a *threshold* of exposure below which there was no effect from the particulate (Schwartz, 1994).

Although UK air is not the same as US air, these studies provide strong evidence that the traffic fume-dominated air pollution in our cities is harmful to our health. A recent government-appointed expert group has concluded: 'The impact of diesel vehicles on urban air quality is a serious one' (Quality of Urban Air Review Group, 1993).

What are the lessons from the history of diesel fumes, cancer and respiratory disease?

1. Evidence from laboratory studies can be a good predictor of effects in humans; and 'negative epidemiology' has to be 'adequate and convincing—an ideal situation that is rarely reached' (according to L Tomatis, ex-Director of the International Institute for Research on Cancer), to take precedence over good, positive animal data.
2. Waiting for 'convincing' human evidence is costly, in terms of deaths, ill health and treatment but despite the lessons of smoking and asbestos, the benefit of the scientific doubt is still given to substances, not people.
3. Substances that are harmful to more highly exposed workers are likely to be harmful to the less exposed public, in the absence of a *threshold* effect, and the much larger numbers at risk in the public domain can mean that the overall health hazard for the public is greater than for workers.

Benzene

Benzene is a chemical that causes leukaemia, and which is present in cigarette smoke, some workplaces, and in petrol and diesel exhaust fumes. There are also very small amounts in food and water. The history of occupational cover-up from benzene is depressingly similar to asbestos and diesel fumes, but it is the extrapolation of the occupational risks of benzene to public risks which is relevant to the traffic fumes debate. Over 85% of benzene emissions come from vehicle exhaust fumes (GB Department of the Environment, 1994).

Personal exposure depends on where we live and work, and whether or not we smoke. A non-smoker living in an unpolluted rural area and not working with benzene is likely to get one-tenth of the dose, compared to a 20 cigarettes-a-day smoker living in a city. Urban living gives roughly the same benzene exposure as 12 cigarettes a day. People who work with benzene can be exposed to high levels, and a worker exposed to say 1000 ppb will breathe in some 10 000 μkg a day of benzene compared to about 650 mg a day that a non-smoking city dweller might take in. There is no known level of benzene that does not give a risk of leukaemia, so benzene is likely to cause leukaemia in the public, although their much lower exposure means that the number of cases should be small, despite the greater numbers at risk.

The government's 'Expert Panel on Air Quality Standards' has recently looked at the danger to the public from benzene in vehicle exhausts, and concluded that there should be an 'Air Quality Standard' of 5 ppb of benzene, when measured continuously over a year, to be reduced to 1 ppb as soon as practicable. Current exposures are around 4–5 ppb at a kerbside in Central London, and 0.5–1.0 at a rural site in Harwell, Oxfordshire. (GB Department of the Environment, 1994). This quality standard is based on the results of health studies of benzene-exposed workers subsequently adjusted for the main differences between occupational and environmental risks, which are:

– the much longer duration of exposure of the public i.e. 24 hours a day, not 8 hours; and
– the much greater differences in individual susceptibility to harm in the general public, where the very young and the old, and people already stressed from other diseases, are likely to be much more sensitive to the harmful agent than relatively healthy adult workers.

Unfortunately, scientists do not know how to adjust the evidence from studies of workers to account for these important differences, especially when they do not know where the 'thresholds' of harm may be. However, a public exposure limit was needed, so the Expert Panel made a large but fairly arbitrary reduction in the workers' exposure limit. If the resulting target limit of 1 ppb is to be maintained in the face of rising traffic volumes, then traffic fumes will need to be reduced, especially on days that produce high pollution. For example, the traffic pollution

of December 1991 produced a 'peak' exposure to benzene of 15 ppb in London. 'As both traffic levels and weather patterns that cause these high pollution episodes are predictable, it should be possible to restrict the use of motor vehicles at these times', concluded the expert group (GB Department of the Environment, 1994, p. 7).
What are the relevant lessons from benzene?

– Although it is the *lifetime duration of exposure* to benzene which is thought to be most relevant to the leukaemia it causes, high *peak exposures* can raise the long run average exposure significantly, and they may increase the overall risk of leukaemia by overwhelming defence mechanisms, so it is worthwhile trying to restrict peak exposures.
– Despite the risk of leukaemia from benzene in traffic fumes being low, it is significant enough to justify curbing exposure to traffic fumes, particularly on high pollution days.

Occupational asthma

Recognition of occupational asthma progressed in the usual way, with respiratory sensitizers moving from 'unknown' to 'known' causes of disease via the following steps:

– 'there is no hazard'
– 'only smokers are at risk'
– 'only high levels of exposure cause problems'
– 'some substances can *trigger* existing asthma'
– 'one or two substances can *cause* asthma in sensitive workers'
– 'many substances can cause asthma in many workers'

Substances that pollute the workplace can both cause asthma by themselves, and react together with allergens in the general environment and in households to both trigger and cause asthma following exposure both inside and outside workplaces. This complexity of disease processes may therefore offer particularly valuable insights into the general problem of air pollution and asthma. The relevant lessons from occupational asthma would seem to be:

– Workplace pollution can trigger, cause and exacerbate asthma.
– Workplace pollution can sensitize people to levels of allergens inside and outside work to which they would normally have no response.
– Some people can tolerate asthma-causing chemicals at work for many years without ill effect, but once they develop asthma, it can then be triggered by minute levels of exposure to the chemicals which had hitherto been harmless.
– If exposure lasts for more than a few months, it can cause permanent asthma which can persist long after exposure to the sensitizing agent has been stopped.
– Only a proportion of people (5–10%) are usually affected, reflecting genetic

predisposition, although if exposure is high enough 100% can react to some substances.

– Some people can have both the allergic and the non-allergic asthma, being sensitive to both irritants and allergens.

Traffic pollution and health—the current state of knowledge

Table 4.4 summarizes the health effects of the main pollutants from vehicle pollution. We have clearly come a long way in the process of moving from 'unknown' to 'known' causes of ill health since the Ministry of Transport told the Clean Air Council in 1979 that: 'the effects of pollution from motor vehicles can be summarized : There is no evidence that this sort of pollution has any adverse effects on health' (Read, 1994).

The relationship between traffic fumes and asthma is particularly controversial. Although there have been several studies linking asthma with air pollution and traffic fumes, there is as yet no clear evidence that air pollution *causes* asthma, even though it clearly triggers asthma and increases its severity in some people. This means that air pollution is already responsible for some extra deaths from asthma. In addition to the increased death rates from heart and lung disease from particulates, traffic-related pollutants (particulates, nitrogen dioxide and ozone) are all associated with a 'fall in lung function and an increase in respiratory problems in healthy people as well as those with asthma' (Walters, 1994). However, the complexity of the asthma disease processes and of indoor and outdoor air pollution means that convincing evidence that air pollution causes asthma could well take several more years to prove 'beyond all reasonable doubt'.

Approaches to scientific uncertainty: the 'profligacy', or the 'precautionary' principle?

In dealing with scientific uncertainty in either occupational or environmental risk we have to choose between giving the benefit of scientific doubt to people and the planet, or to the substance or process that may give rise to harm, whilst waiting for further research to hopefully reduce uncertainty.

There are two basic approaches to scientific uncertainty, depending on the direction in which the benefit of the doubt is given.

The 'Profligacy Principle' is applied when substances are given the benefit of the doubt, whereas the precautionary principle is applied when people, or the planet, are given that benefit. Table 4.5 summarizes key features of two approaches the 'problem recognition' stage, the 'response' stage and the results. Application of the profligacy principle leads to long delays in problem recognition, which often stokes up the pressure for a quick and public response, resulting in high health and economic costs to victims and the community. Asbestos, rubber industry fumes, ground water contamination and acid rain are known examples

Table 4.4 Health effects of vehicle pollution

Pollutant	Source	Health effect
Nitrogen dioxide (NO_2)	One of the nitrogen oxides emitted in vehicle exhaust. Combines with VOCs to create ozone.	May *exacerbate asthma* and possibly increase susceptibility to infections.
Volatile organic compounds (VOCs)	A group of chemicals emitted from the evaporation of solvents and distribution of petrol fuel. Also present in vehicle exhaust.	Benzene has most given cause for concern in this group of chemicals. It is a cancer causing agent which can cause leukaemia.
Ozone (O_3)	Secondary pollutant produced from nitrogen oxides and volatile organic compounds in the air.	Irritates the eyes and air passages. *Increases the sensitivity of the airways to allergic triggers in people with asthma.* May increase susceptibility to infection.
Acid aerosols	Airborne acid formed from common pollutants including sulphur and nitrogen oxides	May *exacerbate asthma* and increase susceptibility to respiratory infection. *May reduce lung function in those with asthma.*
Sulphur dioxide (SO_2)	Mostly produced by burning coal. Some SO_2 is emitted by diesel vehicles.	May provoke wheezing and *exacerbate asthma.* It is also associated with chronic bronchitis.
Particulates PM_{10}, total suspended particulates, black smoke	Includes a wide range of solid and liquid particles in air. Those less than 10 μm diameter (PM_{10}) penetrate the lung fairly efficiently and are most hazardous to health. Diesel vehicles produce proportionally more particles than petrol vehicles.	Associated with a wide range of respiratory symptoms. Long-term exposure is associated with an increased risk of death from heart and lung disease. Particulates can carry carcinogenic materials (PAHs) into the lungs.
Polycyclic aromatic hydrocarbons (PAHs)	Produced by incomplete combustion of fuel. PAHs become attached to particulates.	Includes a complex range of chemicals, some of which are carcinogens. It is likely that exposure to PAHs in traffic exhaust poses a low cancer risk to the general population.
Carbon monoxide (CO)	Comes mainly from petrol car exhaust.	Lethal at high doses. At low doses can impair concentration and neuro-behavioural function. Increases the likelihood of exercise related heart pain in people with coronary heart disease. May cause heart disease and present a risk to the foetus.
Lead	Compound present in leaded petrol to help the engine run smoothly.	Impairs the normal intellectual development and learning ability of children.
Asbestos	May be present in brake pads and clutch linings, especially in heavy duty vehicles. Asbestos fibres and dust are released into the atmosphere when vehicles brake.	Asbestos can cause lung cancer and mesothelioma, cancer of the lung lining. The consequences of the low levels of exposure from braking vehicles are not known.

Source: Amended from Read (1994) *Vehicle Pollution and Health*, Ashden Trust.

Table 4.5 Two 'problem/response' approaches to occupational/environment hazards in the context of uncertainty

PROBLEM RECOGNITION	RESPONSE	RESULTS
A. The 'Profligacy Principle' approach Assume harmless—until there is high level of proof ('beyond all reasonable doubt') of substantial damage, usually to humans. Takes a long time—e.g. 100 years (asbestos; acid rain).	Very little—until problem is widely acknowledged then voluntary before mandatory controls. But can be quick—driven by public/political response to harm. (e.g. 2–10 years).	• High human/environmental costs • Pipeline effect (50–100 years) • High economic costs (retrofit, refurbishment) • Conflict/mistrust between scientists/public • Uneven distribution of costs between victims/'problem' industries/society
B. The 'Precautionary Principle' approach Assume harmful—confirmed by low level of proof ('balance of probabilities') of likely damage, based on non-human and human evidence. Could take much shorter time, e.g. 2–10 years.	Begins earlier, avoids profligate investment in the 'harmful' substance; and encourages 'eco-efficiency'. Can be longer, e.g. 5–15 years.	• Low human/environmental costs • Low economic costs • Encourages innovation in exposure control/eco-efficiency • Less conflict between private/public sectors • Greater trust/public confidence in scientists • More even distribution of costs

of the profligacy principle in action–global warming is likely to be another candidate. However, the alternative precautionary approach has been developed to protect workers at risk from health hazards (Gee, 1980, 1987), and Appendix 1 summarizes this approach. Applying the precautionary principle in practice can predict harm well in advance of 'official' recognition of the harm, thereby reducing risks to those exposed. For example, the precautionary trade union approach was applied to the cancer dangers of both diesel fumes and manmade mineral fibre, and to the need for a two- to fivefold reduction in the exposure limit for radiation, some eight to ten years before official recognition of these dangers (General and Municipal Workers Union, 1980–82).

A parallel approach has been developed in order to protect the planet from irreversible damage. It does not claim always to predict harm (though in practice it usually does) but it is based on the view that the cost of a 'false negative' (that is, when something that is 'safe' turns out not to be so, like asbestos, or CFCs, for example) is less than the costs of a 'false positive' (that is, when something that is assumed to be harmful turns out not to be so). The cost of a false positive is usually the minor misallocation of resources, whilst the cost of a false negative is often catastrophic damage; as with asbestos (about 3000 deaths a year now in the UK alone, and clean up costs in the billions of dollars), nuclear power generation (Chernobyl), CFCs (ozone depletion), or 'safe' engineering (Bhopal).

This *precautionary* approach to the problem of causation, evidence and proof was developed in Germany and applied internationally to the North Sea in 1984. The traditional approach, the profligacy principle, assumes that emissions to the environment were harmless until proven harmful by 'convincing' evidence. This was supported by research that tried to show that the eco-system could assimilate emissions without unacceptable effects (Joint Group of Experts on the Scientific Aspects of Marine Pollution, 1990).

By 1984 it had become obvious that this *profligate* approach to the environment was facing similar difficulties to those found in occupational risk assessment:

- scientific uncertainty, where the complex interactions in nature, involving different pathways, exposures, target groups, and forms of harm, are impossible to identify and research fully;
- the difficulty of knowing how close we are to the threshold of harm in a species or eco-system when we do not know how stressed a system already is, or where the threshold or critical load is. For example seals, dab fish and zooplankton already seem to be affected by pollution in the North Sea but we do not know how near we are to causing critical damage;
- the logical impossibility of proving a negative like 'there are no harmful effects'–as Karl Popper put it: 'seeing just white swans doesn't help you to prove that there are no black swans' (Popper, 1972);
- the likelihood of irreversible effects, so that, as with cancer, once the threshold of serious harm is reached, the damage becomes impossible to reverse; and

– where damage is reversible, the long time period, often generations, needed to rectify damage: for example, the 100 plus years needed to rectify ground water contamination, restore the ozone layer, or stabilize CO_2 emissions.

At the North Sea conference in 1987 government ministers therefore agreed to reduce at source, 'polluting emission of substances that are persistent, toxic, and liable to bioaccumulate'. . . . especially when there is reason to assume that certain damage or harmful effects on the living resources of the sea are likely to be caused by such substances, even when there is no scientific evidence to prove a causal link between emissions and effects' (Haigh, 1994).

This approach was extended beyond the sea to the whole environment in 1990, at the Bergen conference, where ministers declared that: 'Environmental measures must anticipate, prevent, and attack the causes of environmental degradation. Where there are threats of serious or irreversible environmental damage, lack of scientific certainty should not be used as a reason for postponing measures to prevent environmental degradation' (O'Riordan and Cameron, 1994).

The government has signed the Rio Declaration on Environment and Development, which endorses the precautionary principle in the following words: 'Where there are threats of serious damage, lack of full scientific certainty shall not be used as a reason for postponing cost effective measures to prevent environmental degradation' (Principle 15, Rio Declaration on Environment and Development, 1992).

It is clear that at the moment, the government is not applying the precautionary principle to air pollution, even though it would be cost effective to do so.

In practice the two approaches to uncertainty are not alternatives—elements of both can coexist along a multidimensional continuum which contains assumptions about the resilience of people on the planet, estimates of the relevant costs and benefits of action and inaction, and value judgements about the equitable distribution of doubt. But before looking at the costs and benefits of applying the precautionary principle to traffic fumes, we need to address the question of apportioning the 'benefit of the doubt' and the costs of being wrong.

In the face of uncertainty, who or what gets the benefit of the doubt?

In responding to uncertainty, key questions to ask are:

– Which level of proof is more appropriate to public policy issues such as traffic fumes and health:
    – the high 'beyond all reasonable doubt' level or
    – the lower, 'balance of probabilities' level of proof?
– What are the costs of uncertainty, i.e.
    – what are the costs of scientists saying a substance or activity is harmless which later turns out to be harmful? (false negatives)

- what are the costs of us acting as though a substance or activity is harmful which later turns out to be harmless? (false positives)
- Who bears these costs?
- Who or what should get the benefit of scientific doubt?
  - harmful agents or substances, or
  - people and the environment?

Which level of proof?

In law, society uses two levels of proof. In the criminal courts, where employers face charges of breaking health and safety laws, the high level of 'beyond all reasonable doubt' is used. In the civil courts, where workers with occupational asthma try to get compensation by proving that their employers were negligent, a lower level, the 'balance of probabilities', is used.

Society uses a high level of proof in the criminal courts so as to minimize the dangers of innocent people being found guilty—a false positive. The 'cost' of this high level of proof is that some guilty people are judged to be innocent—a false negative. In the civil courts however, society uses the lower level of proof because one party is already damaged and the 'cost' of a false negative would be injured workers not getting compensation for their wrecked livelihoods. The 'cost' of using the lower level of proof in the civil courts is hence that some workers will receive compensation for injury from their employer's insurance company when their injuries were not really caused by their employer's neglect. In this case the cost of being wrong falls mainly on employers and their insurance companies. This is seen as a fairer distribution of the costs of being wrong than that which would result from using a higher level of proof, where the cost of being wrong would be borne by individual workers, who are already suffering from ill health.

But which level of proof is more appropriate to questions of public health policy? It is my view, and one reflected in the precautionary principle, that the lower, 'balance of probabilities' level of proof, as used in the civil courts, is more appropriate to questions of public health policy, than the 'beyond all reasonable doubt' level used in the criminal courts.

Good science requires a high level of proof. 'A' cannot be said to cause 'B' until all other possibilities have been exhausted. Unfortunately, as part of the human evidence for this level of proof, science requires some parties to the issue, namely members of the public, to become ill and in some cases, to die. If the issue is complex, as air pollution is, it can take many years of exposure, and research into damaged people, before evidence becomes 'convincing'. It is scientists who are gathering the evidence about pollution and ill health, but while their methods are appropriate to their work, the question of what society should do in the face of uncertainty, and how many people should be paying the cost of providing human evidence, are questions of public policy, not questions of science.

It should be remembered that millions of people have been exposed to air pollution without scientists having to prove, on *any* level of proof, that it was harmless. In other words, we have given traffic fumes the luxury of the criminal defence, that is, innocent until proven guilty. Should not the burden of proof be the other way round, with strong evidence of harmlessness being made available before people are widely exposed, as with public policy on new chemicals and pharmaceuticals?

What are the costs of uncertainty and who bears these costs?

We know that the costs of some false negatives, for example, 'asbestos is fairly harmless at today's level of exposure', can be very large, involving not only deaths for particular groups, but huge clean-up costs for the rest of society. Most other occupational and environmental hazards have had a similar, if less catastrophic, history, as we have seen with smoking, passive smoking, diesel fumes, benzene and occupational asthma. It is possible, however, to get very costly false positives as well, for example, the costs of radical surgery following a diagnosis of say, breast cancer which, on diagnosis, was a borderline decision, but which later turned out not to be cancer. The cost of false positives depends on what the preventive action is. Drastic and irreversible action, such as breast removal, or the immediate closure of industries can make false positives very expensive, but early preventive action is rarely like this. In the case of traffic fumes, the cost of acting to curb traffic and its fumes can be small in comparison with its benefits, as we will see below.

In addition, both the *severity* and *distribution* of the costs of being wrong are also important. In the case of traffic fumes, the costs of the false positive, such as traffic curbing, when fumes turn out not to cause much ill health, are not very severe (inconvenience at most) and are spread widely across society. In contrast, the cost of the false negative (that is, not curbing traffic when fumes turn out to be harmful) can be severe, even life-threatening, and they are distributed unevenly, being borne by specific and vulnerable groups in society, such as the elderly, the sick and children, many of whom gain little or no benefit from car traffic.

Who should get the benefit of the scientific doubt?

What happens when even the application of the precautionary principle does not justify reducing exposures to, say, traffic fumes, because the uncertainties are so large that even this lower level of proof is not reached? It seems clear to me that if the costs of being wrong are large and unfairly distributed, in comparison to the costs of precaution, then the benefit of the scientific doubt should be given to people and the planet, and exposure reduced. (This is not as utopian as it sounds. The British Nuclear Fuels Compensation Scheme for Radiation Cancer in its Employees, which the author helped to negotiate, allows some compensation to be paid where there is more than a 15% probability that the cancer was radiation induced.) As it happens, the current economic costs of traffic fumes are so large, as we will see below, that even a crude cost/benefit analysis would justify reducing traffic fumes without having to invoke this residual, 'benefit of doubt', argument.

'Dominant' and 'strategic' exposures

Cancer, heart disease, stress and asthma are examples of 'multi-causal' disease processes which have several routes to the disease involving interactions between different inter-dependent causes. It follows that removing just one of these causes could prevent the disease appearing—but which cause or exposure should be targetted for removal? In many cases the 'target' cause would be the 'dominant' one in the disease process, for example possibly 'Allergic' sensitivity in childhood asthma (Table 4.6).

However, in some cases this may not be the most useful exposure to target. A 'strategic' exposure is one which depends least on individual behaviour change, following Legge's dictums on the prevention of lead poisoning at work (Legge, 1934); is most widespread; provides the most equitable sharing of costs; can be most easily implemented, and has the largest supplementary gains, such as traffic fumes in childhood asthma (Table 4.6). Identifying 'strategic' exposures requires some analysis of costs and benefits of action and inaction, to which we now briefly turn.

The costs and benefits of curbing traffic growth and fumes

A comprehensive balance sheet of the costs and benefits of transport, air pollution and health is beyond the scope of this paper. While there are clearly

Table 4.6 'Dominant' and 'strategic' exposures in multi-causal hazards—an illustrative example for childhood asthma

Genetics +	Host state +	Home exposures +	Outdoor exposures	= Harm
e.g. Allergic (25%)	e.g. Veg. deficit (15%)	Pets, Mites (15%), Ovens, Boilers, *Passive smoking* (20%)	*Traffic fumes* (15%), Industrial pollution, Pollen (10%)	= ASTHMA IN CHILDREN

A 'Dominant' exposure is the most important toxicological factor in a multi-causal chain of exposures, e.g. 'Allergic sensitivity'; in the above four factor model, percentages are illustrative only.

A 'Strategic' exposure is the factor which:
* depends least on individual behaviour ('Legge's Lead Dictums')
* is most widespread
* provides most equitable cost sharing
* can be most easily implemented
* has largest supplementary gains
e.g. 'Traffic fumes', above.

some considerable benefits from the use of cars and lorries, recent studies have shown the enormous and increasing health, environmental and economic costs of road transport. These comprise not only road accidents and damage to health, but also noise, congestion and damage to buildings, vegetation and water quality. It follows that any policy to reduce traffic fumes because of their health effects, will produce much wider benefits overall. The Department of Applied Economics at the University of Cambridge, for example, has concluded that the economic benefits of reducing traffic flow by 25% far outweigh the costs, and are likely to be around 1% of GDP, i.e. £4.5 billion (Johnston, 1995). And the Royal Commission on Environmental Pollution has recently estimated that some of the 'external' costs of road transport are between £10 billion and £18 billion, which is 2–4% of GNP (GB Royal Commission on Environmental Pollution, 1994). (Table 4.7.)

Conclusion—some recommendations for action on traffic growth and fumes

It is clear from the above discussion that there is sufficient evidence, on health grounds alone, to justify curbing traffic growth and associated fumes. This is no longer a particularly radical position. The Royal Commission on Environmental Pollution has concluded: 'Despite uncertainties about the effects of transport pollutants, there is a clear case, especially on health grounds, for taking further action to reduce emissions' (GB Royal Commission on Environmental Pollution, 1994).

It is now widely recognized that most congestion and the predicted future growth in demand for car space, cannot be met by just building more roads. Yet the UK invests less in its railways per head than any other major European country, coming tenth in the league table, and spending less than a third of the European average. The UK spent $8.3 per head on rail infrastructure in 1993,

Table 4.7   Estimates of environmental costs of the transport system (1994/95) £ billion a year

Costs attributable to road transport are shown in parentheses	Lower end of range	Upper end of range
Air pollution	2.4 ⎫	6.0 ⎫
Climate change	1.8 ⎬ (4.6)	3.6 ⎬ (12.9)
Noise and vibration	1.2 ⎭	5.4 ⎭
Accidents	5.5 (5.4)	5.5 (5.4)
Total quantified environmental costs	10.9 (10.0)	20.5 (18.3)
	(2% GDP)	(3.5% GDP)

Other environmental costs not counted above include: losses of land, severance of communities, loss of access to land, loss or disruption of habitats, visual intrusion, congestion (not 'external' to users).
Source: Great Britain Royal Commission on Environmental Pollution (1994).

compared to $50 per head in France, $30 in Germany and $25 in Italy. In the UK, the fares on public transport are higher than in other European countries. In London, they are almost twice the European average.

It is therefore clear that an integrated transport policy that was biased in favour of people's health and public transport, rather than towards cars and lorries, would be of considerable net benefit to society. Such a policy could include the following 20 steps:

1. More research into emissions under actual driving conditions; air quality, particularly for respirable PMs and via continuous monitoring at a larger number of sampling points; personal exposure particularly that of children; health effects particularly a comprehensive integrated approach funded jointly by the Departments of Health, Environment and Transport and of the sort recently recommended by the Institute of Environment and Health in Leicester (Medical Research Council, 1994).
2. Better, simpler and enforceable air quality standards.
3. More accurate and more useful public warnings on air quality.
4. Restrictions on traffic on high pollution days.
5. Improved emission standards particularly for diesel vehicles.
6. Random roadside tests to identify the worst polluting vehicles.
7. Improved fuel technology.
8. Alternative fuels, including compressed natural gas, electric powered vehicles and bio-fuels.
9. Exhaust pipes that point upwards rather than at child height.
10. Vapour recovery systems on petrol pumps to reduce exposure to volatile organic compounds (VOCs) including benzene.
11. The creation of more pedestrian areas and restricted access of heavy vehicles in towns and cities.
12. Speed restrictions on sensitive stretches of motorways.
13. A target for curbing all over traffic growth similar to that in the Netherlands, as recommended by the RCEP.
14. A change in approach so that traffic demand is managed rather than met with increasing supply of road space.
15. Substantial improvement in the quality and scale of integrated public transport, together with improved security on public transport and better provision for pedestrians and cyclists.
16. Traffic calming as a duel strategy to reduce traffic speed and encourage pedestrians and cyclists.
17. Increased provisions for cycling.
18. Advanced traffic management systems including automatic driver guidance and integrated signal control.
19. Road pricing as part of a comprehensive package of dealing with traffic growth and not something done in isolation.

20. Increasing the price of fuels and private transport so that more of their 'external' costs are captured in market prices. (This would need to be part of a comprehensive reform of the tax and pricing systems which would refocus the market towards greater 'eco-efficiency' and employment (Gee, 1994).)

Appendix 1 – 'The Trade Union Approach to the Hazards of Toxic Substances', David Gee for the General, Municipal, Boilermakers and Allied Trades Union – 1980

1. Assume that substances are more likely to be harmful than harmless as in Guidance Note EH. 18 from the Health and Safety Executive.
   This then:
   (i)   avoids unnecessary exposure;
   (ii) requires adequate pre-market testing;
   (iii) means that some negative test findings don't invalidate the basic assumption of harmful potential. This reverses the current position where industry does not see positive e.g. from animals as invalidating their assumption of safety.
   (iv) control technology becomes less expensive as demand for it increases.
2. Consider all available types of evidence:
   (i)   Human data   (a) scientific—epidemiology
                       (b) workers experience
   (ii) Short-term tests
   (iii) Animal data
   (iv) Similarity of chemical/physical structure
   Good positive evidence from any of (i)(b) to (iv) to be given greater weight than negative human data, where effects are serious/irreversible.
3. Evidence should be weighed against the 'balance of probabilities' level of proof instead of the 'beyond all reasonable doubt' level. Waiting for 'scientific proof' will be too late and too costly for workers and the community.
4. Risks and benefits would have to be assessed by an administrative procedure that includes all affected interest groups. Benefits would need to be demonstrated. Residual risks would need to be shared by employers and the rest of society through no fault insurance schemes, rather than by victims of occupational disease alone.
5. (i) Control limits should be based on the exposure levels that a majority of users can achieve, with the 'dirty' end of a user group being given temporary exemptions to work to higher limits. This reverses the present position where the 'dirty end' dictates the control limit, with the majority of the user group being expected to get as low 'as is reasonably practicable', which is difficult to enforce.
   (ii) There are no known safe levels for carcinogenic substances.

(iii) Risks should be fixed on the basis of what each particular industry can achieve, not on the basis of comparisons of risks in other industries.

6. Substances would be banned, authorized or controlled depending on the risks and costs in each case. New laws on both carcinogenic substances and other toxic substances are needed.

7. Broadly similar control limits on industries and substances in all countries, plus information and international enforcement are necessary to avoid the export of hazardous substances and plants.

References

ARCI (1898) *Annual Reports of the Chief Inspector of Factories and Workshops, 1802–1974.* HMSO, London. The observation of Miss Deane (1898) and other women inspectors are quoted in Yeadle S (1993) *Women of Courage: 100 years of Women Factory Inspectors, 1893–1993.* HSE/HMSO, London

D'Ambrosio SM, Samual MJ, Dutta-Chowdhury TA, Wani AA (1987) O6-methylguanine-DNA methyltransferase in human fetal tissues: fetal and maternal factors. *Cancer Research*, 47, 51–55

Doll R (1955) Mortality from lung cancer in asbestos workers. *British Journal of Industrial Medicine*, 12, 81–86

Finkel A (1987) *Uncertainty, variability and the value of information in cancer risk assessment.* DSc dissertation. Harvard School of Public Health (Harvard University), Massachusetts

Gee D (1980) *The Trade Union Approach to the Hazards of Toxic Substances.* GMWU, Surrey

Gee D (1987) *The identification and control of toxic substances: a trade union view.* Unpublished paper presented at the Plastics and Rubber Institute Conference, September 1987, University of York, York

Gee D (1994) *Economic Tax Reform: Briefing Number 8 (November) for the Parliamentary Environment Group, London.* Papers and proceedings from Economic Tax Reform focusing the market on Eco-efficiency and Employment (1994). WBMG Environmental Communications, London

General and Municipal Workers Union (1980–82) *A Summary of the Evidence and Precautions on MMMF.* General and Municipal Workers Union, Esher

Great Britain Department of the Environment Expert Panel on Air Quality Standards (1994) *Benzene.* HMSO, London

Great Britain Health and Safety Commission (1993) *Annual Report of the Health and Safety Commission.* HMSO, London

Great Britain Royal Commission on Environmental Pollution (1994) *Eighteenth Report: Transport and the Environment.* HMSO, London

Haigh N (1994) The introduction of the precautionary principle. In O Riordan T, Cameron J (eds), *Interpreting the Precautionary Principle.* Earthscan Publications, London, p. 244

Hammond EC, Selikoff IJ, Seidman H (1979) Asbestos exposure, cigarette smoking and death rates. *Annals of New York Academy of Sciences*, 330, 473–490

Harris CC (1989) Interindividual variation among humans in carcinogen metabolism, DNA adduct formation and DNA repair. *Carcinogenesis*, 10, 1563–1566

International Agency for Research on Cancer (1989) *IARC Monographs on the Evaluation of Carcinogenic Risks to Humans. Volume 46: Diesel and Gasoline Engine Exhausts and some Nitroarenes.* International Agency for Research on Cancer, Lyon

Johnston N (1995) Modelling passenger demand energy consumption and pollution

emissions in the transport sector. Cambridge University Department of Applied Economics. Working Paper no. 95/257. Cambridge
Joint Group of Experts on the Scientific Aspects of Marine Pollution—GESAMP (1990) *The State of the Marine Environment: UNEP Regional Seas Reports and Studies Number 115*. United Nations Environment Programme (96)
Legge TM (1934) *Industrial Maladies*. Oxford University Press, Oxford
Medical Research Council/Institute for Environment and Health (1994) *Air Pollution and Health: Understanding the Uncertainties*. Institute for Environment and Health, Leicester.
O'Riordan T, Cameron J, (eds) (1994) *Interpreting the Precautionary Principle*. Earthscan Publications, London
Petruzzelli S, Camus AM, Carrozi L *et al.* (1988) Long lasting effects of tobacco smoking on pulmonary drug-metabolizing enzymes: a case-control study on lung cancer patients. *Cancer Research, 48*, 4695–4700
Phillips D (1994) Can vehicle pollution cause cancer? In Read C, *How Vehicle Pollution Affects our Health*. Ashden Trust, London
Pope CA, Schwartz J, Ransom MR (1992) Daily mortality and PM10 pollution in Utah Valley. *Archives of Environmental Health, 42*, 211–217
Popper K R, (1972) *Conjectures and Refutations*. Routledge and Kegan Paul, London
Quality of Urban Air Review Group (1993) *Second Report: Diesel Vehicle Emissions and Urban Air Quality*. Quality of Urban Air Review Group, Birmingham
Read C (1994) *Vehicle Pollution and Health, London*. Ashden Trust, London
Rio Declaration on Environment and Development (1992) *Earth Summit 1992*. Regency Press, London
Schwartz J (1994) What are people dying of on high pollution days? *Environmental Research, 64*, 26–35
Schwartz J, Dockery DW (1992) Increased mortality in Philadelphia associated with daily air pollution concentrations. *American Review of Respiratory Disease, 145*, 600–604
Swedish Environmental Protection Agency (1994) *ENVIRO (December)*, Stockholm
Transport 2000 (1994) *Transport Trends and Transport Policies: Myths and Facts*. Transport 2000, London
US National Institute for Occupational Safety and Health (1988) *Current Intelligence Bulletin No. 50. Carcinogenic Effects of Exposure to Diesel Exhaust*. NIOSH, Cincinnati, USA.
US National Research Council (1982) *Diesel Technology-Impacts of Diesel-powered Light-duty Vehicles*. National Academy of Sciences, Washington, DC
US National Research Council (1993) *Issues in Risk Assessment I: Use of the Maximum Tolerated Dose in Animal Bioassays for Carcinogenicity*. National Academy Press, Washington DC
US National Research Council (1994) *Science and Judgements in Risk Assessment*. National Academy Press, Washington DC
Walters S (1994) What are the respiratory health effects of vehicle pollution? In Read C, *Vehicle Pollution and Health, London*. Ashden Trust, London

5
Research methods in air pollution epidemiology

Klea Katsouyanni

University of Athens Medical School, Greece

Introduction

Air pollution epidemiology is the study of the occurrence and distribution of health outcomes in association with community exposure to air pollution. A few decades ago there would have been no need to consider specific research methods in air pollution epidemiology because the discipline consisted of studying such high levels of air pollution that effects were evident even with the crudest study design. The most famous such episode to be studied was the London smog of December 1952. In the 1960s and 1970s the effects of air pollution exposure (especially acute effects) were further quantified and thresholds were identified on the basis of these studies of severe air pollution episodes. Since then, legal and other control measures have led to lower air pollution levels, especially in northern Europe and North America, and for a while the prevailing attitude was that the attained moderate air pollutant levels were not harmful to human health.

Since 1985, however, results from several studies have indicated that lower levels of air pollution than those previously considered safe have serious adverse health effects (Utell and Samet, 1993). As evidence has accumulated, these results have gained credibility to the extent that national and international institutions are revising air quality guidelines and standards based on the results of these more recent epidemiological studies (WHO, 1994). At the same time, it is recognized that we are dealing with a 'weak' effect in terms of the magnitude of relative risks, but an important effect in attributable risk terms since air pollution exposure is, typically, ubiquitous.

Although there is increasing agreement that air pollution, at levels measured today, affects health, there is still much to be understood concerning the effects of specific pollutants, biological mechanisms involved and identification of

Health at the Crossroads: Transport Policy and Urban Health.
Edited by Tony Fletcher and Anthony J. McMichael © 1997 John Wiley & Sons Ltd

sensitive groups of individuals. Some examples of specific questions of interest today are:

1. What are the health effects (especially long-term) of exposure to photochemical smog?
2. Is there interaction between coexistent air pollutants?
3. Are air pollution health effects modified by other environmental factors?
4. Which are the sensitive groups of individuals contributing to the increased mortality and emergency admissions found in various studies?

The extent of potential confounding, time-considerations (e.g. lags and latencies) in air pollution effects, individual variation in air pollution exposure and exposure misclassification are some factors which make the study of these issues complex. Selected qualities and problems which characterize air pollution epidemiology are described below.

Study designs in air pollution epidemiology

Design options in epidemiology may be classified according to different criteria, for example: the conditions of observation (experimental *vs* observational); unit of data collection and analysis (group *vs* individual); or time dimension (cross-sectional *vs* longitudinal).

Experimental study designs such as clinical, field and community intervention trials are not often employed in air pollution epidemiology. The main advantage of this type of study is the control and consequent accurate measurement of exposure. However, the fact that only short-term, reversible effects can be studied, and that sensitive individuals should (for ethical reasons) not be included in the sample, restricts its applications.

Semi-experimental studies have been prominent in air pollution epidemiology. Air pollution episodes may be considered as 'natural' (i.e. outside human control) semi-experiments; however, since their occurrence is often linked to specific meteorological conditions, the health effect of the pollution exposure is difficult to separate. Changes in air pollution exposure may also result from human action like changes in industrial process technology, closing down or starting a plant, migration to and from polluted areas, and specific air pollution control measures. These events afford good research opportunities. Most of the designs applied under these 'semi-experimental' situations can be classified, however, as one or a combination of the observational study design categories which are presented below.

The classification used here is based on the level of data aggregation, on the use of incidence *vs* prevalence and on whether the selection of the study population is based on exposure or disease status. However, a particular study often does not fall into one distinct class, but it may be a combination of designs—or may be regarded as a different design type when looked at from a different perspective.

One important and pervasive problem in air pollution epidemiology is exposure assessment. When exposure is measured by fixed site monitors there can be no estimate of the individual variation in exposure, nor, commonly, any assurance that these measurements are representative of the mean population exposure. Attempts to construct an individual exposure index based on time-activity pattern information are hindered by the lack of relevant databases. The use of personal monitors—the closest proxy of received exposure–is difficult and expensive for use on a large scale. Although there is continuous improvement towards more accurate exposure measurements, the problem of exposure assessment is to some extent inherent in air pollution epidemiology.

Studies using aggregated data

The special characteristics of air pollution exposure have fostered study designs which have been extensively used in air pollution epidemiology, but which occupy very little space in standard epidemiology textbooks. The typical ubiquity of exposure leads to designs with aggregated data, the so-called ecological designs. Ecological studies, typically, are not extensively treated in epidemiological textbooks (Rothman, 1986), as they are usually thought of as hypothesis-generating, descriptive studies, that are subject to substantial confounding and other biases (which is their most important methodological problem). However, confounding can be reduced if data on potential confounders are available. The potential for confounding also depends on the unit of aggregation; smaller and more uniform units may minimize confounding. Furthermore, one type of ecological design with an important (historical and current) role in the detection of effects of short-term exposure to air pollution, namely the temporal or time-series study, using a short time period (usually one day) as the aggregation unit, is often ignored in texts and papers dealing with the classification of studies. Because most time-series studies are done within a single population, the problem of confounding is greatly reduced.

Although the unit of aggregation may be diverse (e.g. occupations, families) the following sections will deal mainly with geographic (or spatial) and chronological units of aggregation.

Geographical or spatial studies using aggregated data

A method to test long-term air pollution health effects which is conceptually straightforward, and usually cheap and easy, is to compare the frequency of a health outcome across different areas with varying levels of exposure.

The main advantages of this design are:

1. The possibility of using routinely collected data on the health outcome(s).
2. The greater exposure contrast that exists between, rather than within, areas.

The main problems concern control of confounding, which is, as mentioned above, a major issue in ecological studies (Rothman, 1986). Some of the older studies were unable to measure adequately the potential confounding variables (Winkelstein *et al.*, 1967; Lambert and Reid, 1970; Colley and Reid 1970) but more recent studies combine other design approaches in order to achieve increasing sophistication in the assessment of confounding variables. One such approach is to conduct prevalence studies in each area and thereby record information on all relevant confounders (Ware *et al.*, 1986). Another approach is to conduct a prospective study within a set of contrasting populations and to measure the incidence of disease- or cause-specific mortality as well as the levels of potential confounders in each population (Dockery *et al.*, 1993).

Temporal studies using aggregated data

In this design, the relationship between an exposure and an outcome variable, each measured over the same time units (days, weeks, etc.) during a specified period, is investigated. The measurements of each variable thus constitute a time-series.

This type of study, originally developed within the social sciences, has been extensively used to assess short-term effects. During the last decade many time-series studies have been published and their results have collectively contributed to our understanding of short-term air pollution effects on health (Hatzakis *et al.*, 1986; Derriennic *et al.*, 1989; Pope *et al.*, 1992; Schwartz and Dockery 1992a, 1992b; Schwartz *et al.*, 1993; Schwartz 1993; Sunyer *et al.*, 1993; Touloumi *et al.*, 1994).

Time-series studies are relatively cheap as they usually use routinely collected data on both the health outcome (e.g. total or cause-specific mortality counts, number of hospital admissions) and the exposure. Although aggregated data are used, this design is relatively free of confounding effects because the same population is used as exposed and control populations, and the only potential confounding variables are those which vary with the time units of aggregation. Such variables are usually meteorological and chronological (season, day of week etc.), and are generally easily measured and recorded. Other problems specific to this design (e.g. autocorrelation) are addressed by the use of complex time-series statistical analysis methods. The use of very long series of daily data (typically data for several years) gives enough power to detect weak effects.

In-depth studies aimed at identifying those population subgroups more at risk gave rise to a time-series design where individual health outcome data were collected for a sample of days chosen to maximize contrast in exposure (Katsouyanni *et al.*, 1990, Schwartz 1994a, 1994b). This enabled identification of age groups more at risk and causes of death which exhibit the most pronounced increase on high air pollution days.

Studies with data at the individual level

Cross-sectional studies

A typical cross-sectional study entails the study of exposure and health outcome in a sample of individuals (taking account of potential confounding factors). In air pollution epidemiology such cross-sectional studies have rarely been conducted because of lack of individual exposure assessment. Rather, cross-sectional surveys have been used to collect data on the prevalence of a health outcome and to improve the information on the prevalence of confounding variables in the broader framework of ecological comparisons (as described above).

Panel studies

A panel study is a prospective study following closely a cohort of individuals for a relatively short time-period. The method is mainly used to investigate short-term effects of air pollution and the health outcomes measured include self-reporting of symptoms, medication use and indices of respiratory function. Several panel studies have followed groups of sensitive subjects, such as asthmatics and a typical size for such panels is around 100. The time unit of observation is often a day or a number of hours. Individual assessment of exposure can be attempted (Frezieres *et al.*, 1982; Perry *et al.*, 1982; Clench-Aas *et al.*, 1991, Roemer *et al.* 1993).

Panel studies data are complicated to analyse statistically. Individual experiences may be compared separately but data may also be pooled and averages formed for each time period of follow-up. In the latter case, the analytical approach actually treats the panel study as a temporal study using aggregated data. In all cases autocorrelation is an important problem. Medication use is a significant confounder which may mask or complicate the analysis (Korn and Whittemore, 1979; Schwartz *et al.*, 1991).

Cohort studies (long-term)

Few cohort studies have been performed to evaluate the long-term health effects of air pollution (Detels *et al.*, 1979; Van der Lende *et al.*, 1981; Krzyzanowski *et al.*, 1986; Carrozzi *et al.*, 1990; Dockery *et al.*, 1993). In these studies the cohorts were chosen from different areas known to have different air pollution levels. Exposure assessment for individuals was usually not attempted and air pollution has been measured 'ecologically' by fixed site monitors. Although health outcomes and data on confounders have been collected at an individual level, the final inference from these studies is based on comparison of a few points, similar to that used in the geographic studies using aggregated data.

Case-control studies

Case-control studies have been rarely used in air pollution epidemiology, other than to investigate the long-term effects of air pollution on the development of lung cancer and chronic obstructive pulmonary disease (Haenszel and Taeuber, 1964; Lyon *et al.*, 1981; Vena, 1982; Jedrychowski *et al.*, 1990; Xu *et al.*, 1989; Katsouyanni *et al.*, 1991; Tzonou *et al.*, 1992). Case-control studies have some advantages over cohort studies in air pollution epidemiology. Long-term individual exposure assessment must be reconstructed retrospectively on the basis of measurements from fixed site monitors coupled with the usual time-activity patterns of an individual and his/her residential and occupational history. Exposure assessment on this basis is almost as good as any prospective assessment of individual air pollution exposure, even if the latter is done using personal monitors (an expensive exercise, the use of which will be very limited in duration). Many of the diseases studied in the context of long-term effects of air pollution are rare diseases and the case-control approach therefore would give good opportunities, on a cost–benefit basis, for the next generation of studies, i.e. those which will attempt a more refined individual exposure estimation.

The case-crossover design recently introduced (Maclure, 1991) and used in a different context (Mittleman *et al.*, 1993) may be adapted for use in air pollution epidemiological studies.

Multicentre studies

In recent years the need for European collaborative biomedical projects has been widely recognized and this fact has been expressed in the numerous calls by the Commission of the European Communities (CEC) for joint research proposals and concerted actions. There are some obvious advantages in these multicentre projects: they afford larger and more diverse populations, with a wider variability in the distribution of exposure and associated risk factors. An important positive result of such collaborations is also the transfer of knowhow and the 'assimilation' in research procedures and approaches among the involved research groups. The need to pull together data and results from similar protocols is also evident in the many recent attempts to apply meta-analysis (Schwartz, 1993). The results of meta-analyses are inherently more powerful than the individual results and are useful and informative when the requirements for comparability across the original studies are fulfilled.

In air pollution epidemiology, an approach based on large and diverse geographical areas is particularly suitable for many reasons. At the levels of air pollution observed today powerful techniques are required to identify and quantify the possible health effects. Furthermore, the expected relatively weak associations, to be observed, under these conditions can often be a result of confounding effects. The observation of the same relationship under different circumstances and populations makes causality a more plausible interpretation of any possible association.

Three multicentre air pollution epidemiological studies are ongoing under the CEC's Environment Programme, investigating health effects of air pollution:

1. Effects of short-term changes in urban air pollution on the respiratory health of children with chronic respiratory symptoms (The PEACE (Pollution effects on asthmatic children in Europe) project, coordinated by B. Brunekreef, University of Wageningen, the Netherlands).

   In the framework of this project 28 panels of about 75 asthmatic children age 7–11 years each have been followed for a specified winter period (Brunekreef, 1993). Exposure to air pollution and health status have been closely monitored and the data are now being analysed.

2. Short-term effects of air pollution on health: a European approach using epidemiological time-series data (The APHEA project, coordinated by K. Katsouyanni, University of Athens, Medical School, Greece).

   A very extensive database of epidemiological time-series data (daily number of deaths, daily number of hospital emergency admissions, daily air pollution measurements and data on confounders) from ten European countries representing various environmental and air pollution situations will provide estimates of short-term effects of air pollution. The method of analysis for every centre was standardized and the data are now being meta-analysed (Katsouyanni et al., 1995).

3. Small area variations in air quality and health (The SAVIAH study coordinated by P. Elliott, London School of Hygiene & Tropical Medicine, UK).

   This is mainly a methodological study, to apply, test and evaluate methods in epidemiology, geography, pollution modelling and small area health statistics and their combination in a consistent geographic framework. It will also evaluate the use of low-cost personal passive sampler methods as a means of predicting individual exposure to ambient air pollution.

Conclusion

Epidemiological studies on the health effects of air pollution have proliferated over the last decade, and their results are having a wider impact in regulating air pollution and setting standards. Most studies assessing air pollution health effects are directly or indirectly ecological, but they have gone a long way in addressing the problems of inference based on aggregated data by choosing appropriate units of aggregation and collecting individual data on confounding factors. To address the many remaining questions in air pollution epidemiology, innovative research approaches are needed to effectively combine traditional study designs, achieve better exposure assessment and use larger and more diverse study populations.

References

Brunekreef B (1993) *Effects of Short-term Changes in Urban Air Pollution on the Respiratory Health of Children with Chronic Respiratory Symptoms: Study Procedures.* (Internal report)

Carrozzi L, Giuliano G, Viegi G et al. (1990) The Po River Delta epidemiological study of obstructive lung disease: sampling methods, environmental and population characteristics. *European Journal of Epidemiology, 6*, 191–200

Clench-Aas J, Larssen S, Bartonova A et al. (1991) *The health effects of traffic pollution as measured in the Valerenga area of Oslo.* Lillestrom (Internal document NILU OR 7/91)

Colley JRT, Reid DD (1970) The urban and social origins of childhood bronchitis in England and Wales. *British Medical Journal, 2*, 213–217

Derriennic F, Richardson S, Mollie A, Lellouch J (1989) Short-term effects of sulphur dioxide pollution on mortality in two French cities. *International Journal of Epidemiology, 18*, 186–197

Detels R, Rokaw SN, Coulson AH et al. (1979) The UCLA population studies of chronic obstructive respiratory disease. I: Methodology and comparison of lung function in areas of high and low pollution. *American Journal of Epidemiology, 109*, 33–58

Dockery DW, Pope CA, Xu X et al. (1993) An association between air pollution and mortality in six U.S. cities. *New England Journal of Medicine, 329*, 1753–1759

Frezieres RG, Coulson AH, Katz RM et al. (1982) Response of individuals with reactive airway disease to sulphates and other atmospheric pollutants. *Annals of Allergy, 48*, 156–165

Haenszel W, Taeuber KE (1964) Lung cancer mortality as related to residence and smoking histories. II: White females. *Journal of the National Cancer Institute, 32*, 803–838

Hatzakis A, Katsouyanni K, Kalandidi A et al. (1986) Short-term effects of air pollution on mortality in Athens. *International Journal of Epidemiology, 15*, 73–81

Jedrychowski W, Becher H, Wahrendorf J, Basa-Cierpialek Z (1990) A case-control study of lung cancer with special reference to the effect of air pollution in Poland. *Journal of Epidemiology and Community Health, 44*, 114–120

Katsouyanni K (ed.) (1993) *Study Designs.* Air Pollution Epidemiology Report Series: Report Number 4. Luxembourg Office for Official Publications of the European Communities

Katsouyanni K, Karakatsani A, Messari I et al. (1990) Air pollution and cause specific mortality in Athens. *Journal of Epidemiology and Community Health, 44*, 321–324

Katsouyanni K, Trichopoulos D, Kalandidi A et al. (1991) A case control study of air pollution and tobacco smoking in lung cancer among women in Athens. *Preventive Medicine, 20*, 271–278

Katsouyanni K, Zmirou D, Spix C et al. (1995) Short-term effects of air pollution on health: a European approach using epidemiologic time series data. *European Respiratory Journal, 8*, 1030–1038

Korn EL, Whittemore AS (1979) Methods for analyzing cohort studies of acute health effects of air pollution. *Biometrics, 35*, 795–802

Krzyzanowski M, Jedrychowski W, Wysocki M (1986) Factors associated with the change in ventilatory function and the development of chronic obstructive pulmonary disease in a 13-year follow-up of the Cracow study. *American Review of Respiratory Disease, 134*, 1011–1019

Lambert PM, Reid DD (1970) Smoking, air pollution and bronchitis in Britain. *Lancet, 1*, 853–857

Lyon JL, Klauber MR, Graff W, Chiu G (1981) Cancer clustering around pint sources of pollution: assessment by a case-control methodology. *Environmental Research, 25*, 29–34

Maclure M (1991) The case-crossover design: a method for studying transient effects on the risk of acute events. *American Journal of Epidemiology, 133,* 144–153

Mittleman MA, Maclure M, Tofler GH *et al.* (1993) Triggering of acute myocardial infarction by heavy physical exertion. *New England Journal of Medicine, 329,* 1677–1683

Perry GB, Chai H, Dickey DW *et al.* (1982) Effects of particulate air pollution on asthmatics. *American Journal of Public Health, 73,* 50–56

Pope CA, Schwartz J, Ransom MR (1992) Daily mortality and PM10 pollution in Utah Valley. *Archives of Environmental Health, 47,* 211–217

Roemer W, Hoek G, Brunekreef B (1993) Effect of ambient winter air pollution on respiratory health of children with chronic respiratory symptoms. *American Review of Respiratory Disease, 147,* 118–124

Rothman K (1986) *Modern Epidemiology.* Little, Brown and Co, Boston

Schwartz J (1993) Air pollution and daily mortality in Birmingham, Alabama. *American Journal of Epidemiology, 137,* 1136–1147

Schwartz J (1994a) Air pollution and daily mortality: a review and meta-analysis. *Environmental Research, 64,* 36–52

Schwartz J (1994b) What are people dying of on high air pollution days? *Environmental Research, 64,* 26–35

Schwartz J, Dockery DW (1992a) Increased mortality in Philadelphia associated with daily air pollution concentrations. *American Review of Respiratory Disease, 145,* 600–604

Schwartz J, Dockery DW (1992b) Particulate air pollution and daily mortality in Steubenville, Ohio. *American Journal of Epidemiology, 135,* 12–19

Schwartz J, Wypij D, Dockery D *et al.* (1991) Daily diaries of respiratory systems and air pollution: methodological issues and results. *Environmental Health Perspective, 90,* 181–187

Schwartz J, Slater D, Larson TV *et al.* (1993) Particulate air pollution and hospital emergency room visits for asthma in Seattle. *American Review of Respiratory Disease, 147,* 826–831

Sunyer J, Saez M, Murillo C *et al.* (1993) Air pollution and emergency room admissions for chronic obstructive pulmonary disease: a 5-year study. *American Journal of Epidemiology, 137,* 701–705

Touloumi G, Pocock SJ, Katsouyanni K, Trichopoulos D (1994) Short-term effects of air pollution on daily mortality in Athens: a time-series analysis. *International Journal of Epidemiology, 23,* 957–967

Tzonou A, Maragoudakis G, Trichopoulos D *et al.* (1992) Urban living, tobacco smoking and chronic obstructive pulmonary disease: a study in Athens. *Epidemiology, 3,* 57–60

Utell MJ, Samet JM (1993) Particulate air pollution and health: new evidence on an old problem. *American Review of Respiratory Diseas, 147,* 1334–1335

Van der Lende R, Kok TJ, Reig RP *et al.* (1981) Decrease in VC and FEV1 with time: indicators for effects of smoking and air pollution. *Bulletin of European Physiopathology and Respiration, 17,* 775–792

Vena JE (1982) Air pollution as a risk factor in lung cancer. *American Journal of Epidemiology, 116,* 42–56

Ware JH, Ferris BG, Dockery DW *et al.* (1986) Effects of ambient sulfur oxides and suspended particles on respiratory health of preadolescent children. *American Review of Respiratory Disease, 133,* 834–842

Winkelstein W, Kantor S, Davies EW *et al.* (1967) The relationship of air pollution and economic status to total mortality and selected respiratory system mortality in men. *Archives of Environmental Health, 14,* 162–171

World Health Organization (1994) *Updating and Revision of Air Quality Guidelines for*

Europe: Meeting of the Working Group on 'Classical' Air Pollutants, Bilthoven, The Netherlands, 11–14 October 1994

Xu ZY, Blot WJ, Xiao HP *et al.* (1989) Smoking, air pollution and the high rates of lung cancer in Shenyang, China. *Journal of the National Cancer Institute*, 81, 1800–1806

6
Health effects of air pollution from traffic: ozone and particulate matter

Joel Schwartz

Harvard School of Public Health and Channing Laboratory, Boston, USA

The increase in vehicle miles travelled in the last 30 years has led to increased concerns about traffic-related air pollution. While our knowledge is still incomplete, a reasonable picture is beginning to emerge for a number of the relevant pollutants. The principal pollutants associated with traffic are nitrogen dioxide, ozone, airborne particles, carbon monoxide, lead, and hydrocarbons. This chapter focuses on the pollutants where the clearest data exist, that is, airborne particles and ozone.

Lead is another pollutant for which we have a great deal of knowledge. However, because lead is no longer present in petrol in the USA, and is gradually disappearing from petrol in western Europe, this pollutant will not be discussed, although there are clearly health consequences of the remaining lead in petrol in Europe today.

This chapter discusses recent studies associating acute exposure to air pollution to short-term changes in daily deaths or hospital attendance. In addition, it addresses the question of whether air pollution is responsible for the increase in asthma reported in the Western world.

Investigations of the potential health effects of air pollution date to the Fumifugium of Evelyn in 1661, if not earlier. Evelyn argued that the increased rates of respiratory disease in London were associated with increased coal combustion. Graunt, in 1662, linked variations in weekly bills of mortality in London to variations in the 'airs'. Studies shortly after the Second World War indicated that very large increases in air pollution were associated with large

Health at the Crossroads: Transport Policy and Urban Health.
Edited by Tony Fletcher and Anthony J. McMichael © 1997 John Wiley & Sons Ltd

increases in daily mortality and morbidity (Great Britain Public Health Service, 1954). The London mortality experience in the celebrated London smog of 1952 was important because it provides biological plausibility to all subsequent studies. Given the time pattern of the episode, there really is no other possible explanation for the mortality increase.

Recent studies have focused on common levels of air pollution in the Western world. In contrast to studies of cancer, many of the other health outcomes associated with air pollutants occur at high incidence, and are generally non-specific. Not surprisingly, the relative risks are low. However, in contrast to airborne carcinogens from chemical plants, or exposures from hazardous waste sites, the exposed population is very large. Hence the attributable risks can be substantial, and generally dwarf those associated with other pollution exposures.

Increased mortality and hospital admission rates

The London smog episode, dominated by high levels of particulates and sulphates, occurred during 5–9 December 1952. In the week ending 6 December 1952, 945 people died in the London administrative county. In the next week, there were 2484 deaths (Great Britain Public Health Service, 1954). Hospital admissions for respiratory and cardiovascular disease also increased. In the 160 Great Towns of England excluding London, death counts changed little during this same period (4585 to 4749). No evidence of an infectious epidemic was found. Subsequent analyses of this episode left little doubt that particulate based smog at high concentrations can increase mortality and morbidity. Whether smaller changes in particle concentrations are associated with smaller increases in morbidity and mortality remains a critical issue.

The pioneering study in this regard was that of Bates and Sizto (1987). They reported that ozone and sulphate particulate exposure was associated with increased hospital admissions for respiratory disease in Ontario. Since that time, many studies have examined the short-term effects of air pollution on all respiratory admissions, admissions for chronic obstructive pulmonary disease (COPD), admissions for pneumonia, and emergency visits for asthma. In addition, two papers have examined hospital admissions for cardiovascular disease. Table 6.1 summarizes the results of recent studies that have examined these associations with airborne particles. Most of these results are from two pollutant models including ozone and airborne particles. PM_{10} is particulate matter less than 10 μm in diameter, which is small enough to enter the respiratory tract. The weighted average represents a meta-analysis weighted by the inverse of the variances of each study. Several points are apparent. First, the association with all respiratory admissions, pneumonia admissions, and COPD admissions is consistent across studies. Second, the relative increase in respiratory admissions is greater than the relative increase in mortality that has been associated with the same exposure. Finally, the relative increase for COPD is larger than for all respiratory admissions. In the 1952 London smog disaster, the largest relative increase in mortality was in deaths from COPD.

Several studies, using various research methods, have reported a positive association between asthma episodes in children and particulate air pollution (e.g. Pope 1989, 1991).

Some of these studies also reported associations of particulates with heart disease. The relative risks of heart disease admissions were highest for heart failure, but lower than for respiratory admissions. This is also in accord with the London 1952 episode, where the relative increase in heart disease deaths (and hospital admissions) was less than that seen for respiratory disease. Because cardiovascular deaths and admissions are more common than respiratory ones, the absolute increases were larger in London. This is also true in the hospital admissions data in Table 6.1.

Chi-squared tests were conducted to determine if any of the associations reported in Table 6.1 showed evidence of heterogeneity. That is, was the variation in slope among the studies greater than might be expected due to random variability? Heterogeneity would suggest the existence of effect modifiers or confounding. No evidence for heterogeneity was found for any outcome. This suggests that confounding by other pollutants or weather is not the source of these associations, since the coincident weather patterns and levels of other pollutants varied greatly across the studies. In particular, studies in the western USA (Spokane, Tacoma, Santa Clara) had very low levels of sulphur dioxide, and much less humidity that in the eastern USA locations. Particulate air pollution was highest in the summer in the eastern USA, and in the winter in the western USA.

Table 6.2 shows similar results for ozone. In general, these results are from two pollutant models (particles and ozone). The relative risks are lower, but the same pattern of a larger relative risk for COPD is seen. Neither study found any evidence of an association between ozone and hospital admissions for cardiovascular disease. No significant heterogeneity was found in these associations. However, for all respiratory admissions, there was a marginally significant finding, suggesting that further investigation is warranted. Schwartz (1995b) has reported that ozone results in Spokane were sensitive to the method of statistical control of weather.

While sulphur dioxide was associated with respiratory hospital admissions in some of these studies, those associations generally disappeared after control for either PM_{10} or ozone in most of the locations (Schwartz, 1995a, 1995b). In addition, in Spokane, sulphur dioxide concentrations were so consistently low that the monitoring network was taken down, yet similar associations are seen with PM_{10} and ozone as in locations with sulphur dioxide present. This suggests that the sulphur dioxide associations are due to confounding with the other pollutants. Further support for this comes from the studies in the Utah valley. They show associations between PM_{10} and respiratory hospital admissions in a location with trivial concentrations of sulphur dioxide. In his 1989 paper, Pope

Table 6.1 Relative risk of respiratory admissions for a 100 $\mu g/m^3$ increase in PM_{10}

All respiratory admissions

Location	Relative risk (95% CI)
Buffalo (Thurston et al., 1992) *	1.24 (1.45–1.06)
Ontario (Burnett et al., 1994) +	1.12 (1.15–1.08)
New Haven (Schwartz, 1995b)	1.12 (1.26–1.01)
New York (Thurston et al., 1992)	1.10 (1.20–1.02)
Spokane (Schwartz, 1995a)	1.17 (1.27–1.07)
Tacoma (Schwartz, 1995b)	1.20 (1.35–1.06)
Weighted average	1.13 (1.15–1.10)
Test for heterogeneity	$\chi^2 = 3.83$, df = 5, p = 0.57

* Converted assuming $SO_4/PM_{10} = 0.25$ based on Six City Study data.
\+ Converted assuming $SO_4/PM_{10} = 0.40$ based on sixth day PM_{10} monitoring.

COPD admissions

Location	Relative risk (95% CI)
Barcelona (winter) (Sunyer et al., 1993) *	1.22 (1.33–1.13)
Barcelona (summer) (Sunyer et al., 1993) *	1.16 (1.33–1.13)
Birmingham (Schwartz, 1994b)	1.26 (1.50–1.08)
Detroit (Schwartz, 1994c)	1.20 (1.37–1.09)
Minneapolis (Schwartz, 1994f)	1.57 (2.06–1.20)
Ontario (Burnett et al., 1995)	1.15 (1.22–1.064)
Philadelphia (Schwartz, 1995a)	1.34 (1.68–1.06)
Weighted average	1.19 (1.24–1.15)
Test for heterogeneity	$\chi^2 = 7.3$, df = 6, p = 0.30

* Converted from black smoke assuming $BS/PM_{10} = 1$.
\+ Converted assuming $SO_4/PM_{10} = 0.40$ based on sixth day PM_{10} monitoring.

Pneumonia admissions

Location	Relative risk ((95% CI)
Birmingham (Schwartz, 1994b)	1.19 (1.32–1.07)
Minneapolis (Schwartz, 1994f)	1.17 (1.33–1.02)
Detroit (Schwartz, 1994c)	1.12 (1.21–1.04)
Ontario (Burnett et al., 1995)	1.10 (1.15–1.05)
Philadelphia (Schwartz, 1995a)	1.38 (1.67–1.14)
Weighted average	1.13 (1.17–1.09)
Test for heterogeneity	$\chi^2 = 6.9$, df = 4, p = 0.14

Heart disease admissions

Location	Heart failure	Relative risk (95% CI) Ischaemia	Dysrhythmia
Ontario (Burnett et al., 1995)	1.09 (1.17–1.02)	1.07 (1.12–1.02)	1.04 (1.14–0.94)
Detroit (Schwartz, 1995a)	1.10 (1.16–1.04)	1.05 (1.10–1.02)	1.06 (1.14–0.99)

Asthma emergency room visits

Location	Relative risk (95% CI)
Seattle (Schwartz et al., 1993)	1.45 (1.83–1.14)
Atlanta (White et al., 1994)	1.22 (3.39–0.66)

Table 6.2   Relative risk of respiratory hospital admissions for a 100 mg/m³ increase in ozone

All respiratory admissions

Location	Relative risk (95% CI)
Buffalo (Thurston *et al.*, 1992)	1.12 (1.24–0.99)
Ontario (Burnett *et al.*, 1994)	1.05 (1.07–1.03)
New Haven (Schwartz, 1995b) *	1.07 (1.15–0.99)
New York (Thurston *et al.*, 1992)	1.07 (1.09–1.04)
Spokane (Schwartz, 1995a)	1.54 (2.38–1.00)
Tacoma (Schwartz, 1995b) *	1.20 (1.37–1.06)
Weighted average	1.06 (1.08–1.05)
Test for heterogeneity	$\chi^2 = 9.2$, df = 5, p = 0.10

* Converted assuming peak ozone/mean ozone = 2.5.

COPD admissions

Location	Relative risk (95% CI)
Birmingham (Schwartz, 1994b)	1.07 (1.20–0.96)
Detroit (Schwartz, 1994c) *	1.12 (1.21–1.03)
Minneapolis (Schwartz, 1994f) *	1.07 (1.14–1.01)
Philadelphia (Schwartz, 1995a)	1.11 (1.17–1.04)
Weighted average	1.10 (1.13–1.06)
Test for heterogeneity	$\chi^2 = 1.24$, df = 3, p = 0.74

* Converted assuming peak ozone/mean ozone = 2.5.

Pneumonia admissions

Location	Relative risk (95% CI)
Birmingham (Schwartz, 1994b)	1.04 (1.12–0.97)
Minneapolis (Schwartz, 1994f) *	1.06 (1.13–0.99)
Detroit (Schwartz, 1994c) *	1.11 (1.17–1.05)
Philadelphia (Schwartz, 1995a)	1.04 (1.10–0.99)
Weighted average	1.07 (1.10–1.04)
Test for heterogeneity	$\chi^2 = 3.46$, df = 3, p = 0.33

* Converted assuming peak ozone/mean ozone = 2.5.

examined the number of admissions of children to the hospital for respiratory disease in three winters: 1985,1986, and 1987. In 1986, the steel mill that supplies most of the air pollution in the Utah Valley was closed by a strike. The mill was reopened the following year. Figure 6.1 shows the results of that study. In Salt Lake City, in contrast, where no noticeable change in pollution occurred in 1986, there was no significant difference between 1986 and the other two years in respiratory hospital admissions of children. Following Bates and Sizto's work, the question of associations with daily mortality was also reopened.

Schwartz and Dockery (1992a) examined the correlation between daily deaths in Philadelphia and daily concentrations of total suspended particles (TSP)

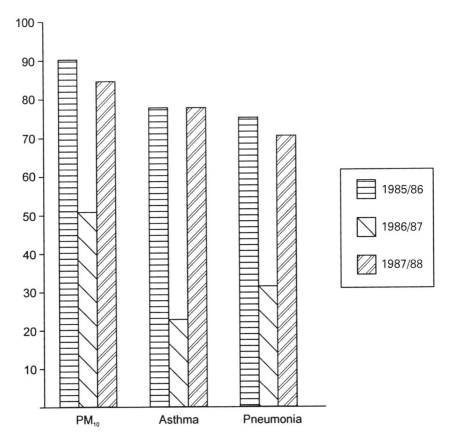

Figure 6.1   PM$_{10}$ and respiratory hospital admissions in Utah Valley in three winters

during the years 1973–1980. After controlling for year of study, continuous time trend, daily temperature, daily humidity, very hot days, very humid days, and season, TSP was a highly significant predictor of daily mortality. While SO$_2$ was also a significant predictor of daily mortality, when both pollutants were considered simultaneously TSP remained significant (with only a minor reduction in its estimated effect size), while the greatly reduced effect of SO$_2$ became insignificant. TSP was highest during the warm months in this study, while mortality peaked in the winter, suggesting that inadequate control for seasonal factors would only bias downward the estimated pollution effect. When quintiles of TSP were used instead of the continuous pollution variable, a dose dependent increase in mortality risk with increasing TSP was seen. This is illustrated in Figure 6.2, which shows the relative risk of all cause mortality adjusted for the other covariates, by quintile of TSP. The risk in the lowest quintile was taken as the reference level. Schwartz and Dockery also examined age and cause specific

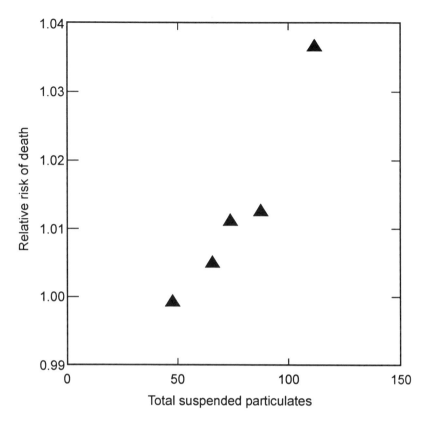

Figure 6.2 Covariate adjusted relative risk of death in Philadelphia by quintile of TSP concentration

risks of particulate exposure. These are illustrated in Figure 6.3, which shows the relative risk of 100 $\mu g/m^3$ of TSP for all cause mortality, mortality in persons aged 65 and older, mortality in persons aged less than 65 years, and mortality from COPD, pneumonia, cardiovascular disease, and cancer. The pattern of much larger relative risks in the elderly, and for COPD deaths, followed by pneumonia and cardiovascular disease, parallels what was seen in London in 1952, when the absolute magnitudes of both the relative risks and pollution exposure were much greater. A reanalysis of these data found that the results were not sensitive to the methods of modelling weather (Schwartz, 1994a).

This finding is consistent with other recent findings. Table 6.3 shows the estimated relative risk of exposure to 100 $\mu g/m^3$ PM_{10} for all cause mortality in recent studies in three continents. These studies, showing similar slopes in areas with different mean temperatures and climatic conditions, and with both winter and summer peaking air pollution, make a strong case for the association. A

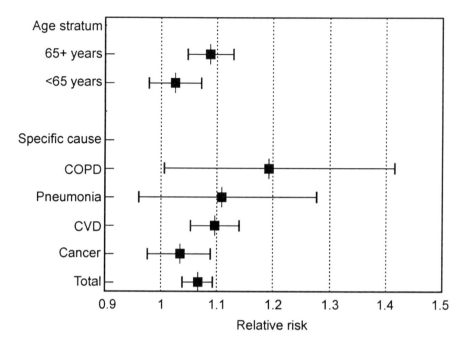

Figure 6.3   Covariate adjusted relative risk of death for a 100 μg/m³ increase in TSP in Philadelphia by age and underlying cause of death groupings

recent meta-analysis found no difference in slopes between locations where airborne particles were high in the winter and locations where airborne particles were high in the summer. Humid and dry locations likewise showed no difference, and the two locations without noticeable SO_2 or ozone exposure also showed mean effects of similar size. This makes confounding by weather, by SO_2 (mostly present in the winter), or by ozone (mostly present in the summer) unlikely. Table 6.3 contains more studies than were reported in that meta-analysis, and so the analysis by winter-versus-summer-peaking particulate air pollution location has been repeated. Little difference is seen between the results, again suggesting confounding by weather is unlikely. A chi-squared test for heterogeneity of the slopes was highly insignificant (p = 0.35).

Recent papers have tried a different approach to avoiding confounding by weather. They have reported results before and after exclusion of extreme weather days, which are the ones most likely to result in confounding. No evidence for confounding has been seen, as indicated in Table 6.4.

Figure 6.4 shows the relative risk of death in each location plotted against the mean temperature in that location. Little evidence is seen for any variation in the PM_{10} effect estimate with temperature. In Figure 6.5, the mean PM_{10} effect size in each location is plotted against the mean SO_2 concentration in that location.

Table 6.3 Relative risk of death for a 100 $\mu g/m^3$ increase in PM_{10}

City	Relative risk	(95% CI)
Amsterdam	1.08	(1.16–0.99)
Athens	1.08	(1.10–1.06)
Birmingham	1.11	(1.20–1.02)
Chicago	1.08	(1.10–1.01)
Cincinnati *	1.1	(1.17–1.05)
Detroit *	1.12	(1.16–1.05)
Erfurt	1.12	(1.17–1.04)
Kingston, TN	1.16	(1.57–0.88)
Los Angeles	1.05	(1.10–1.00)
Minneapolis *	1.09	(1.15–1.04)
Philadelphia *	1.12	(1.17–1.07)
Provo	1.15	(1.23–1.09)
Santiago	1.11	(1.15–1.08)
Santa Clara	1.08	(1.16–1.02)
Steubenville *	1.08	(1.10–1.04)
St Louis	1.16	(1.34–1.01)
São Paulo	1.14	(1.21–1.07)
Overall	1.09	(1.10–1.08)
Winter cities only	1.09	(1.11–1.07)
Test for heterogeneity	$\chi^2 = 16.4$, df $= 15$, p $= 0.35$	

* Converted from TSP assuming $PM_{10}/TSP = 0.60$

Table 6.4 Sensitivity of PM association to exclusion of extreme weather days

City	Outcome	RR before exclusion	RR after exclusion
Philadelphia	Pneumonia	1.32	1.35
Cincinnati	Death	1.1	1.1
Birmingham	Pneumonia	1.19	1.17
Minneapolis	Pneumonia	1.17	1.18
Spokane	All respiratory	1.17	1.18
Detroit	Ischaemia	1.05	1.05

Erfurt is excluded because of its extreme values. There is little suggestion that the PM_{10} effect size is larger in locations with more SO_2, as might be expected if the associations were due to confounding with SO_2. Including Erfurt (Figure 6.6), with SO_2 levels more than an order of magnitude higher than those in the lower SO_2 communities, again shows little dependence of the PM_{10} effect on SO_2 concentration.

Figure 6.7 (p. 73) shows the PM_{10} effect size plotted against the mean ozone concentration in the study location. No general trend is seen in the data except for Los Angeles, which had a lower PM_{10} coefficient and very high ozone levels. When the plots are done against the ratio of mean PM_{10} concentration to mean

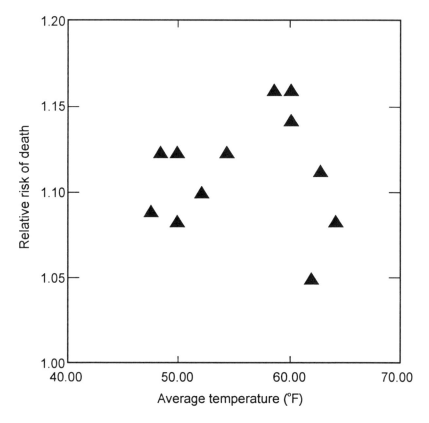

Figure 6.4   Covariate adjusted relative risk of death for a 100 $\mu g/m^3$ increase in PM_{10} plotted versus the average temperature in the study location

SO_2 (or O_3) concentration (Figures 6.8 and 6.9, pp. 74–75), again little evidence of confounding, is seen.

Ozone has also been examined as a predictor of daily mortality. The results of those studies, shown in Table 6.5, are more mixed, and do not provide a convincing argument for an effect.

A number of studies have looked for long-term differences in age adjusted mortality rates between locations with different air pollution concentrations. Most of these analyses have been ecological, with no control for individual risk factors (e.g. Ozkaynak *et al.*, 1986). However, two recent prospective cohort studies have examined the association between air pollution and life expectancy. The Harvard Six City Study looked at 14-year survival in a cohort of 8000 adults chosen to be representative of their communities. Air pollution concentrations varied across the six communities, and after control for age, sex, smoking, body mass, hypertension, diabetes and occupational exposure, a significant gradient in

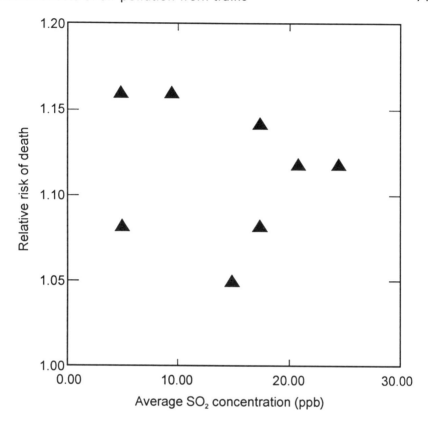

Figure 6.5 Covariate adjusted relative risk of death for a 100 $\mu g/m^3$ increase in PM_{10} plotted versus the average SO_2 concentration in the study location. Erfurt is excluded to better allow examination of the variation with SO_2 in the other locations

Table 6.5 Relative risk of death for a 100 $\mu g/m^3$ increase in ozone

Location	Relative risk (95% CI)
Detroit	1.01 (1.02–0.99)
Eastern Tennessee	0.97 (1.15–0.81)
Los Angeles	1.00 (1.02–0.98)
São Paulo	1.01 (1.13–0.88)
St Louis	1.01 (1.09–0.94)
Overall	1.008 (1.017–0.999)
Test for heterogeneity	$\chi^2 = 3.47$, df = 3, p = 0.33

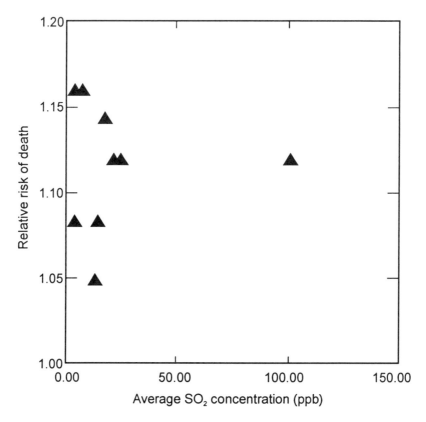

Figure 6.6   Covariate adjusted relative risk of death for a 100 μg/m^3 increase in PM$_{10}$ plotted versus the average SO$_2$ concentration in the study location

mortality was found across location when ordered by long-term average particulate concentration. The association became stronger as the particulate index was changed from TSP to PM$_{10}$, and from PM$_{10}$ to PM$_{2.5}$. No evidence of an association was seen for ozone (Dockery *et al.*, 1993). In a cohort of over 550 000 persons across 150 communities, a similar gradient was seen between sulphate concentration and mortality on follow-up, after control for individual risk factors (Pope *et al.*, 1995). These findings in prospective cohort studies add considerable weight to the evidence, because the likely confounders are quite different from those in daily time-series, yet positive associations are reported.

Exposure considerations

Unless air pollutants are extraordinarily toxic, very short-term exposure at current concentrations is unlikely to produce adverse effects, even in sensitive

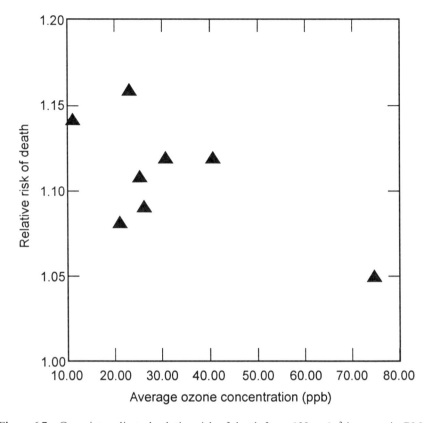

Figure 6.7 Covariate adjusted relative risk of death for a 100 μg/m^3 increase in PM$_{10}$ plotted versus the average O$_3$ concentration in the study location

populations. Since most people spend over 90% of their time indoors, this means that outdoor air pollutants must penetrate indoors in order to produce an adverse response. We can use our knowledge of such penetration to help us understand what may be behind the observed associations.

This paper has documented that airborne particles are associated with adverse effects. The measured particle concentration is likely to be only a proxy for exposure to some component of particulate air pollution. What can our knowledge about indoor penetration and concentrations tell us about this?

Early suspicion focused on the strong acidity of some particulates. Some studies have suggested a stronger association between aerosol acidity and mortality (Thurston *et al.*, 1989) and hospital admissions (Thurston *et al.*, 1992) than for particle measures. However, this judgement was based predominantly on minor differences in statistical significance (e.g. t values of 2.36 *vs* 2.26 in the Toronto hospital study) and other studies have failed to find any association with

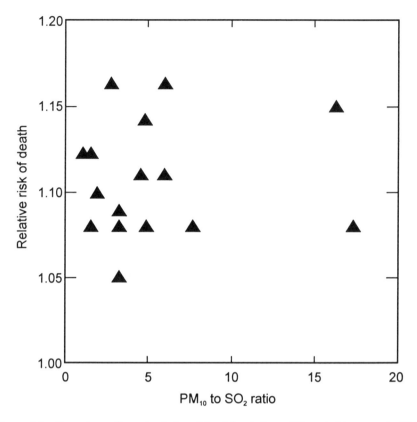

Figure 6.8 Covariate adjusted relative risk of death for a 100 $\mu g/m^3$ increase in PM_{10} plotted versus the ratio of PM_{10} to SO_2 concentration in the study location

particle acidity in studies where associations were found with other particle measures (Dockery *et al.*, 1992). Particle associations have been seen in locations where aerosol acidity never exceeded the detection limit (Pope *et al.*, 1992).

When we consider indoor penetration, however, the acidic aerosol story becomes problematic. While fine aerosol sulphates readily penetrate indoors, they are rapidly neutralized by indoor ammonia. Brauer *et al.* (1989) reported that indoor concentrations of H^+ were 27% of outdoor in non air-conditioned homes, and substantially less when air conditioning was operating. In a study by Suh *et al.* (1992) average indoor H^+ concentrations were only 17% of outdoor levels, and indoor concentrations of ammonia above 15 ppb resulted in essentially complete neutralization of H^+. In a later study (Suh *et al.*, 1994) Suh estimated that across the common range of indoor ammonia concentrations, the half-life for indoor H^+ ranged from one to thirty minutes. At an air exchange rate of one per hour and an ammonia concentration of 20 ppb (the means for the

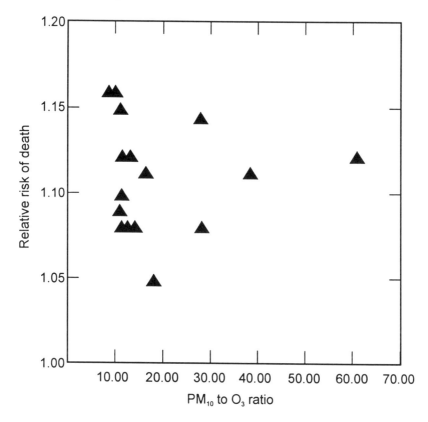

Figure 6.9 Covariate adjusted relative risk of death for a 100 $\mu g/m^3$ increase in PM_{10} plotted versus the ratio of PM_{10} to O_3 concentration in the study location

study), the estimated indoor to outdoor H^+ ratio was about 0.10. While children playing outdoors during the summer may have some acid exposure, it is unlikely that the elderly, who account for the majority of the mortality and morbidity associated with particulate air pollution, have noticeable exposure.

The case for fine particulates appears stronger. Particles with an aerodynamic diameter of 2.5 mM or less penetrate easily into homes, and have settling rates measured in days to weeks. Suh *et al.* (1992) reported that in non-air-conditioned homes, the slope of the indoor–outdoor sulphate ratio was 0.94. Anuzewski *et al.* (1995) reported that short-term nephelometry (light scattering) measurements indoors versus outdoors had slopes of about 0.90. It should be noted that total personal exposure to particles includes indoor sources, such as wood or paraffin fuelled heating devices, environmental tobacco smoke, and vacuum cleaner dust. However, the issue is not what is the association between particles from any source and health outcomes; it is what is the association with particles from outdoor sources.

Coarse particles (i.e. those greater than 2.5 mM in aerodynamic diameter) have poor indoor penetration rates and settle out quickly. This suggests that the associations seen with airborne particles are likely due to the fine particles, or some more common aspect of them than acidity. However, PM_{10} is highly correlated with $PM_{2.5}$. In the Harvard Six City Study, for example (Schwartz, 1994a–f), the correlation in daily concentration exceeded 0.90. Hence, it is an excellent proxy for fine particle exposure. Black smoke will also be a good proxy for fine particles in locations where most of the fine particles are black. Cities with substantial diesel exhaust may fall in this category.

The situation implicating ozone with adverse health effects is less strong. In homes without air conditioning, indoor concentrations of ozone are typically about half of those outdoors (Hayes, 1991). In air conditioned office buildings and homes, ozone concentrations are usually quite low. Ozone concentrations tend to peak later in the day when people spend the most time outdoors, particularly children. Hence, hospital admissions associated with ozone exposure are particularly strong for children, whereas the much weaker association with heart disease morbidity and mortality in the elderly may reflect this outdoors–indoors exposure.

Finally, studies of indoor exposure also are informative about the alternative hypothesis that the observed associations are due to sulphur dioxide. Sulphur dioxide has a penetration rate close to one; however, it is highly reactive on surfaces inside the home, with a correspondingly short half-life. Suh (1993) has reported that typical summer indoor to outdoor ratios are only about 0.20. Winter ratios are lower. Since sulphates are a major constituent of fine particles, the correlation between outdoor sulphur dioxide and outdoor fine particle concentrations is quite high. In the Harvard Six City Study, the correlation was 0.55, for example (Schwartz, 1994a–f). Hence sulphur dioxide may well be another proxy for exposure to fine particles.

General comments on air pollution studies

All of the studies cited above have been controlled for season and weather. Most of them have investigated nonlinear temperature effects. The Buffalo and New York results are an exception. While the particle results are generally insensitive to weather models, the ozone results are more affected (Schwartz, 1995b). Therefore, the results in Buffalo and New York for ozone must be viewed with more caution. Multiple methods have been used in these studies to control for long wavelength and other seasonal patterns, and it seems unlikely that these results are biased by lack of control. Given the consistency and coherency of the results for morbidity and mortality, a causal interpretation seems justified.

Trends in asthma and air pollution

Considerable attention has focused on the increasing trends in asthma prevalence and morbidity in the western world in the last two decades. Many in Europe have speculated that these increases may be related to air pollution. However, in the USA air pollution has been decreasing during the period. Nevertheless, similar trends of increasing asthma morbidity are seen in the USA. This is indicated in Figure 6.10, which shows national asthma hospital admission rates of persons under 15 years of age plotted over time from 1968 to 1989. Concentrations of carbon monoxide and nitrogen dioxide are also plotted. CO is shown, not

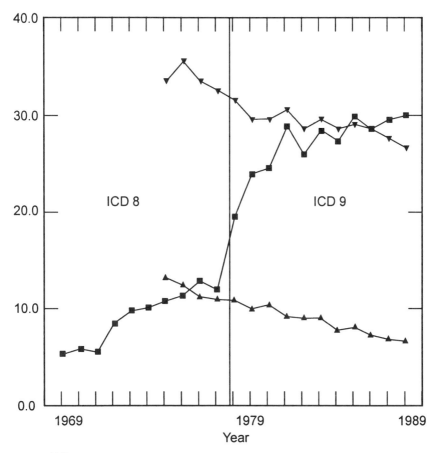

▼ NO₂ (ppb)

▲ CO (ppb)

■ Asthma admissions per 10 000

Figure 6.10 Rate of hospitalization for asthma of children aged 15 and under in the USA, and average CO and NO₂ concentrations in the USA, both plotted versus year

because it is a suspected factor in asthma, but because it serves as an excellent marker for total traffic-related pollutants. Motor vehicles are the predominant source of nitrogen dioxide. Both of these pollutants show major decreases during the period that asthma hospitalization rates were increasing. Concentrations of other pollutants, such as TSP, ozone, and SO_2 were also declining during that period. This is shown in Figure 6.11. The reason for the falling levels of traffic-related pollution in the USA is not a reduction in traffic, but rather the

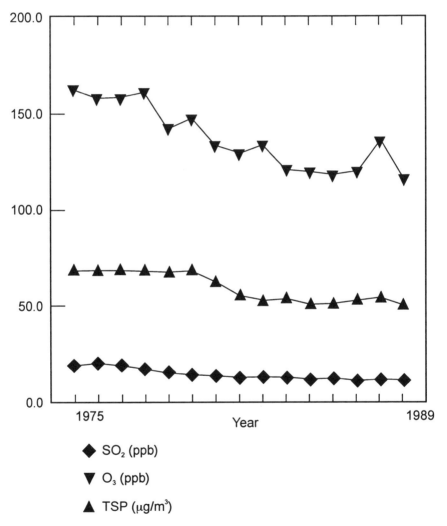

◆ SO_2 (ppb)

▼ O_3 (ppb)

▲ TSP ($\mu g/m^3$)

Figure 6.11   Average TSP, SO_2 and O_3 concentrations in the USA plotted versus year

requirement for catalytic converters on automobiles from 1974, and light trucks from 1980. This is also responsible for the decline in ozone levels. The divergence in the two trends weakens the ecological argument for an association. This is in contrast to the issue of whether air pollution *exacerbates* asthma—for which considerable evidence is building up, both for hospital emergency visits (Table 6.1) and for increased symptoms and reduced peak flow in diary studies (Dockery *et al.*, 1989; Korn and Whittemore 1979; Ostro *et al.*, 1991; Pope *et al.*, 1991; Pope and Dockery 1992; Roemer *et al.*, 1993; Krupnick *et al.*, 1990).

A number of studies have examined whether long-term differences in air pollution concentrations were associated with differences in the prevalence of respiratory disease. Of these studies, the strongest results are those that link long-term differences in airborne particles with differences in chronic bronchitis in adults (Euler *et al.*, 1987, 1988; Schwartz, 1994b–f; Portney and Mullahy, 1990; Xu and Wang, 1993), and bronchitis in children (Dockery *et al.*, 1989).

Conclusion

A coherent and consistent pattern of associations between airborne particles and both mortality and hospital admissions exists. The associations are restricted to deaths and admissions from respiratory and cardiovascular disease. They are also supported by many studies reporting that respiratory symptoms and illness are associated with airborne particle exposure. For ozone, a consistent pattern of exacerbation of respiratory disease is seen, with hospital admission data supported by studies on symptoms and pulmonary function. The evidence for an association between ozone and mortality is weak, perhaps because of the lack of association with cardiovascular disease.

In contrast to studies showing that air pollution exacerbates pre-existing illness, relatively little evidence exists to suggest that air pollution is a risk factor in developing asthma. However, a small but consistent literature exists suggesting that it is a risk factor for developing bronchitis.

References

Anuszewski J, Larson TV, Moseholm L, Koenig JQ (1995) Simultaneous indoor and outdoor particle light-scattering measurements at nine homes using a portable nephelometer. *Environmental International*, 21 (in press)

Bates DV, Sizto R (1987) Air pollution and hospital admissions in Southern Ontario: the acid summer haze effect. *Environmental Research*, 43, 317–331

Brauer M, Koutrakis P, Spengler JD (1989) Personal exposures to acidic aerosols and gases. *Environmental Science and Technology*, 23, 1408–1412

Burnett RT, Dales RE, Raizenne ME *et al.* (1994) Effects of low ambient levels of ozone and sulfates on the frequency of respiratory admissions to Ontario hospitals. *Environmental Research*, 65, 172–194

Burnett RT, Dales RE, Krewski D et al. (1995) Associations between ambient particulate sulfate and admissions to Ontario hospitals for cardiac and respiratory diseases. *American Journal of Epidemiology, 141*, 15–22

Dockery DW, Speizer FE, Stram DO et al. (1989) Effects of inhaled particles on respiratory health of children. *American Review of Respiratory Disease, 139*, 587–594

Dockery DW, Schwartz J, Spengler JD (1992) Air pollution and daily mortality: associations with particulates and acid aerosols. *Environmental Research, 59*, 362–373

Dockery DW, Pope CA, Xu X et al. (1993) An association between air pollution and mortality in six US cities. *New England Journal of Medicine, 329*, 1753–1759

Euler GL, Abbey DE, Magie AR, Hodgkin JE (1987) Chronic obstructive pulmonary disease symptoms effects of long term cumulative exposure to ambient levels of total suspended particulates and sulfur dioxide in California Seventh-Day Adventist residents. *Archives of Environmental Health, 42*, 213–222

Euler GL, Abbey DE, Hodgkin JE, Magie AR (1988) Chronic obstructive pulmonary disease symptom effects of long term cumulative exposure to ambient levels of total oxidants and nitrogen dioxide in California Seventh-Day Adventist residents. *Archives of Environmental Health, 43*, 279–285

Evelyn J (1661, reprinted 1969) Fumifugium, or the inconvenience of the aer and smoake of London dissipated. In Lodge JP Jr (ed) *The Smoake of London: Two Prophecies.* Maxwell Reprint Company, Elmstead, NY

Fairley D (1990) The relationship of daily mortality to suspended particulates in Santa Clara County, 1980–1986. *Environmental Health Perspectives, 89*, 159–168

Graunt J (1939) *Natural and Political Observations Made upon the Bills of Mortality, London, 1662.* Johns Hopkins Press, Baltimore

Great Britain Public Health Service (1954) *Mortality and Morbidity During the London Fog of December 1952: Report Number 95 on Public Health and Medical Subjects.* HMSO, London

Hayes SR (1991) Use of indoor air quality model (IAQM) to estimate indoor ozone levels. *Journal of the Air and Waste Management Association , 41*, 161–170

Korn EL, Whittemore AS (1979) Methods of analyzing panel studies of acute effects of air pollution. *Biometrics, 35*, 795–802

Krupnick AJ, Harrington W, Ostro BD (1990) Ambient ozone and acute health effects: evidence from daily data. *Journal of Environmental Economics and Management, 18*, 1–18

Ostro BD, Lipsett MJ, Wiener M, Selner JC (1991) Asthmatic responses to acid aerosols. *American Journal of Public Health, 81*, 694–702

Ozkaynak H, Spengler JD, Garsd A et al. (1986) Assessment of population health risks resolution from exposures to airborne particles. In Lee SD, Schneider T, Grant LD et al. (eds) *Aerosols: Research Risk Assessment and Control Strategies.* Lewis Publishers, Chelsea (Michigan)

Pope CA (1989) Respiratory disease associated with community air pollution and a steel mill, Utah Valley. *American Journal of Public Health, 79*, 623–628

Pope CA (1991) Respiratory hospital admissions associated with PM10 pollution in Utah, Salt Lake, and Cache Valleys. *Archives of Environmental Health, 46*, 90–97

Pope CA, Dockery DW (1992) Acute health effects of PM10 pollution on symptomatic and asymptomatic children. *American Review of Respiratory Disease, 145*, 1123–1128

Pope CA, Dockery DW, Spengler JD, Raizenne ME (1991) Respiratory health and PM10 pollution: a daily time series analysis. *American Review of Respiratory Disease, 144*, 668–674

Pope CA, Schwartz J, Ransom M (1992) Daily mortality and PM10 pollution in Utah Valley. *Archives of Environmental Health, 42*, 211–217

Pope CA, Thun MJ, Namboodiri MM et al. (1995) Particulate air pollution as a predictor of mortality in a prospective study of US adults. *American Journal of Respiratory*

Critical Care Medicine, 151, 669–674

Portney P, Mullahy J (1990) Urban air quality and respiratory disease. *Regional Science and Urban Economics, 20,* 407–418

Roemer W, Hoek G, Brunekreef B (1993) Effect of ambient winter air pollution on the respiratory health of children with chronic respiratory symptoms *American Review of Respiratory Disease, 147,* 118–124

Saldiva PHN, Pope CA, Schwartz J *et al.* (1995) Air pollution and mortality in elderly people: a time series study in Sao Paulo, Brazil. *Archives of Environmental Health, 50,* 159–163.

Schwartz J (1991) Particulate air pollution and daily mortality in Detroit. *Environmental Research, 56,* 204–213

Schwartz J (1992) Particulate air pollution and daily mortality: a synthesis. *Public Health Reviews, 19,* 39–60

Schwartz J (1993) Air pollution and daily mortality in Birmingham, Alabama. *American Journal of Epidemiology, 137,* 1136–1147

Schwartz J (1994a) Air pollution and daily mortality: a review and meta-analysis. *Environmental Research, 64,* 36–52

Schwartz J (1994b) Air pollution and hospital admissions for the elderly in Birmingham, Alabama. *American Journal of Epidemiology, 139,* 589–598

Schwartz J (1994c) Air pollution and hospital admissions for the elderly in Detroit, Michigan. *American Journal of Respiratory Critical Care Medicine, 150,* 648–655

Schwartz J (1994d) Nonparametric smoothing in the analysis of air pollution and respiratory illness. *Canadian Journal of Statistics, 22,* 471–487

Schwartz J (1994e) Particulate air pollution and daily mortality in Cincinnati, Ohio. *Environmental Health Perspectives, 102,* 186–189

Schwartz J (1994f) PM10, ozone, and hospital admissions for the elderly in Minneapolis-St. Paul, Minnesota. *Archives of Environmental Health, 49,* 366–374

Schwartz J (1994g) What are people dying of on high air pollution days? *Environmental Research, 64,* 26–35

Schwartz J (1995a) Air pollution and hospital admissions for respiratory disease. Unpublished paper

Schwartz J (1995b) Short term fluctuations in air pollution and hospital admissions of the elderly for respiratory disease. *Thorax, 50,* 531–538

Schwartz J, Dockery DW (1992a) Increased mortality in Philadelphia associated with daily air pollution concentrations. *American Review of Respiratory Disease, 145,* 600–604

Schwartz J, Dockery DW (1992b) Particulate air pollution and daily mortality in Steubenville, Ohio. *American Journal of Epidemiology, 135,* 12–19

Schwartz J, Marcus A (1990) Mortality and air pollution in London: a time series analysis. *American Journal of Epidemiology, 131,* 185–194

Schwartz J, Morris R (1995) Air pollution and hospital admissions for cardiovascular disease in Detroit, Michigan. *American Journal of Epidemiology, 142,* 23–35

Schwartz J, Slater D, Larson TV *et al.* (1993) Particulate air pollution and hospital emergency visits for asthma in Seattle. *American Review of Respiratory Disease, 147,* 826–831

Spektor DM, Lippmann M, Lioy PJ *et al.* (1988) Effects of ambient ozone on respiratory function in active, normal children. *American Review of Respiratory Disease, 137,* 313–320

Spix C, Heinrich J, Dockery D *et al.* (1993) Air pollution and daily mortality in Erfurt, East Germany, 1980–1989. *Environmental Health Perspectives, 101,* 518–526

Suh HH (1993) *Characterization of Acid Aerosol and Gas Exposures in Non-Urban Environments.* Harvard School of Public Health, (PhD Thesis)

Suh HH, Spengler JD, Koutrakis P (1992) Personal exposures to acid aerosols and ammonia. *Environmental Science Techniques*, *26*, 2507–2517

Suh HH, Koutrakis P, Spengler JD (1994) The relationship between airborne acidity and ammonia in indoor environments. *Journal of Exposure Analysis and Environmental Epidemiology*, *4*, 1–23

Sunyer J, Saez M, Murillo C *et al.* (1993) Air pollution and emergency room admissions for chronic obstructive pulmonary disease: A 5-year study. *American Journal of Epidemiology*, *137*, 701–705

Thurston GD, Ito K, Lippmann M, Hayes C (1989) Reexamination of London, England, mortality in relation to exposure to acidic aerosols during 1963–1972 winters. *Environmental Health Perspectives*, *79*, 73–82

Thurston GD, Ito K, Kinney PL, Lippmann M (1992) A multi-year study of air pollution and respiratory hospital admissions in three New York State metropolitan areas results for 1988 and 1989 summers. *Journal of Exposure Analysis and Environmental Epidemiology*, *2*, 429–450

Thurston GD, Ito K, Hayes CG *et al.* (1994) Respiratory hospital admissions and summertime haze air pollution in Toronto, Ontario: consideration of the role of acid aerosols. *Environmental Research*, *65*, 271–290

Touloumi G, Pocock SJ, Katsouyanni K, Trichopolous D (1994) Short-term effects of air pollution on daily mortality in Athens: a time series analysis. *International Journal of Epidemiology*, *23*, 957–967

White MC, Etzel RA, Wilcox WD, Lloyd C (1994) Exacerbations of childhood asthma and ozone pollution in Atlanta. *Environmental Research*, *65*, 56–68

Xu X, Wang L (1993) Association of indoor and outdoor particulate level with chronic respiratory illness. *American Review of Respiratory Disease*, *148*, 1516–1522

Discussion

Ross Anderson

St George's Hospital Medical School, London, UK

Joel Schwartz has provided us with a clear presentation of some of the complex epidemiological evidence which associates air pollution with increased mortality and morbidity. He has concentrated mainly on the short-term effects—for which most evidence is available—but has also touched upon the equally important question of chronic effects and the role of air pollution in the changing epidemiology of asthma.

Short-term effects on morbidity and mortality

Episodes of air pollution associated with major health effects are now infrequent and our understanding of the short-term effects of current levels of air pollution rests on the relationship between daily variations in air pollution and health indicators such as lung function, symptoms, use of services and mortality. This more powerful statistical approach is capable of detecting effects which can no longer be observed using traditional episode analysis, but entails complex methods for dealing with confounding, autocorrelation and other factors which could lead to misleading results.

There has been considerable resistance to accepting the findings of such studies, because many have come from areas with pollution levels which are low by historical standards. However, the remarkable consistency of results, as demonstrated in this paper, has persuaded many sceptics that this is a real phenomenon. It should be noted that these studies employ very crude methods of exposure assessment (often a single city monitor) which makes it likely that there will be some misclassification of exposure at the individual level; the effect of this will be to underestimate the exposure–response relationship. The evidence to date therefore indicates that air pollution levels which currently exist in many parts of the world, including Europe, continue to have adverse acute health effects. There remain, however, at least four important questions.

One of these concerns the identification of the responsible component(s) of the pollution mix. Without this information, our efforts to monitor and control the important pollutants will have an uncertain basis. The pollutants customarily studied are but indicators of a very complex cocktail and may not in themselves be important. The various pollutants tend to covary and their individual effects are difficult to disentangle statistically within one area. This is why one-pollutant situations such as occurred in Utah are important. This is also why studies using standard techniques among cities with different pollutant mixes (as in the EC Short term effects of air pollution on health: a European approach 'APHEA' project) are required.

Another question concerns the role of different sizes and compositions of particulate matter. It is clearly important to establish whether the newer forms of pollution from traffic are more toxic than the older type associated with the burning of coal.

Another important area of ignorance concerns the mechanisms by which air pollution harms health. Without this knowledge, the biological plausibility of the epidemiological evidence will continue to be questioned. The differences described in Schwartz's chapter between particulates and ozone in their effects on hospital admissions and mortality suggest that they may be exerting their effects through different mechanisms.

A further question concerns exposure–response relationships. Knowledge of the shape of the relationship and the existence of a threshold is needed for rational policy-making and impact assessment but it is very difficult to obtain with existing methods.

Asthma and air pollution

One of the issues raised in Joel Schwartz's chapter is that of air pollution and asthma. It is very plausible that asthma, a condition characterized by susceptibility of the airways to inhaled irritants, might be affected by air pollution. There is understandable concern that the increase in traffic pollution may be linked to what appears to be a global increase in asthma and allergies. As Schwartz has pointed out, there is no obvious correlation in time between air pollution and asthma admissions in the USA. The available evidence from the UK presents a similar picture. In the UK, evidence from numerous surveys of childhood asthma suggests that asthma prevalence has increased by about 50% over the past 20–30 years. There has been a much larger increase in general practitioner consultations and hospital admissions, but the major part of this could be explained by changes in medical practice.

While asthma has been increasing, there has been a marked decline in emissions and in ambient levels of sulphur dioxide and particulate matter. So, to implicate pollution in an increase in asthma it is necessary to postulate that the increase in asthma is specifically related to the increase in traffic emissions such as particulates from diesel vehicles, oxides of nitrogen and the secondary pollutant, ozone. One problem with this argument is that we know little about trends in the exposure of the population to these pollutants. While emission inventories show

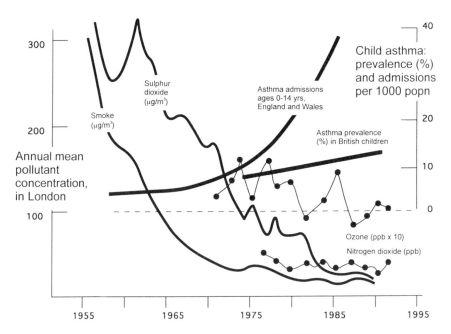

Figure 1   Time trends in major air pollutants in London, UK, and in asthma prevalence and hospitalizations in British children over the past few decades. NB. Since 1960 in the UK, the emissions of nitrogen oxide and fine particulates from traffic exhaust have increased approximately fourfold (not shown in figure). *Figure prepared by the editors from multiple sources supplied by R. Anderson*

an increase in oxides of nitrogen, measured ambient concentrations in most urban centres such as London, are showing little or no change. Ozone levels have been falling in both urban and rural sites. Black smoke concentrations have fallen to historically low levels in urban areas. It could be argued that there is something different about the newer particulates, but Schwartz suggests that the adverse effects of particulates (on mortality) may be more of a generic particle effect than one which depends on the source of the particle.

Other evidence casts doubt on the theory that air pollution plays a major role in the epidemiology of asthma. Studies of short-term effects of air pollution on asthmatics have not been consistent in their findings, and where positive associations have been observed the size of effect has been modest. Where air pollution episodes have been associated with adverse health effects, these have mainly been in older people with chronic obstructive lung disease but not in asthmatics and, notably, not in children with asthma. The seasonal pattern of asthma bears little relationship to the seasonal patterns of pollution.

Studies which have compared the prevalence of asthma between polluted and non-polluted areas have not been conclusive. In Britain there does not seem to be any geographical correspondence between air pollution and childhood asthma, nor does there seem to be a substantial difference in prevalence between urban and rural children.

In interpreting these observations it is important to note that many other equally plausible (though as yet unproven) explanations exist for trends and variations in asthma. On the basis of existing evidence it is difficult to say more than that air pollution is likely to play a fairly small part in the aggravation of asthma, and it is unlikely to be a factor in the causation of asthma itself.

7
Scientific basis for establishing air quality standards; their role in quantitative risk assessment and in monitoring the effectiveness of intervention strategies

Isabelle Romieu

Pan American Center of Human Ecology and Health, Mexico

In many countries, the increase in air pollution from the expanding use of fossil energy sources and the growth in the manufacture and use of chemicals has been accompanied by mounting public awareness and concern about its detrimental effects on health and environment. Air quality guidelines (AQG) have been developed by the World Health Organization (WHO) in order to provide nations with recommended air pollution levels that should not be exceeded to protect public health from adverse effects (WHO, 1987). Nations can then adopt exposure standards based on their specific situation, and intended to be enforceable. This chapter reviews the scientific basis for the establishment of air quality guidelines and standards of major outdoor pollutants, and discusses their role in quantitative risk assessment and their usefulness in monitoring the effectiveness of intervention strategies.

Process of establishing air quality standards

Air quality standards (AQS), as defined in different countries, seek to regulate

Health at the Crossroads: Transport Policy and Urban Health.
Edited by Tony Fletcher and Anthony J. McMichael © 1997 John Wiley & Sons Ltd

allowable pollutant concentrations within the atmosphere, to avert adverse effects on the health and welfare of the public (Padgett and Richmond, 1983). They are based on a technical review of the published scientific evidence which identifies and quantifies associations between exposure to airborne pollutants and the resulting effects on humans (leading to the setting of primary standards), as well as the effects on crops, materials, and natural ecosystems (secondary standards). In addition to utilizing these scientific estimates of risk, ambient air standards are also based on 'best judgements' and 'adequate margins of safety' necessary to protect the segment of population that is at greater risk (Garner, 1986).

Air quality guidelines and standards should focus on air pollutants of special environmental and health significance, taking into account (1) the severity and frequency of adverse health effects, especially if effects are irreversible, (2) ubiquity and abundance in the environment, (3) environmental transformation or metabolic alteration, (4) persistence in the environment, and (5) size of the exposed population and, in particular of high risk groups (WHO, 1987).

Review of scientific information

The first phase in the establishment of air quality guidelines or standards is an extensive review of the scientific literature in order to determine the sources and health impacts of air pollutants in different groups of the population. However, data are often scarce and the quantitative relation uncertain; scientific judgement and consensus therefore play an important role in establishing acceptable levels of population exposure (WHO, 1987).

The standard setting process begins with an extensive review of all published scientific information concerning a specific pollutant, including sources of the pollutant, its atmospheric transformation, and the evidence for a causal relationship between a given exposure and the one or more health effects with which it is associated. Judgements about the value of information from a particular epidemiological study are influenced by such factors as the adequacy of study design, the size of the study, the precision of health and exposure data, the appropriateness of the data analysis (Evans, 1978), the control of potential confounding factors, and the generalizability of the results (Padgett and Richmond, 1983).

A major challenge for epidemiological studies is the assessment of exposure to air pollution (Lippman and Lioy, 1985), particularly to individual pollutants or classes of pollutants, with enough precision to permit quantitative estimation of risk. Such assessment must take into account indoor as well as outdoor exposure. Assessment of the health effects themselves poses a technical challenge, because each disease caused by air pollution has other causes as well. Numerous factors other than air pollution must therefore be accounted for if causal relationships between air pollution and disease are to be clearly established. The various air pollutants may have interactive effects and are often correlated with each other.

Also, it is likely that air pollution insult at community concentration levels will not be instantaneous, and some degrees of lagged effects have to be studied. Because of these several difficulties, associations observed in air pollution studies are usually weak, and interpretation often relies on expert judgement.

The issue of causal inference has received considerable attention from epidemiologists. Criteria for causal inference in epidemiology have been developed by Hill (1965) and include: (1) temporal sequence; (2) consistency; (3) strength of the association; (4) biological gradient or dose response; (5) specificity of effect: a cause is specific to an effect if the introduction of the putative causal factor is followed by the occurrence of that effect only, and if removal of the factor is followed by the absence of the effect. However, this principle does not take into consideration that multiple causes and effects are the rule rather than the exception. Specificity of an association supports a causal interpretation, but lack of specificity does not negate it; (6) biological plausibility: there must be a plausible physiological pathway between dose and response. However, the postulated biological plausibility is limited by the bounds of actual scientific knowledge, and the observation of an association between an exposure and a health effect may lead to further biological research in order to establish the plausibility of the association; (7) coherence: concordance with the prevailing medical wisdom, including support among various health endpoints: if an agent is associated with excess mortality, it should also be associated with excess morbidity; (8) experimental manipulation: does reduction of the dose weaken or eliminate the effect? Case studies of pollution campaigns may be useful in this regard; (9) analogy: is the association consistent with a similar, previously established cause-and-effect relationship? (Lipfert, 1994). Usually, only a subset of these principles are fulfilled, and hence scientific judgement plays an important role in the assessment of causality.

Establishment and revision of national air quality standards: experience of the US Environmental Protection Agency (USEPA)

The main elements of the review process of establishing and revising national ambient air quality standards (NAAQS) of the USEPA are presented in Figure 7.1 (Padgett and Richmond, 1983). Scientific research provides the basis for the content of the criteria document. After public and scientific peer review, the criteria document is summarized in a 'staff paper' which reflects the staff interpretation of the key studies and scientific evidence described in the criteria document and identifies critical elements to be addressed on the standard-setting process. The staff paper addresses issues such as: which effects are significant for standard-setting; what are the lowest levels at which effects have been convincingly demonstrated; what are the various factors which should be considered in selecting a standard that provides an adequate margin of safety (Richmond, 1981)? The staff paper helps to bridge the gap between science contained in the

90

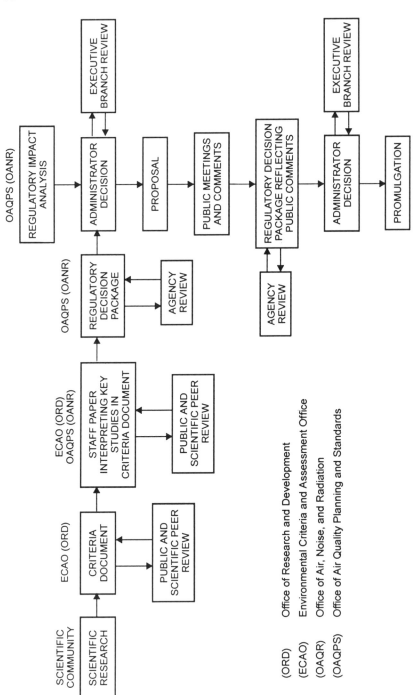

Figure 7.1 An overview of NAAQS (National Ambient Air Quality Standards) standard setting process. Source: Padgett and Richmond (1983)

(ORD)   Office of Research and Development
(ECAO)   Environmental Criteria and Assessment Office
(OAQR)   Office of Air, Noise, and Radiation
(OAQPS)   Office of Air Quality Planning and Standards

criteria document and judgements required by the administrator in setting ambient standards. Regulatory impact analysis is also undertaken to estimate the national cost of meeting alternative standards, the economic impact on various industries and communities, to compare the costs and benefits of alternative standards. All these elements and the associated proposal are submitted for public comments before the setting of NAAQS (Padgett and Richmond, 1983). Primary US EPA standards are required to be solely health based, and designed to protect the most sensitive group of individuals, but not necessarily the most sensitive members of that group, against adverse health effects. Costs incurred to attain an ambient air standard are not considered in setting primary standards (Padgett and Richmond, 1983). Although guidelines and standards are based on the current best scientific judgement, periodic revision is needed, in the light of accruing scientific data and changing social procedures.

Major issues to be considered in the setting of air quality standards are:

1. The concept of 'adverse effect': the scientific literature is the key to the identification of adverse health effects, but frequently the literature is not sufficient to clearly establish whether an observed effect is in fact adverse or at what level of exposure the effect occurs. For example, many air pollutants cause a temporary degradation in lung function. When this degradation is sufficiently high, there is little doubt that the resulting effect on human health is adverse. However, there is considerable disagreement among scientists as to how much degradation one must experience before this effect could be considered adverse.
2. The identification of population groups that may be particularly susceptible to the effects associated with a given pollutant. It is important not to overlook potential sensitive groups.
3. The identification of the lowest level of exposure at which health effects occur. For most air pollutants, the available scientific data to determine at what levels of exposure various health effects occur is incomplete or contradictory. There is great uncertainty in extrapolating results from animal studies to human populations. Safety considerations limit the research which can be accomplished with susceptible individuals in controlled exposure studies, and in epidemiological studies it is often difficult to account for all confounding factors that may interfere in the relation between air pollution and health effects.
4. The fact that guidelines have been established for single chemicals. Chemicals, in mixture, may have additive, synergistic or antagonistic effects; however, knowledge of these interactions is still slight. With a few exceptions, such as the combined effect of sulphur dioxide and particulates, there is insufficient information at present to establish guidelines for mixtures (WHO, 1987).
5. The imprecise concept of 'adequate margin of safety'. The concept refers to the broad objective of protecting the health of sensitive population groups

and the population as a whole (Padgett and Richmond, 1983). Some factors that are considered in deciding the margin of protection are related to the scientific uncertainty because of limitations in the extent or quality of the database. Effects observed in laboratory animals in the absence of human studies generally require a larger uncertainty factor, because humans may be more susceptible than laboratory animal species. Also, a pollutant level producing slight alteration in physiological parameters (of uncertain health significance) requires a smaller uncertainty factor than a pollutant level that produces a clearly adverse effect. Scientific judgement about uncertainty factors will also take into account the toxicology of pollutants, including the type of metabolites formed, variability in the metabolism or response in humans suggesting hypersusceptible groups, and the likelihood that the compound or its metabolites will accumulate in the body (WHO, 1987).

Health effects of air pollutants: interpretation of European Air Quality Guidelines in non-European countries

In 1987, the WHO Regional Office for Europe (EURO) issued a report that established air guidelines for Europe (AQGE). These AQGE were based on general health effects from studies conducted mostly in North America and Europe. Although health effects are expected to be similar in non-European countries, some factors present in these countries may affect human response to air pollutants. These factors include: climatic factors such as temperature, humidity, and altitude; non-anthropogenic particulate matter such as desert sandstorms; specific country conditions such as endemic diseases, nutritional status of the population, access to medical care, local habits and lifestyle, genetic factors; and the prevalence of susceptible groups such as young children, asthmatics, elderly and subjects with pre-existing heart or pulmonary diseases. The potential impact of these factors on the health effects of air pollutants are presented in Table 7.1. For example, high altitude will exacerbate the effect of particulate matter by the mechanism of increased ventilation and the enhanced deposition of the particle in the deeper part of the lung. Similarly, local habits and lifestyle such as time spent outdoors, exercising and manual labour, cooking and heating habits influence the effective exposure to particulates (WHO, 1993). It is recommended that in the setting of country-specific air quality standards, these modulating factors be taken into account since they condition the human health response to air pollutants. Also, at the country level, decision-makers must take into account the trade-off between the health benefits derived and the cost to society of the increased emission controls that would be required if air pollutant standards were set at a specific value.

Table 7.1 Factors modulating the health effect of air pollutants

Outdoor pollutant	Extremes of temperature		Extremes of humidity		High altitude	High natural TSP	Endemic disease	Inadequate medical care	Nutritional deficiency and debilitating disease	Genetic factors	Local habits	Life style	Susceptible groups
	High	Low	High	Low									
PM_{10}	+	(+)	(+)	+	+	+	?	+	+	+	+	+	a-f
Ozone	+	0	(+)	0	(+)	?	(+)	+	+	?	+	+	a,c,d
SO_2	+	+	+	+	?	+	+	+	+	?	+	+	a,b,c,f
NO_2	(+)	+	?	(+)	(+)	(+)	+	+	+	?	+	+	a,b,c,c
CO	(+)	0	0	0	+	0	+	+	+	+	+	+	h,d,e,f
Pb	0	0	0	0	(+)	(+)	+	+	+	+	+	+	h,d,e

One of the following symbols was chosen to be added to each cell:

+ increase can exacerbate the effect
(+) increase probably enhances the effect
0 increase produces no effect
(−) increase probably mitigates the effect
− increase can mitigate the effect
? insufficient evidence to establish a consensus of the panel

(a) Asthmatics. (b) Elderly. (c) COPD. (d) Myocardial pathology. (e) Children infants and/or fetus. (f) Pulmonary fibrotic disease.

Source: WHO (1993)

Quantitative risk assessment

In recent years, the need to quantify the health risk associated with exposure to environmental and occupational toxicants has generated a new interdisciplinary methodology (particularly in North America) referred to as risk assessment.

Risk assessment for NAAQS

Risk assessment can be used to determine whether an exposure standard provides an adequate margin of safety in relation to adverse health effects. In this context, the objectives of a risk assessment are: to assess the risk (probabilities) of the occurrence of adverse health effects in relation to a specified level of exposure, and, for a given population, to calculate the expected numbers of specified health events based on the current state of knowledge; and to describe qualitatively the nature and the severity of the particular adverse events were they to occur (Padgett and Richmond, 1983). The output of this form of risk assessment is necessary for the regulatory decision-making process (Figure 7.2). Risk assessment is followed by risk management which refers to the selection and implementation of the most appropriate regulatory action based upon the results of risk

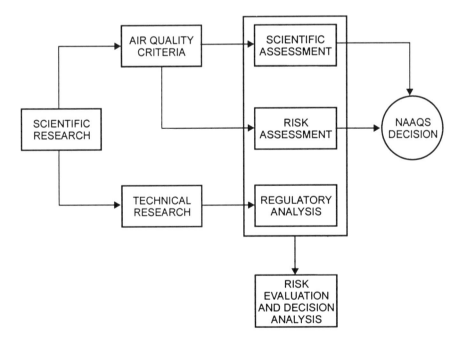

Figure 7.2   Conceptual overview of a NAAQS (National Ambient Air Quality Standards) decision-making process using formal risk analysis. Source: Richmond *et al.* (1982)

assessment, available control technology, cost–benefit analysis, acceptable risk, acceptable number of cases, policy analysis, and social and political factors (see also McMichael, Chapter 3, this volume).

To develop a risk assessment analysis in relation to an exposure 'standard', the input (exposure) variable corresponds to the standard specified in a convenient, measurable manner. The output variables' 'adverse effects' have to be precisely defined and include a complete description of all health effects associated with a pollutant. The objective is to obtain the probability distribution ($f(d/s)$) of each health effect (d) given the particular level of exposure (s) in the population as a whole or in specific subgroups. Experts derive from the scientific literature the probability distributions for different outcomes at specific levels of air pollutants. These probability assignments are based on scientific information. For example, what percentage of a population exposed to 0.12 ppm ozone level will suffer various degrees of forced expiratory volume (FEV) reduction. The experts participating in the evaluation should represent a wide spectrum of views and must be well-respected in their area of expertise. Based on the expert estimations, probability distribution of outcome (d) will be determined for a given standard (s). The number of people with adverse health effects at a given pollutant concentration can thus be calculated as well as the effects on sensitive groups. However, since in environmental assessment, the 'objective' health-effects data are often inadequate, the knowledge and experience of experts is often a very important source of information (Winkler and Sarin, 1981).

Three distinct types of risk measures have been proposed: benchmark risk and head count risk, each based on a decision analytic approach, and the reference concentration methodology.

The benchmark risk is defined as the probability that the maximum or n-th highest time-averaged concentration of a pollutant over a specified period of time (fixed by the form of a standard being analysed) will exceed the concentration that adversely affects a specified fraction of the sensitive group if the whole group were exposed to pollutant levels just meeting the standard. A specific example is the risk that the maximum 1-hour average ozone concentration in Los Angeles will exceed the ozone concentration that causes a 15% reduction in pulmonary function response in 10% of the asthmatics living in Los Angeles. This example illustrates a 10% benchmark for a 15% reduction in FEV_1 response (Richmond et al., 1982).

The headcount risk involves dealing more completely with the relationship between exposure and human response than is necessary in estimating benchmark risks. It is defined as the probability that a specific number of incidents of an adverse health effect will occur or a specified number of persons will suffer an adverse health effect over a specified period of time when a given air quality standard is just attained. Risk should be expressed as distributions of estimates showing a range of probabilities (Richmond, 1988).

The reference concentration is defined as an estimate (with uncertainty spanning perhaps an order of magnitude) of a daily exposure to the human population (including sensitive groups) that is likely to be without an appreciable risk of deleterious effects during a lifetime. The requirements for estimating it are toxicity data, uncertainty factors, and possible modifying factors. The uncertainty factor is invoked to account for the variation in sensitivity among human sub-population (Shoaf, 1991).

Air quality guidelines and standards and risk assessment

The US National Research Council (1983) described four components of quantitative risk assessment in relation to the impact of a specific exposure on health: hazard identification, exposure assessment, dose–response assessment, and risk characterization. Hazard identification is the determination of whether a particular chemical is or is not causally linked to particular health effects. Dose–response assessment is the quantitative relationship between the magnitude of exposure and the occurrence of human health effects. Exposure assessment is the determination of the extent of human exposure in including the evaluation of exposure and the number of people exposed. Risk characterization is the description of the nature, and often the magnitude of human risk, including attendant uncertainty. Essentially, risk assessment is an integration of dose–response assessment and exposure assessment (Shoaf, 1991).

Ideally, guideline values should represent concentrations of chemical compounds in air that would not pose any hazard to the human population. However, because of the lack of information, compliance with the AQG do not provide absolute safety (WHO, 1987). Epidemiological data on the adverse effects of air pollutants are still sparse. Therefore risk characterization may be deficient. Standards are often set using extrapolation from animal data or experimental control human health studies without a clear idea of the shape of the dose–response relationship between air pollutants and specific health effects. The fact that guidelines are established for single chemicals restricts their utility to protect the health of the population since it is likely that mixtures of air pollutants will have synergistic effects. In addition the concept of 'adequate margin of safety' is limited in the absence of epidemiological data and relies on imprecise concepts such as scientific judgement. Finally, averaging time used in setting the guideline may not be adequate in relation to health effects, especially in areas where subjects are chronically exposed.

All these limitations emphasize the shortcomings of the use of AQG to assess quantitatively the health risk in the population. It is assumed that individuals exposed to air pollutant levels not exceeding the guideline or standards should not experience adverse health effects. However, cumulative exposure could reach a critical level, even though the air pollutant concentration did not exceed the standard. For example, ozone ambient level may not exceed the USEPA standard of 1-hour daily maximum of 120 ppb, but a subject may accumulate a large exposure if living in an area where ozone ambient level is elevated for several hours a day. Thus, estimation of an individual exposure to a contaminant only based on the number of violations to the regulatory norm of a specific pollutant would tend to underestimate the exposure, and therefore it is not adequate for quantitative risk assessment. In conclusion, although air quality guidelines and standards are developed to provide a basis for protecting the population from adverse health effects from exposure to air pollutants, they do not provide sufficient information on subject exposure and potential adverse health effects to be useful in quantitative risk assessment. They can only be useful for obtaining a qualitative estimation of risk among the population exposed to air pollutants.

Place of air quality guidelines and standards in monitoring the effectiveness of intervention strategies

Air quality standards are used to monitor the quality of the ambient air in relation to the regulated air pollutants. They provide the authorities with guidance for the implementation of control strategies and of legislative procedures against specific sources in case of non-compliance.

Different countries have defined their own air quality indicators that are used to communicate daily air quality to the public. For example, in Mexico information on daily air quality is provided in terms of 'IMECA' (indice de calidad del aire) with a cut-off point of 100 corresponding to the Mexican standard for each regulated air pollutant (for example, 100 IMECA correspond to the norm of 1-hour daily maximum of ozone of 110 ppb, and to the norm of 275 $\mu g/m^3$ 24-hour average of total suspended particulate) (Comision Metropolitana, Mexico, 1992). When the IMECA is less than 100, the air quality is defined as good; between 100 and 200, the air quality is defined as regular; between 200 and 300 as bad; and over 300 as very bad. However, the index provided to the population corresponds only to the highest air pollutant level and does not consider the concomitant elevation of various air pollutants.

Intervention strategies are implemented when air pollutant levels exceed air quality standards and the effectiveness of the intervention is then based on the compliance with these standards. Air pollution control strategies can then be defined for short-term and long-term periods.

Short-term period: when the air pollutant levels or indices acutely exceed certain pre-specified levels, intervention strategies are implemented to decrease air pollution levels. For example, in Mexico, intervention plans are redefined for three IMECA levels. The first phase of the contingency plan occurs when the IMECA reaches 250 points; the second phase when the IMECA reaches 350; and the third phase when the IMECA reaches 450 points (Comision Metropolitan, Mexico, 1992). During each phase, specific control measures are programmed and the effectiveness of the control is monitored by the evolution of the air quality index. If the first phase contingency plan is not sufficiently effective, supplementary actions are implemented in order to decrease air pollution levels. This includes the participation of various federal and state institutions.

Long-term period: when air quality standards are used to monitor and compare the air quality over long periods (such as years). Results are often presented as the number of violations to the norm during a given time. These estimates can be used to evaluate the effectiveness of intervention measures.

The use of standards—or guidelines—to monitor intervention strategies is useful because it allows a clear goal to be reached. Standards—or guidelines—are easy to interpret and to communicate to the public. They convey a clear message and can be used as tools for qualitative risk evaluation and for setting goals of risk management and to compare intervention strategies. For example, the number of violations to the ozone standard can be compared over different years corresponding to the implementation of different control measures. It is necessary also to consider meteorological and other factors that may interfere with air pollution levels and which may vary over the years. It is also of great value for regulation purposes to determine compliance of fixed sources of air pollutants and to establish legal penalties. However, a major problem of using standards to monitor intervention strategies is that it is based only on a single number and it does not give a quantitative evaluation of the effectiveness of control measures. Violations to the standard may be of different amplitudes and this will not be picked up if we consider only the number of violations. Therefore it is necessary to quantify air pollution levels.

In conclusion, air quality standards and guidelines have been developed to provide a basis for protecting public health from adverse effects of air pollution. Given our limited knowledge on the adverse health effects of air pollutants and the unavoidable uncertainty involved in the development of these norms, it is difficult to use them for quantitative risk assessment. However, they provide a useful tool to monitor air quality and can help decision-makers to plan and monitor air pollution control strategies.

References

Comision Metropolitana para la Prevencion y Control de la Contaminacion Ambiental en el Valle de Mexico (1992) *Manual para la Aplicacion del Programa de Contingencias Ambientales.* CMPCCA, Mexico

Comision Metropolitana para la Prevencion y Control de la Contaminacion Ambiental en el Valle de Mexico (1993) *Informe Mensual de la Calidada del Aire.* CMPCCA, Mexico

Evans AS (1978) Causation and disease: a chronological journey. *American Journal of Epidemiology, 108*, 249–258

Garner JHB (1986) *Air Quality Criteria Development.* (Unpublished document)

Hill AB (1965) The environment and disease: association or causation? *Proceedings of the Royal Society of Medicine, 58*, 295–300

Lipfert FW (1994) *Air Pollution and Community Health: A Critical Review and Data Sourcebook.* Van Nostrand Reinhold, New York

Lippmann M, Lioy PJ (1985) Critical issues in air pollution epidemiology. *Environmental*

Health Perspectives, 62, 243–258

Padgett J, Richmond H (1983) The process of establishing and revising national ambient air quality standards. *Journal of the Air Pollution Control Association*, 33, 13–16

Richmond HM (1981) A framework for assessing health risks associated with national ambient air quality standards. *The Environmental Professional*, 3, 265–276

Richmond HM (1988) *Development of Probabilistic Health Risk Assessment for National Ambient Air Quality Standards*. (Unpublished paper presented at APCA International Specialty Conference on Regulatory Approaches for Control of Air Pollutants, Atlanta, Georgia, 17–20 February 1987)

Richmond HM, McCurdy T, Jordan B (1982) Risk analysis in the context of national ambient air quality standards. In *Proceedings of the 75th Annual Meeting of the Air Pollution Control Association, New Orleans, Louisiana, 20–25 June 1982*. APCA, Pittsburgh

Shoaf CR (1991) Current assessment practices for noncancer end points. *Environmental Health Perspectives*, 95, 111–119

United States National Research Council Agency (1983) *Risk Assessment in the Federal Government: Managing the Process*. National Academy Press, Washington DC

Winkler RL, Sarin RK (1981) Risk assessment: consulting the experts. *The Environmental Professional*, 3, 265–276

World Health Organization (1993) *Report of the Expert Committee on the Interpretation of WHO Air Quality Guidelines*. (Unpublished paper)

World Health Organization Regional Office for Europe (1987) *Air Quality Guidelines for Europe*. WHO Regional Publications, European Series No 23. WHO Regional Office for Europe, Copenhagen

Discussion

Bert Brunekreef

University of Wageningen, Netherlands

In discussing Isabelle Romieu's chapter, it is useful to distinguish clearly between air quality guidelines and air quality standards. The guidelines are, at least in theory, based on scientific judgement alone, whereas the standards include considerations of cost and technical feasibility. Because of this, air quality standards can never be interpreted *directly* as concentrations that separate 'safe' from 'unsafe' conditions. Depending on the considerations that form the background, a standard may have been set at a level at which adverse health effects actually can be expected to occur, or at a level much lower than the level of concern.

An air quality guideline can, loosely, be defined as the concentration at which, based on the available scientific evidence and expert judgement, adverse effects on health do not occur. There are some important caveats: 'adversity' is not a clear-cut notion, and it is by no means clear how it should be defined in the framework of setting air quality guidelines, which often are aimed at preventing subtle effects on human health. The WHO Air Quality Guidelines published in 1987 contain a rather detailed discussion of this issue, which illustrates the complexities involved, and provides at least some guidance on how to deal with 'adversity' in setting air quality guidelines.

A more self-explanatory caveat that is nevertheless worth mentioning is that scientific knowledge is never complete. It is clear that methods improve, and that our understanding of biological mechanisms through which air pollution affects human health increases; in reality we study changes as well, however, and to some extent, the reason why we see so many studies being published in recent years suggesting health effects of air pollution at very low levels of exposure is that such levels were not to be found one or two decades ago, at least not in the densely populated areas that are needed for some epidemiological studies.

A third caveat concerns the use of 'margins of safety'. In standard toxicity-testing, factors of 100 or more are routinely used to arrive at 'safe' levels of intake, extrapolating from the lowest observed adverse effect level (LOAEL), or from the highest level at which no adverse effects were observed in some bioassays (NOAEL). For major air pollution components, this approach could never be used for the simple reason that even background levels are often much higher than LOAELs or NOAELs seen in bioassays. For some pollutants such as airborne suspended particulate matter, the main body of evidence stems from epidemiological rather than toxicological studies, and it could be argued that in such cases, we need smaller 'margins of safety' as we do not need to extrapolate from animal toxicity test systems to humans. Nevertheless, the 1987 WHO *Air Quality Guidelines for Europe* contain several examples of guidelines set with no 'margin of safety' (ozone) or very small ones (PM_{10}, NO_2). It is no wonder that the guidelines strongly discourage the use of terminology such as 'margins of safety' or 'protection factors', because when the 'margins' are absent, or the 'factors' less than 2, no safety can be guaranteed, and little protection is being offered. The use of 'uncertainty factors' was proposed as the preferred terminology, and I would argue that 'embarrassment factor' is possibly more appropriate terminology for those guidelines that were set at or ever so slightly below the levels at which adverse health effects had been observed when the guidelines were set (e.g. ozone and particulate matter).

As Dr Romieu correctly points out, epidemiological associations between air pollution and health are often weak, due to exposure misclassification, unspecificity of effect etc. Compliance to air quality standards is normally assessed by measuring relevant components at a limited number of outdoor sites. It is immediately obvious that such measurements do not automatically represent exposure of human beings who spend most of their time indoors, and move through the area while commuting etc. From the researcher's point of view, it is clear that we need to try to strengthen the associations by doing a better job at exposure assessment, for example through application of personal and indoor monitoring.

However, air quality guidelines and standards are not usually set for personal or indoor exposure, because compliance would be impossible to measure. So in our epidemiological studies, we will always need to relate more refined exposure measurements back to the data obtained at 'compliance' monitoring sites because otherwise the health risks of air pollution measured at 'compliance' sites cannot be properly assessed.

A related problem that is not always appreciated is that a significant part of our knowledge on effects of air pollution components on human health does not come from epidemiological studies of effects of real, ambient air pollution mixtures. Controlled human exposure studies have greatly increased our understanding of acute effects of substances such as SO_2, NO_2, O_3 and CO. Some of our insights come from occupational epidemiology studies in which subjects may have been exposed to mixtures of rather different composition from those encountered outdoors; and for some substances such as NO_2, epidemiological studies have focused on the residential indoor environment rather than ambient air. Data from such studies cannot always directly be used for development of ambient air quality guidelines and standards, for two main reasons: firstly, relationships between concentrations measured at ambient 'compliance' sites and personal exposure and dose may be quite different from those between concentrations measured in the other study types and personal exposure and dose; and secondly, pollutants in ambient air never occur in isolation, but always in mixtures, and pollutants such as SO_2 and NO_2 have traditionally been studied not only for their own toxicity, but also as components representing mixtures containing many different substances from fossil fuel combustion, traffic emissions etc. At present, there have been few if any attempts at 'back-extrapolation' from such studies to ambient air quality conditions.

SECTION 2

TRAFFIC AND INJURY

8
Introduction

Tony Fletcher and Anthony J. McMichael

London School of Hygiene & Tropical Medicine, UK

This section addresses a number of issues related to road vehicle-related death and injury. These include the magnitude of the impact and trends and how these differ between the developed market economy countries, post-communist countries and those in the developing world. Finally what can we learn from current research activities, particularly into high risk subgroups?

Brühning's overview of available statistics identifies the basic problems in comparing figures between countries, where differences in injury rate can reflect more the variations in definition and efficiency of data collection than real differences in risk. In particular, motorists' injuries are more completely collected than non-motorized road injuries. Of necessity, greater reliance is placed on fatality statistics and these reveal clear trends for the OECD countries included in the database at the International Traffic and Accident Database in Bergisch Gladbach. Discussions continue over what the best comparative measure of risk for these statistics is. Over the last 20 years, death rates have been falling fairly steadily, whether presented per 100 000 inhabitants or per billion vehicle-kilometres, with the glaring exceptions of Central and Eastern Europe, where the general pattern has been an increase during the later part of the 1980s with peaks reached in 1990–91. Differences in risk remain large between countries of the European Union, both in level of risk and distribution of risk. The UK has relatively low fatality rates, but a high proportion of pedestrian fatalities. Analyses by type of driver, the large urban/rural difference in fatality rate, and measuring the impact of changes such as the introduction of seatbelts all suggest priority areas for further reductions in injury rates.

Taig's discussion of Brühning's chapter identifies the importance of placing the risk of fatality in a wider context. Because the risk of injury from car driving is lower than cycling, people are further encouraged to choose car travel as an alternative. The market is responding to the quite proper desire for motorists to have safer vehicles, and the freedom to drive where and when they wish, but the

Health at the Crossroads: Transport Policy and Urban Health.
Edited by Tony Fletcher and Anthony J. McMichael © 1997 John Wiley & Sons Ltd

market does not necessarily deliver safety to pedestrians and cyclists. In reducing casualties overall, the balance needs to be struck between the freedom of motorists to travel and the necessary restrictions on that freedom inherent in control measures. Good quality comparable statistics play an invaluable role in identifying priorities for action and evaluating the effectiveness of interventions.

Bly, focusing on the UK situation, describes the rise in road injuries and fatalities until the 1960s and the subsequent decline, along with the TRL research programme into primary and secondary accident prevention. Accident surveillance has included both the collection of brief information as completely as possible for all accidents and more labour intensive in-depth studies of accident circumstances. Almost all accidents are caused by human error rather than mechanical failure and research has been carried out on how improved education can reduce accident frequency, focusing on education for schoolchildren and the improved training of novice drivers. Reduction of driving while drunk and reducing average speeds (by improved enforcement of speed limits, for example) have been quite successful in reducing car accidents. Traffic engineering has yielded many benefits, particularly that involving segregating incompatible road users, improving road surfaces and traffic calming. Experience has shown the importance of integrating several different techniques to maximum effect. Secondary safety addresses improvements in vehicle design to reduce severity of injury following impact, for example with anti-lock brakes and safety features for reducing the effect of head-on collisions, the largest category. The European Commission is responsible for safety standards in vehicle design and the Transport Research Laboratory (TRL) contributes to its many expert working groups. Future research on primary prevention will need to deepen our understanding of why people behave as they do. Current research on secondary prevention includes the development of instrumented dummies to understand better the damage incurred by road users from vehicle collisions.

Mohan, in his comments on Bly's chapter, extends the concept of human error to embrace errors in policy-making and inadequate enforcement. Limiting discussion of error to those of individual road users limits our vision for devising preventive strategies. Given that so many people have to drive because of limited alternatives, a limit to education is imposed by their necessarily including many who cannot expect to be optimally 'alert' and 'careful'. Mohan also questions whether the claimed negative cost in terms of time, as a consequence of speed reduction, has been exaggerated. The focus on car design is of less relevance in developing countries where fatalities involving collisions with buses and trucks are much more important. He concludes with a call for more research into accident causation and prevention in less motorized countries.

Taig's discussion of Brühning's chapter identifies the importance of placing the risk of fatality in a wider context. Because the risk of injury from car driving is lower than cycling, people are further encouraged to choose car travel as an alternative. The market is responding to the quite proper desire for motorists to have safer vehicles, and the freedom to drive where and when they wish, but the market does not necessarily deliver safety to pedestrians and cyclists. In reducing casualties overall, the balance needs to be struck between the freedom of motorists to travel and the necessary restrictions on that freedom inherent in control measures. Good quality comparable statistics play an invaluable role in identifying priorities for action and evaluating the effectiveness of interventions.

Jacobs reminds us that most road deaths occur in poorer countries and fatality rates in developing countries tend to be an order of magnitude higher than in industrialized countries, and have become a major proportion of all deaths. Furthermore, these rates have been rising, for example quadrupling over the period 1968–85 in several African countries surveyed. Specific investigations of under-reporting indicate that the problem may be even larger. Young people are disproportionately affected. Local in-depth studies have identified in some areas lack of respect for traffic rules and high alcohol use. For monitoring road accidents, the TRL has developed the Microcomputer Accident Analysis Package which has been adopted nationally or locally in over 14 countries, and has proved very valuable for generating comparable statistics and identifying hazardous locations and monitoring road safety measures. Various examples are given in relation to improvements in engineering and planning, vehicle safety, education and training and enforcement. It is to be welcomed that some donor agencies are now incorporating a road safety component in highway development projects.

9
Injuries and deaths on the roads—an international perspective

Ekkehard Brühning

Bundesanstalt für Straßenwesen, Bergisch Gladbach, Germany

This chapter will first give an overview of international safety levels for selected highly motorized countries. Differences in definitions and under-reporting are some of the problems for international comparisons. Second, it will focus on some road safety problems. Measures taken in the past have proved that road safety can be influenced. Therefore, it is absolutely necessary to identify priority areas for future action.

The data provided below were drawn from the International Road Traffic and Accident Database (IRTAD) run under the auspices of OECD with BASt (German Federal Highway Institute) acting as database host. Data are made available to those subscribing to the database through floppy disks and continuous on-line access.

International road traffic safety levels

How to compare traffic safety internationally

International comparisons of traffic safety should be based on traffic fatality figures. Other characteristics like the number of injury accidents cannot be compared internationally since the individual definitions of injuries differ widely (see below). The international fatality figures have to be adjusted to the 30-day-definition.

Clearly absolute figures on fatalities alone do not suffice for an international comparison. Therefore, absolute numbers have to be translated into rates which are based on population or take road usage and exposure to accidents into account:

Health at the Crossroads: Transport Policy and Urban Health.
Edited by Tony Fletcher and Anthony J. McMichael © 1997 John Wiley & Sons Ltd

1. the mean risk of inhabitants being involved in fatal accidents is calculated on the basis of the home population (killed per 100 000 inhabitants); and
2. the mean risk resulting from road usage and mobility is quantified on the basis of vehicle kilometres (killed per 1 billion vehicle kilometres).

In contrast to the two rates above, a comparison based on the number of motor vehicles should be avoided since the number of motor vehicles does not describe adequately the accident exposure of road users. In addition to these rates, it is also useful to derive percentages, for example the percentage of killed occupants of cars (this includes taxis and private motor vehicles) relative to the total number of killed road users. This provides a description of the accident structure.

Not all exposure data are readily available. In general, population data do not pose any problems as they are used in all countries. However, the availability of vehicle kilometrage figures is very limited in some countries. One of the future IRTAD Special Reports will give an overview of different methods used to compile the data (including fuel consumption, odometer readings based on samples and traffic counts).

Traffic safety levels in European OECD countries

Population-related risk

The mean risk of being fatally injured in a traffic accident in European OECD countries has clearly diminished since the early seventies even though vehicle ownership and use have been increasing over the same period. Although the overall trend of risk rates has been downwards for a long time internationally, there is a considerable variance across the European Union with the highest national rates some four times higher than the lowest. For example, in 1992 the mean risk rates ranged among 7.5 in Great Britain and 32.9 (killed/10^5 inhabitants) in Portugal.

Figure 9.1 illustrates that, at the beginning of the 1990s, the European countries under comparison can be grouped into those with low, medium, or high risk rates. A structural break has emerged in East Germany: until 1989—resulting from the comparatively low motorization and other system related factors—the global population-based risk of being fatally injured had been similar to highly motorized European countries with the most favourable accident statistics: Great Britain, Sweden and the Netherlands. With German reunification in 1990, however, the risk values were about twice as high in the new German federal states as in the year before. In 1991 even worse figures were recorded with East Germany exceeding the other European countries under comparison. Since 1992 road deaths have decreased, but 1994 figures are still 68% above the 1989 level.

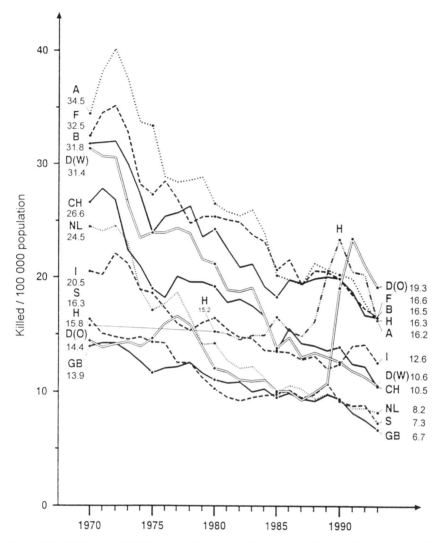

Figure 9.1   Killed per 100 000 population (selected countries). Country legend: A, Austria; B, Belgium; CH, Switzerland; D(0), East Germany; D(W), West Germany; F, France; GB, Great Britain; H, Hungary; I, Ireland; NL, Netherlands; S, Sweden

Fatality rates

As described above, fatality rates are obtained by relating the total number of killed road users to the total kilometrage. However, kilometrage data are not available for all highly motorized countries.

Figure 9.2 illustrates that there is a long-term trend of decreasing fatality rates

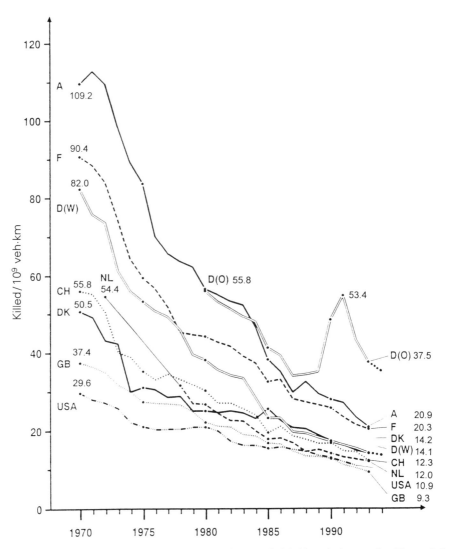

Figure 9.2   Death rates since 1970 (selected countries) (abbreviations as for Figure 9.1)

among the OECD countries under comparison. Considerable differences, however, are emerging at an international level. In 1993 Great Britain recorded the most favourable figure (9.3 killed per 10^9 veh·km) whereas other European countries, such as France and Austria, account for more than 20 killed per 10^9 veh·km. The mobility-related fatality rate in East Germany increased sharply after 1989 from 35.0 killed per 10^9 veh·km in 1990. In 1991 it reached its peak with a high of 53.4—the highest fatality rate recorded in the countries under comparison.

However, an important fall in fatality rates was recorded in 1992 and in 1993 with a further decrease in 1994.

For reasons of data availability, Southern European countries cannot be included in this comparison. It may be assumed, however, that the rate would be extremely high in Portugal and Spain. The risk of being killed related to vehicle kilometrage—where known—is four times higher in the 'most dangerous' country than in the 'safest' country. Reasons for such variation include differing degrees of motorization, types of travel, types of vehicles, weather, topography, etc. as well as inherent differences in national levels of traffic safety. However, it can be concluded that there is a long-term trend of decreasing fatality rates for most Western European countries and the USA.

Traffic safety in Eastern European countries

The political changes of the past years in the former socialist countries have particularly affected road traffic. The newly gained freedoms to travel, the opening-up of markets towards the West and increasing passenger car ownership are only a few of the factors affecting road traffic conditions in those countries.

The following brief overview is part of a report on traffic safety in five Eastern European non-OECD countries (Brühning, 1992). Poland and Hungary represented Eastern countries that had been rather open towards the West even before 1989. As a result of the reshaping of the political landscape in Eastern Europe, the Czech and Slovak Federal Republic (CSFR) is no longer in existence. Therefore, traffic situations in the Czech Republic and Slovakia were analysed separately. Estonia was taken as an example for the Baltic states. In addition, developments in these selected countries were compared with trends occurring in East Germany.

Population-related risk

The differences in risk values among the above-mentioned countries were rather marginal in 1985. As soon as 1989, however, the risk values of Hungary, Poland and Estonia were about twice as high as in the former CSFR or East Germany. In the following years, the number of killed road users and hence the risk values increased considerably in all the countries. With German reunification in 1990 the population-related risk of East Germany doubled (see Figure 9.1) and continued to rise in 1991. The development in Hungary followed the same pattern as East Germany.

Fatalities peaked not only in East Germany and Hungary but also in other Eastern European countries in the years 1990 and 1991. Since then figures have been showing a downward trend. However, these countries are still recording very unfavourable accident statistics.

Changes in accident structure

Not all aspects of traffic accidents in Eastern European countries have been equally affected by the overall rise in traffic accidents.

1. As far as vulnerable road users are concerned, the surge in passenger car fatalities was balanced by a fall in pedestrian fatalities. Following the same pattern the percentage of killed occupants of motorized two-wheelers has been decreasing constantly since 1989.
2. At the same time, the percentage of killed road users in rural areas has been increasing in the Eastern countries and East Germany, i.e. the number of fatalities is rising faster outside urban areas than in built-up areas. The percentages, however, vary considerably between the Eastern countries.

Crucial areas of road safety at the international level

National characteristics and problems are apparent when focusing on accident structure and special aspects of traffic safety. Figure 9.3 illustrates the percentage of fatalities according to road usage. In all countries passenger car fatalities account for the highest percentage related to all killed road users. Considerable differences are emerging at an international level. Among Western European countries Great Britain records the highest percentage of pedestrian fatalities, whereas Germany accounts for a high share of passenger car fatalities. Traffic safety measures prove to be very effective in terms of numbers for those areas with high fatality records.

Figure 9.4 represents the fatality rate by age bands. It becomes evident that great progress has been made as far as children are concerned. However, young people are one of the high-risk groups with the 18–20-year-olds being particularly at risk as occupants of passenger cars. In West Germany, young people are five times as likely to die in a road accident than mature road users aged 25–64 years. As illustrated in Figure 9.5, access to a driving licence is reflected in the risk run by 16–18-year-olds to be killed in an accident. In the USA, figures are on the rise for the 16-year-olds, whereas Great Britain records a leap for the 17-year-olds. In Germany, fatality rates peak for 18-year-olds.

Urban areas, country roads and motorways are marked by a completely different accident typology. Therefore, the risk of being involved in a fatal accident differs according to road network areas. Among the highly motorized Western nations, country roads account for more than half of all road fatalities. In Western Germany 62% of all fatalities are recorded on country roads (55% in Great Britain). The percentage of country-road fatalities has been rising over a long period. The improvement in overall traffic safety levels is due to progress made in urban areas and on motorways.

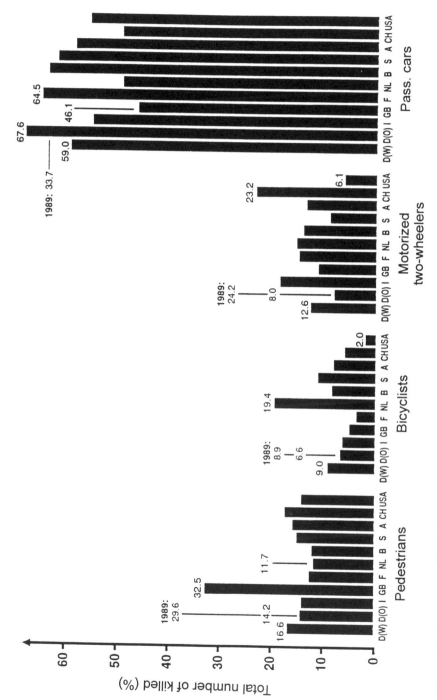

Figure 9.3 Percentage of killed in 1993 by traffic participation (selected countries) (abbreviations as for Figure 9.1)

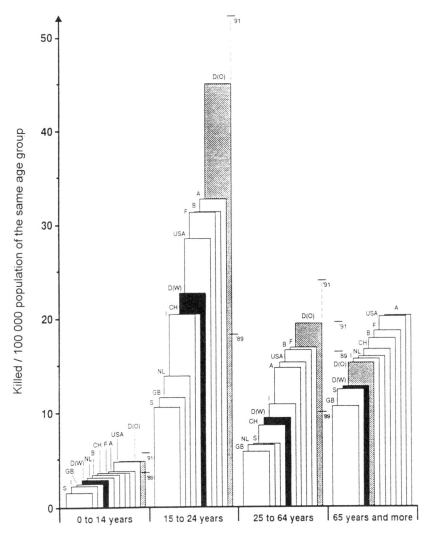

Figure 9.4   Killed per 100 000 population in 1993 (selected countries) (abbreviations as for Figure 9.1)

- In most countries the majority of all severe country road accidents involve a single vehicle (running off the roadway); in West Germany this accounts for 36% of all country road fatalities. Often collision with a tree affects the severity of the accident.
- Accidents on country roads are also characterized by a high proportion of accidents involving alcohol (in West Germany 19% of all country road fatalities).

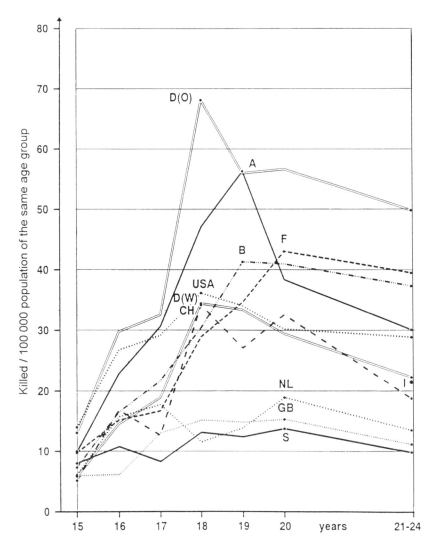

Figure 9.5   Killed aged 15 to 24 years per 100 000 population in 1993 (selected countries) (abbreviations as for Figure 9.1)

- Young people account for a remarkable proportion of all country road fatalities (in West Germany 33%) as they are often on the road at night. The majority of severe country road accidents involve novice drivers (aged 18 to 24 years).

  Vulnerable road users represent another important group: pedestrians and bicyclists account for 38% of all road user fatalities in West Germany, and 48% in Great Britain (see Figure 9.3).

Detailed analyses of the structure of accidents show crucial areas of traffic safety that are eligible for introducing improved safety measures (see below).

Accident and injury definitions: limitations of international comparability and the scope for harmonization

Comparison of accident data at an international level requires the terminology and definitions to be agreed upon by all countries.

The IRTAD Special Report 'Definitions and Data Availability' (IRTAD, 1992) states as follows: Today the only reliable category for comparison of traffic accident data is that of 'killed' as most of the countries adhere to the definition given in the Convention of Road Traffic (European Commission for Europe (ECE), 1968): 'Any person who was killed outright or who died within 30 days as a result of the accident'. For those countries that do not comply with this definition correction factors are applied to improve comparability of the data. Other terms commonly used in accident statistics such as 'injured', 'slightly injured' and 'seriously injured', however, do refer to widely differing national definitions. Therefore, these categories are not considered in IRTAD. Even the definitions of 'traffic accident' and 'injury accident' show some differences when being compared internationally.

With an emerging need for comparison of data on seriously injured road users it was decided to introduce a new variable in IRTAD. This newly integrated category called 'hospitalized' is defined as: 'Non-fatal accident victims admitted to hospital as in-patients'. The majority of the IRTAD member countries are able to provide data on hospitalized accidents. The introduction of the 'hospitalized' category will allow international comparison of data on injured. Unfortunately, the British definition of seriously injured differs slightly from the 'hospitalized' term. International harmonization of definitions is difficult to achieve. As has been the case with the introduction of the 30-day follow-up for recording of fatalities the 'hospitalized' definition might be adopted by those countries which still adhere to differing definitions.

Under-reporting of accidents

Accident data as recorded by the police should allow for an objective assessment of accident trends, the identification of priority areas, the effectiveness of countermeasures, etc.

Both under-reporting and under-recording of traffic accidents are a problem for reliable analyses based on police data. The IRTAD Special Report '*Under-Reporting of Road Traffic Accidents Recorded by the Police at the International Level*' (IRTAD Special Report, 1994) gives an overview of recent findings from

international research on under-reporting:
The level of under-reporting is considerable and depends on a number of factors.

* national factors are connected to how accidents are defined, how serious the least reportable injury is etc. Differences in the local tradition for reporting accidents to the police and how the recording procedure is organized are other important factors explaining the differences between countries. It is therefore not advisable to compare gross figures subject to under-reporting between countries;
* accidents with motor vehicles involved have a rather high rate of reporting, 50–80%, except for rear end accidents resulting in whiplash injuries which have a rate of 30–50%;
* single bicycle accidents have a very low reporting rate. Pedestrians sliding, stumbling, falling, etc. are not reported to the police at all, because it is not defined as a traffic accident by law; and
* serious injuries are more often reported to the police than slight injuries. British research reports indicate the following rates:
  – Fatal injuries: 95–100%
  – Serious injuries: 70–90%
  – Slight injuries: 60–80%
  German research indicates the following rates:
  – Fatal injuries: 95%
  – Inpatients: 50–60%
  – Outpatients: 40–50%

The IRTAD Special Report on under-reporting came to the following conclusions:

* the level of reporting of single bicycle accidents is almost negligible. This applies also to collisions between bicyclists. Since the number of such accidents is quite considerable in many countries, it should be discussed more thoroughly if such accident types should be included in the legal term 'road traffic accident'. By including them, the total rate of reporting will be misleading;
* correction factors have been developed for the different types of traffic accidents. By using these on the official figures originating from police reports, it would be possible to get an improved picture as to the magnitude of accidents and casualties; and
* hospital data give the best picture as to the personal injury aspect of the traffic safety problem, while police reports give the most reliable and detailed accident data.

Unfortunately, it is not possible to link hospital data and police-recorded accident data in some countries because of national laws protecting the privacy of individual citizens.

If the level of under-reporting did not differ from year to year, it would only pose a minor problem for reliable and meaningful analyses as it could be treated as a kind of systematically occurring error in statistics. However, the above-mentioned IRTAD Special Report indicates that the rate of reporting can vary over time, as it was observed for rear-end accidents in Norway. This might be due to increased awareness by the public and improved police procedures.

In most countries the level of reporting of fatal accidents is about 95% or even higher. Therefore, under-reporting is negligible as far as international comparisons are concerned. However, on the national level, under-reporting does affect the assessment of accidents involving personal injury (fatalities and injured):

1. the accident risk is being under-estimated;
2. the public is not aware of the risk run by non-motorists; and
3. priorities for action are not being identified correctly. For example, bicyclists as vulnerable road users are not being informed of their high accident risk. In addition, there are not enough funds available to finance effective counter-measures.

Improving traffic safety

Potential for accident prevention

Since the advent of road transport, death on the road has been a fact of life. It has been tried to define a basic safety level as a social goal commonly agreed upon. There is no natural basic level of mortality above 0 that could be applied to road death. Therefore, let us consider two different approaches to assessing safety potentials.

What will happen if the trend of decreasing fatality rates continues? In 1970/1972 fatalities peaked in West Germany and Great Britain (19 193 and 7763 road deaths respectively). Since then fatality rates have been showing a downward trend as illustrated in Figure 9.1, an average annual decrease of 4.6 % and 3.5% respectively. Assuming the trends persist, annual deaths per year in West Germany and Great Britain should fall to 5000 and 3000 respectively.

What will happen if the accident risk of all people older than 15 years is the same as for 45–54-year-olds? As Figure 9.4 shows, young people and the elderly have a much higher fatality rate than the middle age bands. Provided that there are no higher rates in other age groups than the 45–54-year-olds have, the 1993 death tolls in West Germany and Great Britain would be reduced from 6926 and 3814 to 4380 and 2600 respectively.

Realization of preventive measures

The favourable trend observed over the last two decades depends on a variety of factors. Ten years ago, a German study concluded that important changes had been taking place in all traffic areas including road construction, road infrastructure, traffic regulation, vehicle safety, traffic education and emergency systems. Due to the large number of measures, it is very difficult separately to assess the impact of each measure. However, this can be done for measures influencing road traffic in general. For example, it was possible to prove the effectiveness of increased seatbelt wearing following the introduction of legislation in August 1984 (see Figure 9.6, from Ernst and Brühning, 1990). It was estimated that the 1985 death toll would have been 75% higher if subsequent countermeasures—seatbelt wearing, traffic increase on motorways, improvement of emergency system—had not taken place (Brühning *et al.*, 1986).

Examples of future measures to improve traffic safety

In future, the effectiveness of all safety measures has to be evaluated in order to identify new potential for improving traffic safety. Above all, such an approach should be made for the above-mentioned crucial areas of road safety that have not gained from the overall improvement: for example, accidents on country roads are only one of the areas for innovative action.

Occupants of cars account for the highest percentage related to all fatalities (West Germany 59%, Great Britain 46%). Active safety (e.g. Active Braking Systems (ABS)) as well as passive vehicle safety can still be improved. Stricter requirements should be placed on manufacturers in the following areas:

1. protection of occupants from partial frontal impact, not just full frontal impact;
2. improved side impact protection;
3. reduction of severity of injury to unprotected road users struck by cars (Bamberg and Zellmer, 1994);
4. redesign of large passenger cars to reduce crash severity for small cars; and

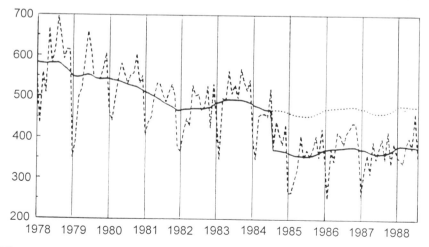

Figure 9.6   Car passenger fatalities taking account of seatbelt legislation (August 1984) figures and trend in West Germany, on a monthly basis

5. improving rear under-run protection for trucks.

These and other technological improvements are discussed in more detail by Bly (*see* Chapter 10).
With a view to active vehicle safety, two-wheelers have to be improved (e.g. brakes).
Road traffic laws offer wide scope for preventive measures. For example, motorway accidents occurring at night or on wet roads could be reduced by introducing special speed limits.
The number of male offenders among the young drivers has to be curbed. According to recent research studies a description of special high-risk groups (lifestyle, leisure, region) is now possible.
The aforementioned examples should provide a perspective on future traffic safety work. There is still a huge potential for safety measures—a challenge for researchers, advisory bodies, decision-makers and local authorities.

References

Bamberg R, Zellmer H (1994) *Benefits of the Introduction of the EEVC WG 10 Proposed Pedestrian Impact Requirements.* (In Preprint of the International Conference on Road Safety in Europe and SHRP, Lille)
Brühning E (1992) Traffic safety in Eastern and Western Europe at the beginning of the nineties. In *Proceedings of the International Conference Road Safety in Europe*, Berlin
Brühning E, Ernst R, Gläser KP *et al.* (1986) Zum rückgang der getötetenzahlen im Straßenverkehr—entwicklung in der Bundesrepublik Deutschland von 1970 bis 1984. *Zeitschrift für Verkehrssicherheit, 4*, 154–163
ECE (1968) *Statistics of Road Traffic Accidents in Europe*, Annex 1. United Nations.
Ernst R, Brühning E (1990) Fünf jahre danach: wirksamkeit der gurtanlegepflicht für Pkw-Insassen ab 1.8.1984—eine zeitreihenanalytische untersuchung. *Zeitschrift für Verkehrssicherheit, 1*, 2–13
Hutchinson TP (1987) *Road Accident Statistics.* Rumsby Scientific Publishing, Australia
International Road Traffic and Accidents Database (1992) *Special Report: Definitions and Data Availability.* BASt, Germany
International Road Traffic and Accidents Database (1994) *Special Report: Under-Reporting of Road Accidents Recorded by the Police at the International Level.* Public Roads Administration, Norway

Discussion

Anthony R. Taig

AEA Technology, Risley, UK

Dr Brühning's chapter has provided an excellent perspective on the risks associated with roads in Europe. The aim of these comments is to promote discussion on some of the key issues which I feel need to be addressed to help us decide on the priorities for future action. I thus make no apology for raising questions without trying to provide the answers, as I focus on three main themes:

1. What should we be aiming to achieve?
2. Whose job is it to drive progress? and
3. Where should attention be focused?

What?

An obvious primary goal is to reduce the annual toll of injuries and deaths. But this cannot be the whole picture: while concern over the environmental impacts of motor traffic is rising, the serious risk of death or injury is an important factor encouraging cyclists and pedestrians to shift to using cars, even for very short journeys, across much of Europe. From the viewpoint of casualty reduction, this is a good thing: the risk of using a car is much lower than that of cycling or walking. From the wider health, social and environmental viewpoint it is a tragedy.

I would therefore like to suggest that, while reducing casualties is a vital objective, we need equally clear partner objectives to enable us safely to use roads in socially and environmentally friendly ways.

Who?

The attention given to safety in the development and marketing of cars today reflects the importance of safety in the eye of the motorist. As drivers, we can choose our preferred make and model of car, we can maintain it in good condition, and we decide how to drive. In other words, we have control over the major factors which determine our safety—all we need is a safe road to drive on, and we can determine our own risk on the road. Viewed from another perspective, the market (that is car makers and maintainers) can deliver us the safety we want, in proportion to our willingness to pay for it.

The degree of control, or market ability to satisfy our demand for safety, is much less for vulnerable road users. Guidance and warnings for pedestrians and cyclists abound, but the perfectly behaved pedestrian or cyclist is still at substantial risk from the behaviour of motorists. And there are large, very important sections of the community, for example children, disabled and elderly people, from whom we cannot and should not expect perfect evasive action.

Thus, to a large extent, the market delivers safety to motorists. But there is no market mechanism to deliver safety to pedestrians and cyclists; indeed their safety conflicts with the freedom of motorists to drive where and as they wish. Thus most governments recognize a particular responsibility:

1. to protect the vulnerable road user; and
2. to encourage the market to protect the motorist (and to protect the consumer from distortion or deception in that marketplace).

Where?

The scale of health impacts in terms of road accident casualties can be usefully represented as the product of three factors:

1. the volume of traffic;
2. the likelihood of accidents ('primary' safety factors); and
3. the casualties resulting from accidents ('secondary' safety factors).

The focus in *marketing*, of cars in particular, tends to be on the third—benefits for the car user, without compromising the pleasure and freedom of driving. The first two issues figure prominently in most governments' road safety programmes; action here delivers major health and environmental, as well as safety benefits. But the actions involved tend to be more controversial, involving fiscal, planning, licensing, traffic regulation and enforcement, highway design and other factors which tend to constrain the motorist.

We ought to be looking for balance across these areas to deliver major reductions in injuries and deaths on the roads.

The big question is *Have we got that balance right*? There are plenty of things which could be done, very quickly, through, for example, traffic calming, tougher traffic law and enforcement, changes in driver licensing, to make massive reductions in the toll of road accident casualties. But the price of many of the really effective measures is curtailment of our much cherished freedom and enjoyment of motoring. Is this a price we should be prepared to pay?

Conclusion

A number of important areas for discussion have been raised as a necessary prelude to prioritizing action on road safety. In conclusion, I would like simply to comment on the very high value of good quality statistics such as those presented by Dr Brühning. Without being able to see the scale of risks, and to analyse accurately where they come from, we could neither predict in advance, nor monitor retrospectively, the effectiveness of any of our actions to advance road safety. We will continue to debate the priorities for action in the field on road safety, but I hope nobody will contest the high priority we should give to continuing efforts to improve the quality and consistency of road accident statistics across Europe.

10
Issues in transport injury research

Philip H. Bly

Transport Research Laboratory, Crowthorne, UK

Over the past twenty years, road traffic in the UK has doubled. It is predicted to double again by the year 2020 or 2035, depending on the assumed future rate of economic growth (Great Britain Department of Transport, 1994). Judging from experience in countries ahead of the UK in developing affluence, there will be little sign of any saturation in this growth over the next few decades unless it becomes necessary or acceptable to impose some form of constraint on road travel.

This continued increase in travel by road has obvious implications for problems of congestion, pollution and accident injury. Of these three, accident injury is the problem which has so far been tackled with most success. Figure 10.1 shows the trends in road traffic and in accident casualties since records began in 1926. There is a discontinuity during the Second World War, but broadly injuries at all levels of severity increased with rising levels of traffic until the early 1960s. Since then injuries have declined despite the continuing increase in traffic. The decline in total injury accidents has been relatively modest, but serious injuries (as categorized rather loosely in the national statistics, but referring predominantly to injuries requiring hospitalization) and fatalities have halved over the past thirty years.

In 1987 the government set a specific emphasis on improving road safety by adopting a target for the year 2000 of reducing casualties by one-third relative to the average between 1981 and 1985. So far, we seem set to achieve the target for deaths and serious injuries, though perhaps not for slight injuries. Even so, there are still about 4000 deaths, 45000 serious injuries and 250000 slight injuries (Great Britain Department of Transport, 1993), at a total financial cost of £10 billion, per year, and there is much still to be done.

This chapter Crown Copyright (1995). Extracts from the text may be reproduced except for commercial purposes, provided its source is acknowledged.

Health at the Crossroads: Transport Policy and Urban Health.
Edited by Tony Fletcher and Anthony J. McMichael published 1997 John Wiley & Sons Ltd

P. H. Bly

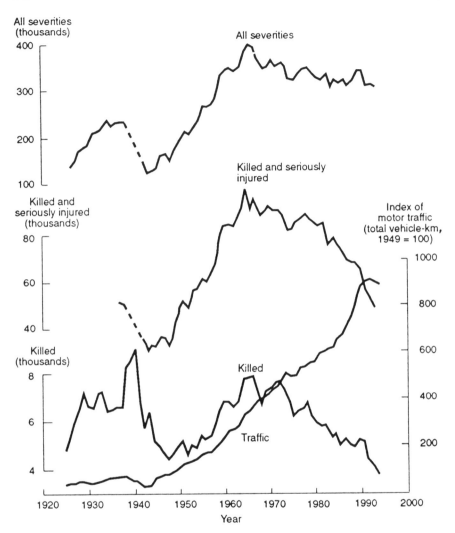

Figure 10.1   Trends in UK road traffic, accidents and injuries, 1926 to date

Approaches to improving safety

Obviously, prevention of accidents is better than amelioration of the effects. Given the more rapid reduction in serious injuries than in slight ones, we seem to have been more successful in the 'cure' than in preventing the disease. Prevention of accidents, whether by training and education, regulation, or by traffic, road or vehicle engineering, is referred to as 'primary' safety. Reduction of the severity of injuries caused by an accident, most obviously through vehicle design, is referred to as 'secondary' safety. These categories are sometimes also referred to as 'active' and 'passive' safety respectively, but there is now scope for confusion with this nomenclature, since some passive safety devices such as airbags or pretensioners are also known as active devices because they are deployed only in an accident.

Another categorization of the different approaches to improving safety is known as the 'Three E's', Education, Enforcement and Engineering, while at Transport Research Laboratory (TRL) the organization of the research programme is grouped for convenience into Road User Safety (that is, behaviour, education and training), Traffic Safety Engineering, and Vehicle Safety Engineering, but with overlap between the separate groupings.

The important point here is that, whatever definitional separations are made, success in improving safety depends crucially on tackling the problems across the broad front, using techniques from within all the different areas of road safety. Road safety research is very much a multidisciplinary effort, with contributions from statistical analysis, the medical profession, psychologists, educators, traffic engineers, road engineers, mechanical engineers, theoreticians and experimentalists, and mathematical and computer modellers of many types.

The decline in serious and fatal injuries over the past three decades, despite the rapid growth in traffic and a substantial increase in general road speeds, is not something which is intrinsic and inevitable in the development of road traffic in the UK. It is, in part, a result of previous actions, and continued success will depend upon our ability to introduce new safety initiatives at the same rate. The year 2000 target is very welcome, and has focused the safety effort in a very beneficial way, but efforts will need to continue beyond the millennium to maintain the downward trend. Indeed, most of the results of present research will not find application until after that date, and there is still a great potential for improvement.

Understanding accidents

As with any other problem, effective solutions depend upon a proper understanding. In this case it is necessary to study the mechanisms of accidents both in order to understand why they happen, and to examine the interactions between people and their surroundings which cause injuries. The difficulty with understanding accidents is that they are relatively infrequent events, unpredictable, and geographically dispersed. Consequently, collection of accident data is expensive, and within a limited resource there is generally a choice between covering a large sample in a rather superficial way, or making a more detailed study of a more limited sample. Both approaches are necessary.

The bedrock of British accident information is the National Road Accident Statistics database, generally known as 'Stats19'. It records a limited number of attributes of injury accidents attended by, or reported to, the police. Given the other duties and priorities of police at an accident, and the often difficult physical conditions, it is important to keep the data collected to a minimum if it is to be reliable, and the assessment of injuries as slight or serious by police with little or no medical training is inevitably somewhat variable. Fatalities (within 30 days of the accident) are recorded very reliably. There is known to be considerable under-reporting: James (1991) estimates that over 30% of injury accidents, including 26% of serious injuries, are not recorded, but it seems likely that the under-reporting is primarily, though not entirely, of the less serious injuries, and there is no reason to believe that either the extent or the nature of the under-reporting is changing with time. Overall, Stats19 records with reasonable accuracy the broad circumstances and nature of the accident, the vehicles and people involved, the wearing of seatbelts, the assessed speed and weather conditions, and the database provides an invaluable cross-section and trend indicator for everyone who works in road safety in the UK.

Similar national databases exist in other countries, and there has been discussion from time to time about standardizing data definition and collection to facilitate amalgamation of data and comparison between countries. Previous attempts to do this have made limited progress, however, since each country is anxious to ensure continuity and consistency in its own data, and the emphasis on what is collected and how it is used varies from country to country. There is probably considerable scope for coordinating some aspects of accident data between countries with similar societies and cultures, but it is clearly important to tailor accident investigation and data collection to the specific needs and characteristics of each country. Even so, a methodical framework is essential, and although the detailed treatment might vary from one place to another, a good underlying methodology can be valuable in a wide range of circumstances. The TRL Microcomputer Accident Analysis Package (MAAP), an analysis system which organizes accident data on a geographical map, was designed for use in developing countries (Hills and Baguley, 1993) but offers such a versatile way of assembling accident data that it is now being used in some UK local authorities, and the interest is spreading (see Jacobs, this volume).

Valuable though Stats19 is, however, it cannot provide sufficient detail for development of the most effective accident or injury prevention measures, and more specific accident studies are required. The most expensive of these are on-the-spot investigations. In the 1970s TRL operated a 'flying squad' of researchers who were notified by police of accidents within a wide radius of the Laboratory, day or night, and who immediately attended the accident while the police were still there and often before there had been any clearance of the vehicles or debris, to make measurements, take photographs, interview witnesses, and assess the likely course and possible causes of the accident. This study was very informative, but very expensive, and because the returns from such immediacy tend to diminish once the main characteristics of a wide range of accidents are understood the study was closed. It seems unlikely that the central causes of road accidents change with time sufficiently quickly to justify frequent repetition of this approach, though it may be desirable to repeat the exercise at long intervals to check whether there are substantial changes in causation. It is probable, however, that indication of such changes would come from more limited studies.

For over ten years, TRL has organized the Cooperative Crash Injury Study on behalf of the Department of Transport, and with some financial support from Ford, Rover and Nissan (Harms, 1993). Expert investigation teams from Birmingham University Accident Research Unit and Loughborough University Institute of Consumer Ergonomics, plus some of the Vehicle Inspectorate's staff, examine the vehicles involved in accidents in their areas and record in great detail the deformation of the vehicles and contact points with occupants or other road users injured in the collision. These contact points are then correlated with the medical details of the casualty's treatment obtained from cooperating hospitals or, in the case of fatalities, with coroner's reports. The database now contains some 7500 vehicles, and represents a mine of information invaluable to improving vehicle safety. It has to be a continuing commitment, however, as the earlier cases become dated and less useful, since vehicle design changes much more rapidly than the human causes of accidents and constant updating is essential. Similar studies are made by some of the major car manufacturers in Europe, but they are restricted to accidents involving their own models, and it is the comparison of crash performance by vehicles of very different design which can offer the most productive lessons. Here again, there is currently interest in standardizing some data definition and collection to facilitate amalgamation of these very expensive databases across different countries and manufacturers, but it will be extremely difficult to achieve compatibility in this very complex area. Even within the single UK study, ensuring consistency between different examiners and institutions is a continuing effort.

TRL also conducts special surveys from time to time to answer particular questions. These are generally based on the assemblage of police and coroners' reports relating to selected types of accident. Recent special studies have investigated heavy goods vehicle accidents and cars under-running the fronts of lorries (Robinson, 1994), pedestrians struck by the fronts of cars (Lawrence *et al.*, 1993), and the involvement of spray from wet roads as a causative factor in accidents (Saville, unpublished). Surveys have also been conducted into behavioural aspects of safety, examining reported accident records rather than individual accidents. For example, 29 500 new drivers were surveyed on a repeated basis in the Cohort Study (Forsyth, 1992a, 1992b) and asked, amongst other things, about traffic regulation violation, 'near misses', and actual accidents.

Road user behaviour

Given that a tiny percentage of accidents are attributable to mechanical defects, human error is a major cause of almost all accidents and reduction of that error has to be a major focus of road safety. It is essential therefore that we understand why we behave as we do, though we should also be realistic about the difficulty of changing human behaviour. There is often a gap between the knowledge of what it is sensible to do, and actual behaviour. But education, training and persuasion can provide people with a better knowledge of the possible consequences of their actions and, on the margins at least, encourage a move to safer behaviour. There has been success on a considerable scale in discouraging drink-driving and encouraging the wearing of seatbelts, for example. But even where changes in behaviour are harder to achieve, it is still important to understand how road users will respond to new legislation or enforcement measures, or to new road environments, signing or lane design, or to new devices in the vehicle to provide the driver with information and enhance safety. Without that understanding, the response to safety initiatives and innovations may be very different from what was intended, reducing their success.

In the past, much of TRL's effort in the behavioural field has been concerned with instilling a proper understanding of safe behaviour from an early age, and educational material has been developed and assessed for schoolchildren at all ages, though with a particular emphasis on primary schoolchildren. This work continues, but the recent emphasis has moved to trying to improve the performance of novice drivers. The incentive for this stems from a European Commission requirement for the UK to introduce a theory part to the driving test. Many other countries already have theory tests, but there is no evidence available to indicate what they achieve. Indeed, there is little hard evidence available to demonstrate that even the practical part of the driving test necessarily produces safer drivers. In the Cohort Study already mentioned (Forsyth, 1992a, 1992b), a sample of the drivers surveyed took part in a retest one year after passing the driving test. The pass rate for this retest of previously successful drivers was very similar to that for the original test, which does not lend much encouragement to the notion that the test distinguishes clearly between competent and incompetent drivers.

If the UK is required to introduce a theory test, this is an opportunity to assess what aspects of a driving test, whether theory or practice, might result in safer driving and to design the test accordingly. Maycock and Lockwood (1993) have shown from a postal survey of 18 500 drivers how accident risk gradually improves with driving experience over the years following passing the test, but that the initial risk is higher the lower the age at passing the test, converging over time to much the same average risk whatever the age of starting to drive. This is illustrated in Figure 10.2. Both this study and the Cohort Study showed that the accident risk (in terms of reported accidents and the more frequent near misses) was initially lower for female and older drivers, but the differences disappeared after the first few years of driving.

The Cohort Study showed that accident rates were lower for those who had previous road experience with motorcycles, and for those who had driven more as learner drivers with friends or relatives, suggesting that there may be value in

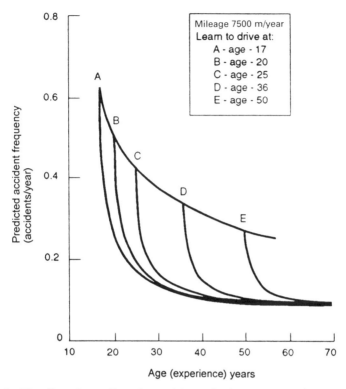

Figure 10.2 The effect of age of learning to drive and subsequent experience on accident frequencies (Maycock and Lockwood, 1993)

some sort of 'apprentissage' scheme aimed at encouraging more on-the-road practice outside formal driving lessons. Unsurprisingly, the study showed that drivers who considered themselves faster than average, or who reported more perceptual errors or violations of traffic regulations, also had higher accident rates, but at least this demonstrates a statistical link between reported behaviour and actual accidents or dangerous situations. It perhaps also illustrates the gap between drivers' awareness of deficiencies and their actual behaviour, and implies the difficulty of making drivers act on their knowledge of unsafe behaviour. The study also showed a link between those who committed errors of awareness and anticipation during the test, yet still passed, and their subsequent accident record, so it gives encouragement to the view that improvements to the test to emphasize particular aspects of behaviour might produce a positive improvement in driver safety. This is especially true of driver perception of hazards, and considerable progress has been made in developing hazard perception testing by use of video recordings which expose the novice driver to a much wider range of hazards than will be met and tested in a whole series of driving lessons. TRL's new driving simulator is extending the realism with which drivers can be exposed to 'on-the-road hazards' and, as the cost of 'virtual reality' in the leisure industry falls, there may be considerable scope for using simulation for both training and testing drivers.

Despite the considerable success over recent years in changing society's attitude to drinking and driving, alcohol is still a contributory factor in 14% of fatal accidents, and there is still more which could be done to help police target offenders more efficiently (Broughton, 1994). With fewer drunk drivers, the problem of drunk pedestrians has become more apparent: in a sample of 1500 pedestrians killed in road accidents, 38% had been drinking, 30% were over the legal limit, and 16% were over 2.5 times the limit (Everest, 1992). The same sanctions are not available against pedestrians as against drivers, however, so there seems little that can be done beyond publicity and education.

A review of international data by Finch *et al.* (1993), and a statistical investigation of accidents on urban roads in the UK (Baruya and Finch, 1994), show a strong link between average speeds and accident rates. In general, a 1 mph reduction in average speed is linked with approximately a 5% reduction of accidents and injuries at all severities, so reduction in speed seems to offer a very powerful lever in improving safety. Against this, of course, it has to be recognized that the gain in safety is made at the cost of some increase in travel time, and a blanket reduction in all speeds is not necessarily acceptable, either socially or in cost–benefit terms. But undoubtedly reductions in speed are likely to be beneficial in many situations. The gains will be in both primary and secondary safety, since lower speeds make accident avoidance more likely for a given driver reaction time, and because kinetic energy increases with the square of the speed so the injuries rise rapidly with impact speed.

More effective enforcement of speed limits would do much to reduce average speeds, though the problem is not simply one of legal limits but also of appropriate speed for the conditions. Technology is providing the means for cheaper and more effective enforcement. Automatic cameras were first used very successfully to identify red light runners, but they are now being used increasingly for speed enforcement (Winnett, 1994). Video analysis systems are becoming available to read the number plates of offending vehicles automatically, so that if the approach became acceptable, legal and widespread, the probability of being fined for speeding could become so great that it would radically alter drivers' habits. Advanced electronics systems, or 'transport telematics', are currently being developed to provide driver information and monitoring beyond anything available so far, and the scope for detecting and penalizing errant behaviour will expand enormously. The constraints will be ones of social acceptability, not technology. It is already technically feasible to set a mechanical limit on a vehicle's speed from the roadside, and this limit could if required be set according to the weather or traffic conditions.

Traffic engineering for safety

The way roads and their surroundings are designed influences both the likelihood and severity of accidents. At the very general level, the skid resistance of the road surface has a direct effect on the probability of accidents, and a recent study has led to a reassessment of the specified surfaces (Roe *et al.*, 1991), estimated to produce a net financial safety benefit of some £300 million annually (Robertson, 1994).

At a more specific level, there has been great progress over the last decade or so in using road design to reduce the likelihood of accidents by:

1. segregating incompatible types of road user, that is, keeping pedestrians and cyclists separate from motorized traffic as far as possible;
2. reducing conflicts between traffic streams engaged in different manoeuvres;
3. and using road profile and layout to reduce speeds in areas where traffic coexists with pedestrians.

During the 1980s TRL helped to design and assess trial safety schemes in seven cities. Banned traffic turns and through-routes kept traffic out of residential areas, parking was carefully controlled and limited to safe places, there were additional speed limits, and pedestrian barriers prevented crossing at unsafe places. Mackie *et al.* (1990) assessed a fall of 13% in injury accidents, and estimated that the schemes gave a first year rate of return of 30 to 40%.

Since those urban safety schemes, action to curb traffic speeds in particular has become much more positive, with a wide range of 'traffic calming' techniques to slow traffic and keep it out of the way of pedestrians in shopping and residential areas. Speed humps are now familiar to everyone, and they have evolved into a wide range of designs appropriate to different situations, with flat-topped speed 'tables' and narrow speed 'cushions' to minimize problems caused to buses and emergency vehicles by some of the earlier designs (Webster, 1993). There is an array of other traffic calming techniques in addition to humps, using chicanes and pinch points, different colours and textures for road surfaces, and a variety of signs and gates. It is the integration of these different measures which is most effective, rather than the individual components. The important aspect is to give a clear indication to drivers that in the protected areas vehicles must be subordinate to the needs of pedestrians (Mackie, 1994). Although speed humps in particular have caused controversy, there has been an increasingly general acceptance that these constraints are necessary to civilize the motor vehicle in sensitive areas.

Safer vehicles

In the above sections on road user behaviour and traffic calming the emphasis has been on primary safety, avoiding accidents altogether, although the speed reduction measures in particular are also effective in reducing the severity of injury should an accident still occur. In vehicle safety, the emphasis tends to be on secondary safety, that is injury minimization, because although primary safety is obviously important, in general the handling and braking of modern vehicles is very good, and there is relatively little scope for improving it in ways which might enable the driver to avoid an impending accident. Anti-lock brakes offer a substantial potential for the driver to retain control of the vehicle under emergency braking, and can undoubtedly prevent some accidents, but their cost-effectiveness is marginal unless their cost can be reduced considerably (Robinson and Riley, 1991). Anti-lock brakes for motorcycles might offer greater potential, but again they would need to be much cheaper for adoption on all but the most expensive machines. Better conspicuity, of both machine and rider, is a cheap and very effective approach to reducing the very high risk of motorcycle accidents.

Figure 10.3 shows the categorization of road accident deaths in the UK. Car occupants account for almost half and pedestrians for a third, so it is obviously sensible to concentrate safety research on these categories. In addition, however, although motorcyclists form a smaller proportion, their risk in relation to distance travelled is ten to twenty times as great as for car occupants, and motorcycle use, although presently very low, tends to swing up and down over periods of a decade or so, so that motorcycle casualties could become more important in the future and it is worth considering what might be done to reduce them.

Figure 10.3 also shows that, of the car occupants, two-thirds die in frontal collisions and a quarter in side impacts. In the 1980s attention concentrated on

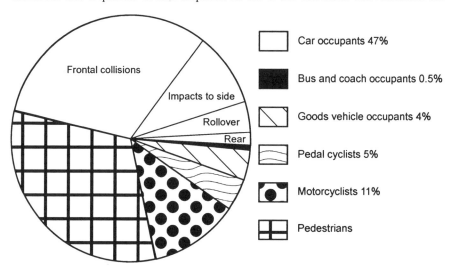

Figure 10.3   Categorization of fatal accidents by mode and, for car occupants, by accident type in UK

side impact protection because there was no safety regulation for this, whereas cars were already subjected to a front impact test, but in recent years attention has swung back to frontal protection.

Vehicle regulation is the responsibility of the European Union rather than the individual nations, and much of the technical advice to the Commission has been provided by the European Experimental Vehicles Committee (EEVC). In the past 15 years TRL has led working groups developing test procedures for side-impact protection, protection of pedestrians in collision with the fronts of cars, and, currently, protection of car occupants in frontal impacts.

The EEVC developed a side-impact test which involves running a mobile barrier, with a front made from cellular aluminium with a stiffness similar to that of a car front, into the side of the car to be tested at 50 kmph (Lowne, 1989). The car contains a specially developed dummy, the European Side-Impact Dummy or EUROSID, which is instrumented to measure accelerations, forces and chest deflection in a way which permits a consistent estimation of the likely injuries caused to a human occupant. The working groups also tested a range of different car models to assess what level of improved protection was realistic. The procedure has been accepted by the European Commission and is currently being finalized as a regulation by the United Nations Economic Commission for Europe.

The pedestrian protection test procedure was developed after detailed examination of injury data from pedestrians hit by the fronts of cars, and on the basis of impact experiments with instrumented dummies and investigations using computer modelling. However, for repeatability the test uses four different impactors on the front of the car rather than impacting a full-scale dummy. The bumper area is hit with an impactor representing the human knee, the bonnet leading edge with an impactor representing the upper leg, the front part of the bonnet with an impactor representing a child's head and the rear part with an adult head impactor. The European Commission is currently considering adopting this test as a requirement for all new cars, and Lawrence et al. (1993) have shown this measure to be highly cost-effective.

Cars are already subjected to a full-frontal 30 mph impact test into a rigid concrete block, but modern cars still show unacceptable amounts of intrusion into the occupant compartment in real accidents, despite their very good performance in the impact test. The problem is that the present test is not representative of most frontal collisions with other cars, where the vehicles tend to be offset from each other so that only part of the front structure is involved in absorbing energy, and because the vehicles are deformable their structure does not collapse in the same way as when it strikes a rigid object. Consequently the EEVC has developed a more realistic test which involves running the car into a deformable barrier, representing the front of another vehicle, with the car overlapping the barrier by only 40% (Lowne, 1994). This produces deformations and dummy measurements very similar to those seen in car-to-car collisions, and should provide better protection than the current test (Hobbs and Williams, 1994), though it should be noted that this protection from intrusion into the occupant compartment is beneficial only if the occupants are wearing seatbelts. The European Commission has agreed that this test will be adopted from 1998, though progress on both this and the side-impact test has been slowed by objections from some manufacturers.

Both pedestrians and motorcycle riders might seem hopelessly exposed in a collision, with little practical protection available. It is true that engineering is unable to offer much to reduce deaths and injuries in high-speed impacts, but most pedestrian injuries occur at impact speeds below 40 kmph, and most motorcycle injuries at speeds below 50 kmph, and in this region there is much that can be achieved. TRL has been alone in developing practical protection for motorcyclists: it has demonstrated the injury-saving potential of leg protection fitted to a wide range of motorcycle designs, and is currently obtaining promising results from airbag protection in frontal collisions (Chinn et al., 1989). Unfortunately, opposition from the industry has been vociferous, and progress in gaining practical adoption of these measures is painfully slow.

Each of the measures described above is likely to achieve a substantial reduction in injuries and deaths. Current estimates are that side-impact protection might save 20–25% of fatalities and serious injuries, pedestrian protection perhaps 25% of serious injuries although only 8% of fatalities which tend to occur at higher speeds where the protection is less effective, and improved frontal protection about a fifth to a quarter of the larger number of frontal casualties. Motorcycle leg protection might reduce serious leg injuries by 40%, and airbags, when fully developed, could reduce head injuries by perhaps a quarter. Taken together, there is scope here for reducing total road accident fatalities and serious injuries by over 20%, and in ways which are very cost-beneficial. This would be a substantial advance.

Conclusions

In the face of rapidly increasing road traffic, and fears of our inability to cope with future congestion and environmental problems, the reduction in road accidents and injuries is a success story indeed. Yet even after the achievements which will follow from safety improvements currently in the pipeline, the casualty toll will remain an unacceptable side-effect of our search for mobility, and we need to continue the efforts to improve safety further if the downward trend is not to reverse at some time in the future.

It is important that the efforts continue in all areas of safety research and policy, since the achievements are based on an integrated and multidisciplinary approach. Rapidly developing telematics will offer totally new approaches, both in controlling vehicles so that they automatically avoid collisions and in deploying protective devices better suited both to the type of accident and the characteristics of the person to be protected. But human behaviour will remain at the centre of safety matters, since we seem to have a propensity to frustrate even the cleverest technology, and an understanding of why we do what we do, within the changing circumstances, will be essential. A better understanding, too, of how the human body responds to the forces acting on it in an impact is very important. At the moment we work through instrumented dummies which we know to be crude in relation to the human frame: they are based on human measurements from accident victims and cadavers, but there are a number of areas, especially head injuries, where we need to know much more about tolerance to injury and the injury mechanisms.

So the challenge remains, and the returns can be great. The satisfaction of designing a successful strategy does not lie in the monetarized net benefits, though such calculations are necessary to establish the priorities. It lies in the avoidance of so much pain and suffering to so many individuals.

Acknowledgements

This chapter describes many aspects of work in TRL's research programme, and the author is grateful for material provided by the researchers involved. Crown Copyright 1995. The views expressed here are not necessarily those of the Department of Transport.

References

Baruya A, Finch DJ (1994) Investigation of traffic speeds and accidents on urban roads. In *Proceedings of the PTRC International Transport Forum*, September 1994. PTRC, London
Broughton J (1994) The actual number of drink/drive accidents. In *TRL Annual Review 1994*. TRL, Crowthorne
Chinn BP, Hopes P, Finnis M (1989) Leg protection and its effect on motorcycle rider trajectory. In *Proceedings of the Twelfth International Technical Conference on Experimental Safety Vehicles, Gothenburg*. NHTSA, Washington, DC
Everest JT (1992) *The Involvement of Alcohol in Fatal Accidents to Adult Pedestrians: TRL Report RR343*. TRL, Crowthorne
Finch DJ, Kompfner P, Lockwood CR, Maycock G (1993) *Speed, Speed Limits and Accidents: TRL report PR58*. TRL, Crowthorne
Forsyth E (1992a) *Cohort Study of Learner and Novice Drivers: Part 1. Learning to Drive and Performance in the Driving Test: TRL Research Report 338*. TRL, Crowthorne
Forsyth E (1992b) *Cohort Study of Learner and Novice Drivers: Part 2. Attitudes, Opinions and the Development of Skills in the First Two Years: TRL Research Report 372*. TRL, Crowthorne
Great Britain Department of Transport (1993) *Road Accidents Great Britain: the Casualty Report*. HMSO, London
Great Britain Department of Transport (1994) *Transport Statistics Great Britain 1994*. HMSO, London
Harms PL (1993) *Crash Injury Investigation and Injury Mechanisms in Road Traffic Accidents*. HMSO, London

Hills BL, Baguley CJ (1993) Accident data collection and analysis: the use of the microcomputer package MAAP in five Asian countries. In *Proceedings of the Conference on Asian Road Safety, Kuala Lumpur*, October 1993

Hobbs CA, Williams DA (1994) The development of the frontal offset deformable barrier test. In *Proceedings of the Fourteenth International Technical Conference on Experimental Safety Vehicles, Munich*. NHTSA, Washington, DC

James H (1991) Under-reporting of road traffic accidents. *Traffic Engineering and Control*, 33, 574–583

Lawrence GJL, Hardy BJ, Lowne RW (1993) *Costs and benefits of the EEVC Pedestrian Impact Requirements. TRL Project Report 19*. TRL, Crowthorne

Lowne RL (1989) EEVC Working Group Report on the EEVC Side Impact Test Procedure. In *Proceedings of the Twelfth International Technical Conference on Experimental Safety Vehicles, Gothenburg*. NHTSA, Washington, DC

Lowne RW (1994) EEVC Working Group 11 report on the development of a frontal impact test procedure. In *Proceedings of the Fourteenth International Technical Conference on Experimental Safety Vehicles, Munich*. NHTSA, Washington, DC

Mackie AM (1994) Safer streets for vulnerable road users—the UK experience. In *Proceedings of the International Conference on Living and Walking in Cities, Brescia, Italy*, June 1994

Mackie AM, Ward H, Walker RT (1990) *Urban Safety Project 3; Overall Evaluation of Area-Wide Schemes: TRL Research Report 263*. TRL, Crowthorne

Maycock G, Lockwood CR (1993) The accident liability of British car drivers. *Transport Reviews*, 13, 231–245

Robertson DI (1994) *Ex Post Evaluation of Selected Transport Research Projects: TRL Project Report 86*. TRL, Crowthorne

Robinson BJ (1994) Fatal accidents involving heavy goods vehicles in Great Britain, 1988–1990. In *Proceedings of the Fourteenth International Technical Conference on Experimental Safety Vehicles, Munich*. NHTSA, Washington, DC

Robinson BJ, Riley BS (1991) *A Study of Various Car Antilock Braking Systems: TRL Research Report 340*. TRL, Crowthorne

Roe PG, Webster DC, West G (1991) *The Relation Between the Surface Texture of Roads and Accidents: TRL Research Report RR296*. TRL, Crowthorne

Webster DC (1993) *Road Humps for Controlling Vehicle Speeds: TRL Project Report 18*. TRL, Crowthorne

Winnett M (1994) Review of speed-camera operations in the UK. In *Proceedings of the European Transport Forum, September 1994, Paper J21i*. PTRC, London

Discussion

Dinesh Mohan

Indian Institute of Technology, New Delhi, India

Dr Philip Bly has attempted a summary of the achievements in road safety over the past few decades and given some guidelines for work in the coming years. Most of the data and experience is based on work done in the UK in general and the Transport Research Laboratories in particular.

The chapter starts by stating that 'almost all accidents are a consequence of human error, and it is important to continue to encourage safer driver behaviour, especially in moderating speeds and in reducing drink-driving'. One can extend this argument one step further and state that *all* accidents are due to human error—harmful policies, hazardous road design, dangerous vehicles, careless and stressed drivers, inadequate enforcement, etc. Therefore, focusing on 'human error' does not help us to think of future strategies in any systematic manner. How important a particular 'error' is depends how far you go back in history before the accident. The longer the time period prior to the accident you examine the more the policy-makers, designers and manufacturers end up sharing the 'blame' with the driver or other road users.

Focusing on the driver also has other limitations. Modern societal systems make it mandatory for most people to participate in road traffic every day. A significant proportion of this population cannot be expected to be 'careful' and 'alert' every day. Every morning some proportion of the road users would be under stress because of some personal tragedy, problems at work or home, or some impending job regarding a great deal of risk. In addition there would be those who have had too much to drink the previous night or are under medication. Children, teenagers, and the elderly also cannot be expected to be ideal road users. Persons suffering from psychiatric disorders cannot be expected to behave perfectly on the road. If one adds up the total of all these groups on the road, it may amount to almost half the population. Therefore, there is a theoretical limit to influence of accident 'prevention' measures focused on modifying behaviour of road users by 'education'.

Reduction of 'human errors' must apply as much to city planners, road and vehicle designers and law enforcers. The present reductions in road traffic injuries and fatalities have come largely from work focused on the car without changing operating realities. A major exception to this trend has been the implementation of 'traffic calming' techniques in Europe. The future of road safety lies more in area-wide measures, changing modal shares in traffic, reducing relative personal travel demand, and focusing on the safety of pedestrians and bicyclists.

Bly mentions that speed reduction offers a 'very powerful lever in improving safety' but it is not acceptable 'either socially or in cost–benefit terms'. It appears that the costs of time have been over-estimated by most researchers. There is some evidence that the so-called 'loss' in time by each road user does not actually add up to huge economic losses in the aggregate. Or conversely, time 'saved' by each individual does not always result in productive activity. The concept of time lost has to be reassessed. It is possible that a blanket reduction in speeds may not result in too much economic loss. It may, on the other hand, reduce tension of road users and make driving more pleasurable. If this turns out to be the case, then cars could have less powerful engines.

Much more work needs to be done to understand traffic flow and crash causation theories. Knowledge in this area for mixed traffic (motorized and non-motorized) is very inadequate. Guidelines need to be developed for safer road layout for situations where bicycle and pedestrian traffic is significant.

Bly has mentioned the improvements possible in car design. Buses and trucks have been given less attention. In large parts of the world, most fatalities are caused by collisions with buses and trucks. It would be important to develop more 'forgiving' fronts for buses and trucks. Bly has also cited some of the work done at TRL to make motorcycles safer. This work is excellent technically but the new designs developed are unlikely to be incorporated in future two-wheelers. It would be more efficient to discourage motorcycle use in the long run by providing better public transport and better land-use planning.

The chapter does not include any discussion on the situation prevailing in the less motorized countries. Since a significant proportion of road accident fatalities and injuries take place there, it is important to develop future strategies for these countries also. This is not going to be very easy as not all solutions developed in the highly motorized countries are applicable in the other countries. It would be desirable to initiate serious theoretical studies for understanding the problems faced in the less motorized countries. Without this understanding it would be difficult to initiate effective countermeasures.

11
Road safety in the developing world

Godfrey D. Jacobs

Transport Research Laboratories, Crowthorne, UK

A recent and independent study by the World Bank (1990) estimates that about 600 000 people lose their lives each year as a result of road accidents and over 15 million suffer injuries. The majority of these, about 70%, occur in those countries of Africa and Asia which the World Bank classifies as low or middle income.

Whereas the road accident situation is slowly improving in high income countries, most developing countries face a worsening situation. As infectious diseases are brought increasingly under control, road deaths and injury increase in relative importance. In Thailand for example, more years of potential life are lost through road accidents than from tuberculosis and malaria combined (Yerrell, 1992); in Mexico, accidents as a cause of death rose from 4% in 1955 to 11% in 1980, with traffic accidents playing the leading role. The question needs to be posed whether or not this is the inevitable price that has to be paid by these countries for the mobility of people and goods which is the hallmark of an industrialized society.

This chapter presents a broad review of the road safety problem in developing countries and outlines recommendations for improvement based on detailed research carried out by the Overseas Centre at the Transport Research Laboratory (TRL) over the last 20 years. The work described forms part of a programme of research at TRL on the highway and transport problems of developing countries under funding from the Overseas Development Administration—which the author gratefully acknowledges.

Background

Studies carried out by the TRL have demonstrated that road accidents in the

Health at the Crossroads: Transport Policy and Urban Health.
Edited by Tony Fletcher and Anthony J. McMichael published 1997 John Wiley & Sons Ltd

Third World are:

1. A serious problem in terms of fatality rates, with rates at least an order of magnitude higher than those in industrialized countries (Jacobs, 1986).
2. An important cause of death and injury.
3. A considerable waste of scarce financial (and other) resources, typically costing at least one per cent of a country's gross national product per annum (Jacobs and Fouracre, 1977).

Rates and trends

The rate used by TRL to compare the seriousness of the road accident problem in different countries throughout the world is the number of deaths from road accidents per annum per 10 000 vehicles licensed. This is far from ideal as an indicator of relative safety in different countries. For example, the injury accidents per million vehicle-kilometre travelled per annum may be a much better parameter to use. Unfortunately, the reporting of non-fatal accidents in most Third World countries is poor and few carry out traffic surveys and censuses which provide information on annual travel by different classes of vehicle.

Results for a number of countries (1990) are shown in Figure 11.1. It can be seen that whilst countries of Western Europe and North America are characterized by a death rate (as defined above) of less than 4, some developing countries have a death rate in excess of 100. In most developing countries there will be an

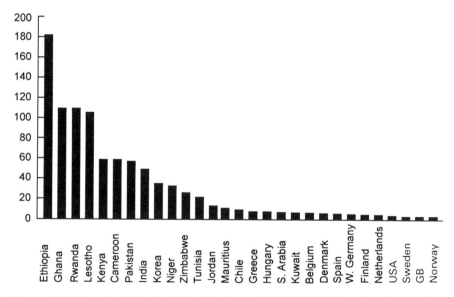

Figure 11.1   Road accident fatalities (deaths per 10 000 vehicles) in selected countries

under-reporting of road accident deaths and an over-estimate of licensed vehicles because as vehicles are scrapped they tend not to be removed from the vehicle register. In a recent study in Bangladesh it was estimated that for the reasons given above, the actual fatality rate may be at least 50% greater than the officially quoted figure of 60.

In 1984, TRL carried out a study in Colombo, Sri Lanka, comparing 'official' road accident statistics from police records with those held by hospitals. It was found that less than 25% of the hospital records (of fatal and serious road accidents) were identified in the police data. Matching of accidents involving children was particularly low. Studies such as these suggest that the road safety problem in developing countries may be much worse than official statistics suggest.

Figure 11.2 shows the percentage increase or decrease in the actual number of road accident fatalities over the period 1968 to 1985 for three groups of countries. It can be seen that over this given time period the number of road accident deaths in 13 European countries actually fell by 25%. Conversely in 6 Asian countries and 8 African countries (for which reasonably accurate statistics were available) there were increases of about 150 and 300% respectively. In these countries therefore there is need for much effort and investment in safety measures to reverse this trend—as has been the case in the developed world.

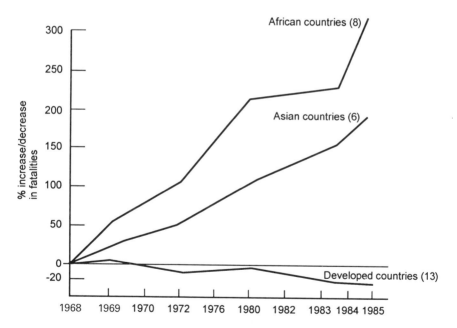

Figure 11.2   Percentage change in road accident fatalities in Asia, Africa and developed countries (1968–85)

The importance of road accidents as a cause of death

In cooperation with the World Health Organization, an early study (Jacobs and Bardsley, 1977) compared deaths from road accidents in selected developing countries with other causes of death, including diseases considered to be of concern in the Third World. Information was obtained from 15 countries which tended to be at the top end of the 'Third World spectrum' (such as Jamaica, Colombia, Peru, Malaysia, Brazil, Venezuela, South Africa, etc.) which could not be said to be representative of the entire Third World. The results nevertheless are of interest in that they show that in these countries road accidents were by no means insignificant as a cause of death. For all age groups combined, road accidents were the tenth most important cause of death (behind causes such as bronchitic, circulatory, parasitic and infectious, enteric, etc.). For the age group 5–64 years, road accidents were the sixth most important cause of death and for the age group 5–44 years they were second in importance (to other accidents, suicides and homicides combined).

In order to investigate how death rates (per head of population) were changing over time, detailed data were obtained for Malaysia, Jordan and Jamaica over the period 1960–72. (These were the only countries for which data were available over such a long period.) Death rates were obtained for road accidents and also for four groups of diseases, namely infectious, intestinal, respiratory and neoplasmic. These groups include diseases such as tuberculosis, dysentery, enteritis, malaria, cholera and smallpox. It was found that, in all three countries, death rates from road accidents and neoplasms increased over time while death rates from infectious, intestinal and respiratory diseases decreased. In Jordan, for instance, over the period 1954–64, the death rate from diseases of the respiratory system decreased by nearly 80% whilst the road accident fatality rate increased by over 160%. Similarly, in Jamaica the road accident fatality rate increased by over 120% between 1958 and 1974 whereas the death rates from respiratory, intestinal and infectious diseases decreased considerably. An examination of the medial records of the three major hospitals in Nairobi, Kenya, also illustrated this trend.

This analysis was used to show that even twenty years ago, road accidents in developing countries were already a growing social problem.

Another important factor affecting the number of people killed in road accidents in developing countries is the level of medical facilities available. Thus in Western Europe with good ambulance services, road accident casualties are very quickly taken to hospital to receive immediate attention. Even before reaching hospital, the availability of trained paramedic services means that expert assistance can be provided at the roadside. Another useful measure of the seriousness of the road accident problem in a country is the Fatality Index (FI), that is, the percentage of all casualties that are fatally injured. In a study carried out by TRL (Jacobs and Hutchinson, 1973) the FI was determined for 32 (mainly) developing countries and was found to range from about 4 (Cyprus, Mauritius) to over 20 (Pakistan, Iraq). Reasons for high FIs were investigated by means of regression analysis and it was found that the level of medical facilities available in these countries (expressed as population per physician and population per hospital bed) were very closely correlated with the FI; the poorer the medical facility as defined above, the higher the FI.

Clearly the level of medical facilities available in developing countries has a significant impact on the number of people dying in road accidents. By improving medical services generally, including ambulances and trained paramedics, the number of people injured in road accidents who subsequently die can be significantly reduced.

The cost of road accidents

Apart from the humanitarian aspects of road safety, it must also be borne in mind that road accidents are responsible in developing countries for a loss of scarce financial resources that these countries can ill-afford to lose. An analysis carried out by TRL (Jacobs and Fouracre, 1977) showed that road accident costs were the equivalent in any country, be it developed or developing, to at least 1% of its annual gross national product. In current prices this suggests that road accidents in Indonesia, for example, may be costing about £600 million per annum, in Pakistan £260 million, in Egypt £200 million, in Chile £150 million, in Kenya £60 million, etc. If one assumes road accidents to cost 1% of GNP in all countries, then for those countries of Africa and Asia below an average GNP/capita of $3500 (figure used by the World Bank to define 'developing' countries), it is estimated that the total annual cost of road accidents is approximately US$25 billion. If the reduction in the substantial pain, grief and suffering caused by road accidents in the Third World is not sufficient motivation, there is also a very strong economic case to be made in the significant loss of resources each year due to accidents.

Unfortunately, road safety is but one of the many problems demanding its share of funding and other resources in developing countries. Even within the boundaries of the transport and highway sector, hard decisions have to be taken on the resources that a Third World government can devote to road safety. In order to assist in this decision-making process it is essential that a method be devised to determine the cost of road accidents and the value of preventing them.

The nature of the road accident problem

Accident patterns

There are some accident characteristics which are common to a number of developing countries and yet are somewhat different from those in developed countries. For example, in the Third World (Figure 11.3 and Table 11.1), a

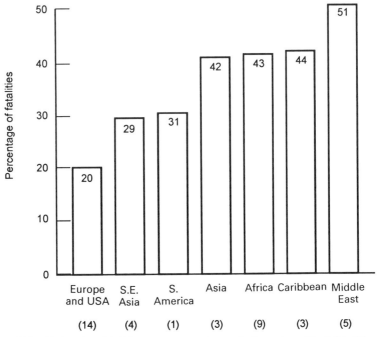

Figure 11.3   Pedestrian fatalities as a percentage of all road accident fatalities. ( ) = number of countries

Table 11.1   Characteristics of fatal accidents

	Percentage of fatalities which:	
Country	were children under 16 years	involved trucks and buses
Botswana (1988)	16	25
Egypt (1984)	12	37
Ghana (1989)	28	50
Pakistan (Karachi) (1988)	14	44
Papua New Guinea (1987)	20	37
Zimbabwe (1989)	11	45
United Kingdom (1988)	9	21

relatively high proportion of fatalities are pedestrians and children aged under 16 years, and many fatal accidents involve trucks, buses and other public service vehicles (Downing, 1991a).

In many cases these higher percentages are an obvious consequence of the differences between the traffic and population characteristics of developed and developing countries. For example, the average percentage of the population aged 5 to 14 years in a sample of 16 developing countries was 28% compared with 15% for 9 developed countries (Downing and Sayer, 1982). As pedestrians, children and professional drivers constitute such a large proportion of the accident problem, it is clear that many Third World countries need to give priority to improving the safety of these particular three groups.

Contributory factors

In most countries, police road accident reports give some information about the factors or causes which contributed to the accidents. In general these data have to be treated with some caution as the police investigating the accidents are unlikely to have been trained as engineers and they may therefore underestimate the contribution made by road engineering problems. Their main aim is usually to determine whether there has been a traffic violation and therefore the emphasis of the investigation is likely to be placed on detecting human error and apportioning blame.

In the UK in the early 1970s, a more reliable approach, namely 'On-the-Spot' investigation, was carried out by a research team from TRL in an area of South East England (Sabey and Staughton, 1975). This study demonstrated the importance of the road user factor which contributed to 95% of the accidents and the strong link between road user error and deficiencies in the road environment, which together contributed to over 25% of accidents (Table 11.2). Constraints of expertise or funding currently prevent a study of this type in developing countries, so police reports are the only source of information available.

Table 11.2 Causes of road accidents as determined by the police in developing countries

	Main cause of accident (%)			
Country	Road user error	Vehicle defect	Adverse road conditions or environment	Other
Afghanistan (1984)	74	17	9	–
Botswana (1982)	94	2	1	3
Cyprus (1982)	94	1	5	–
Ethiopia (1982)	81	5	–	14
India (1980)	80	7	1	12
Iran (1984)	64	16	20	–
Pakistan (1984)	91	4	5	–
Philippines (1984)	85	8	7	–
Malaysia (1985)	87	2	4	7
Zimbabwe (1979)	89	5	1	5
TRRL On-the-Spot Study (1975)*	95	8	28	

*In about 30% of accidents, multiple factors were identified.

From Table 11.2 it can be seen that, in general, the data highlight the seriousness of road user errors in developing countries but give little indication of any road environment factor other than in the case of Iran. It seems likely that the road environment factor has been considerably underestimated by the police in their statistics. The condition of main roads is poorer in developing than in developed countries (see, for example, Harral and Faiz, 1988) and the pace of introducing engineering improvements to reduce road accidents is considerably slower in the Third World.

Road user behaviour and knowledge

Studies of road user behaviour (Jacobs, 1981) at traffic signals and pedestrian crossings in a number of Third World cities indicated that road users tended to be less disciplined than in the United Kingdom. Also, observations in Pakistan (Downing, 1985) demonstrated relatively high proportions of drivers crossing continuous 'no-overtaking' lines (15%) and not stopping at stop signs even when traffic was near (52%). Although the relationship between these differences in behaviour and accidents has not been determined, the results suggest that road safety measures which are not self-enforcing, such as road signs and markings, may be much less effective unless they are integrated with publicity and enforcement campaigns. Poor road user behaviour exhibited by drivers in some developing countries may be due to their lack of knowledge about road safety rules and regulations or their general attitude towards road safety matters. A study of drivers' knowledge in Jamaica, Pakistan and Thailand (Sayer and Downing, 1981) indicated that there were only a few topics where a lack of knowledge was widespread. One such example was stopping distances where 87% of the drivers underestimated the distance required to stop in an emergency when travelling at 30 mph. Answering questions on stopping and following distances also proved to be a problem for professional drivers in Cameroon and Zimbabwe (Downing, 1991b), with truck and bus drivers unable to answer more than half the questions on driving knowledge and skills correctly. Other areas of driver behaviour, such as not stopping at pedestrian crossings, traffic signals and stop signs, were found to be due to poor attitudes rather than to poor knowledge. Although attitudes are notoriously difficult to change, there would seem to be some potential for improving them by introducing publicity and enforcement campaigns.

Another area of concern in some, but not all, Third World countries is the problem of alcohol and road users. From Table 11.3 it can be seen that the blood alcohol levels found in accident fatalities in Trinidad (Simmons, 1990) and Zimbabwe (Sandwith, 1980) were considerably higher than those found in Great Britain (TRL, 1990a). In addition, recent roadside alcohol surveys in Papua New Guinea at weekends between 10 pm and 2 am found that 24% of drivers were over 80 mg/100 ml (the UK legal limit). This is much higher than the figure of 2% found in similar surveys in the UK (Everest, 1991).

Table 11.3 Blood alcohol levels (BAC) in road accident fatalities

		Percentage with BAC exceeding (mg/100 ml)	
Country	Road-user type	0	80
Trinidad (1988)	Driver	–	41
	Pedestrian	–	41
Zimbabwe (1979)	Driver	56	–
	Pedestrian	72	–
Great Britain (1988)	Driver	31*	20
	Pedestrian	37*	28

* = Over 9 mg/100 ml.

Thus, overall there are wide differences between developed and developing countries in the behaviour, knowledge, attitudes and culture of the road users, in the conditions of the roads and the vehicles and in the characteristics of the traffic. Consequently the effectiveness of transferring some developed country solutions to developing countries is uncertain and their appropriateness needs to be considered in relation to the problems and conditions prevailing in individual countries.

Institutions and information systems

Organizational requirements

In road safety matters, as in many other sectors, there is a need to strengthen the various institutions responsible for the various aspects of road safety and to increase their capability for multisectoral action. The whole process of planning and implementing road safety improvements should be multidisciplinary and dynamic. Road safety organizations should be established on a full-time basis and be capable of:

1. diagnosing the road accident problem;
2. drawing up an integrated plan of action including the setting up of goals and objectives;
3. coordinating the work of all organizations involved;
4. procuring funds and resources;
5. producing design guides;
6. designing and implementing improvements;
7. monitoring implementation and evaluating measures; and
8. feeding back information from the evaluations and amending the action plan as necessary.

Road accident databases

One of the key activities listed above was the diagnosis of the road accident problem. The most important source of data for this activity is the police road accident report. In the early 1970s, a survey of road accident information systems in use in developing countries (Jacobs, 1975) indicated that only 15% of the countries had adequate accident report forms and none had computer analysis facilities. Therefore, to help countries improve their accident investigation and research capability, TRL's Overseas Centre, with ODA's support, developed its Microcomputer Accident Analysis Package (MAAP), initially in collaboration with the traffic police in Egypt (Hills and Elliott, 1986) and it is now in use in over 14 countries. It is the nationally adopted system for Botswana and Papua New Guinea, and regionally adopted in most of the other countries; major cities in which MAAP is established include Bandung, Beijing, Karachi and Islamabad. The languages in which MAAP operates include Arabic, Chinese, French and Spanish. It is interesting to note that MAAP is also used by a number of local authorities in the UK.

MAAP is a powerful yet simple system which enables users to:

1. obtain good data for diagnosis, planning, evaluation and research purposes; and
2. set up low-cost engineering improvement schemes similar to those which have proved so successful in developed countries.

It consists of two key components: a police report booklet or form with a recommended structure, although details can vary considerably; and a set of software programs for data entry and analysis. The relatively low-cost and increased availability of microcomputers means that individual highway authorities can analyse their own data to help identify hazardous locations, the nature of the problems, choose appropriate countermeasures and assess their effectiveness, all with increased efficiency and, therefore it is hoped, accuracy.

Road safety improvements

In the Third World, evaluation of improvements is essential because of the lack of data on the benefits (or otherwise) of road safety measures. It is recommended that improvements are introduced on a pilot basis and evaluated before being implemented nationwide.

The Overseas Centre is giving priority to researching road safety countermeasures but, owing to the long-term nature of many of the studies and the limited resources available, there are only a few published results.

In spite of this lack of information the remainder of this paper attempts to give an idea of likely priorities for future road safety action and research by reviewing studies of remedial measures in developing countries with reference to developed country findings where appropriate.

Engineering and planning

Despite the fact that human error is probably the chief causal factor in most road accidents, there is little doubt that engineering and planning improvements can affect road user behaviour in such a way that errors are less likely to occur or, when they do occur, the environment can be made more 'forgiving'. Thus, there has been a growth in emphasis on engineering and planning countermeasures over the past two decades both in Europe and North America.

Engineering and planning can improve road safety through two distinct mechanisms:

1. Accident prevention, resulting from good standards of design and planning of *new* road schemes and related development.
2. Accident reduction, resulting from remedial measures applied to problems identified in the *existing* road network.

It has already been noted that, since the 1970s, industrialized countries have benefited considerably from improvements in engineering approaches to road safety. Developing countries on the other hand, have been slower to adopt these approaches. In many locations, roads are being built or upgraded with little consideration given to road safety, and as a result blackspots are still being created. One factor contributing to this situation could well be the difficulty in acquiring information about the latest techniques and standards. To encourage the transfer of suitable technology in this field, the TRL has published *Towards Safety Roads in Developing Countries* (1991), a road safety guide for planners and engineers. This was produced in association with the Ross Silcock Partnership and is designed to be a first point of reference on road safety issues. It draws upon appropriate material from many existing manuals and standards around the world as well as giving many photographic examples of good and bad practices.

Vehicle safety

Improvements in vehicle design, occupant protection and vehicle maintenance have made a significant contribution to accident reduction in industrialized countries. In developing countries, however, the safety design of vehicles sometimes lags behind that of developed countries, particularly when vehicles are locally manufactured or assembled. Similarly, vehicle condition is likely to be more of a problem when it is difficult to obtain spare parts. Overloading of goods and passenger vehicles is another vehicle factor which commonly contributes to high accident severity and casualty rates.

From Table 11.2 it is clear that the police in some developing countries have blamed a relatively high proportion (up to 17%) of accidents on vehicle defects. Although many of these countries may have inadequate controls to ensure minimum safe standards of vehicle condition, it would seem more appropriate that they should start by introducing low-cost random roadside checks using simple equipment rather than expensive networks of vehicle testing centres with sophisticated technology.

The control of overloading passenger-carrying vehicles combined with improvements in the design of such vehicles would also seem to have some potential for accident and casualty reduction in many countries. For example, in Papua New Guinea (PNG), it is common for passengers to be transported in open pick-ups and, perhaps not surprisingly, an exceptionally high proportion (45%) of the road accident casualties come from such vehicles. To help PNG deal with this problem, the Overseas Centre and Vehicle Safety Division of TRL designed a simple, robust protective cage to protect the occupants. Roll-over trials on TRL's test track demonstrated that the cage provided improved protection and it is planned that the design will be field tested in PNG.

Education and training

Road safety education

It is important for road users to be educated about road safety from as young an age as possible. In developed countries a number of approaches have been tried both through school systems and through parents, and most children receive some advice. However, in developing countries where the child pedestrian accident problem is generally more serious, a study of children's crossing knowledge (Downing and Sayer, 1982) indicated that children were less likely to receive advice (from members of their family, teachers or the police) than in the UK.

There is clearly a need to improve road safety education, but as some countries will have low school attendance figures it is important that education through community programmes is considered as well as through the school system.

It is recognized that road safety education programmes should be graded and developmental (OECD, 1978; Downing, 1987) and that teachers need guidelines on what and how to teach. To meet these requirements, many countries have produced syllabus documents and teacher guides, including a few in the Third World (Leburu, 1990). However, it is in this area that the transferability of developed country solutions to developing countries is less certain and much more research is needed. Further, studies in Europe (Downing, 1987; OECD, 1986), and to some extent surveys in Pakistan and Zimbabwe, have indicated that measures such as producing teachers' guides and making road safety teaching compulsory were not on their own sufficient to improve greatly the quantity and quality of road safety education in schools. For example, in the UK a 'core curriculum' document circulated to all schools was used by fewer than 4%, and in

Zimbabwe a schools 'road safety kit' was used by only 5% of schools. Evidently teacher training and other actions are necessary to promote and increase the provision of road safety education in all countries. Currently TRL is involved in a programme of research in Ghana aimed at developing methods of improving road safety education in developing countries.

Driver training and testing

In developing countries, the problems of poor driver behaviour and knowledge described earlier are likely to be due, to some extent, to inadequacies in driver training and testing.

Professional driving instruction tends to be limited because:

1. driving instructors are not properly tested or monitored;
2. there are no driving or instruction manuals;
3. driving test standards and requirements are inadequate.

Consequently, there is likely to be considerable scope for raising driving standards by improving driver training and testing. One recent contribution by the Overseas Centre in collaboration with the United Nations Economic Commission for Africa (ECA), is a driving guide specifically for truck drivers (TRL, 1990b). This group of drivers tends to have a greater involvement in accidents than in developed countries and inadequate training clearly plays some part in this. The guide was designed to be easy to read (average reading age of 9 years) and its usefulness appears promising, as a study by Downing (1991b) demonstrated that reading sections of the guide helped drivers improve their scores on knowledge tests by up to 25% on some topics.

As well as providing such advice on driving standards, many countries need to improve the licensing, training, testing and monitoring of instructors to ensure that these standards are taught. In training systems where learner drivers are free to choose how they learn, it is important that driving tests demand a high standard of driving especially for the practical 'on the road' assessment. More difficult tests should encourage learners to purchase more lessons from professional instructors.

Enforcement

A large number of studies (OECD, 1974; Spolander, 1977) have examined the effectiveness of enforcement systems in developed countries, particularly with respect to traffic police operations. Many of them demonstrated that a conspicuous police presence led to improvements in driver behaviour in the vicinity of the police, but the evidence for accident reductions was less convincing.

In developing countries, the traffic police are generally less well trained and equipped and often they are non-mobile, i.e. stationed at intersections. Traffic police operating under such conditions are likely to find it difficult to influence moving violations and this was certainly shown to be the case in a study by Downing (1985) of the effects of police presence in Pakistan. However, studies of improved training and deployment of traffic police have indicated large reductions in moving violations (Downing, 1985). Also, following the introduction of highway patrols on intercity roads, a 6% reduction in accidents was achieved in Pakistan, and a similar scheme in Egypt produced accident reductions of almost 50% (Gaber and Yerrell, 1983). Therefore, it would appear that improvements in traffic policing have considerable potential for both improving driver behaviour and reducing accidents provided that the police's capability to enforce moving violations is enhanced.

Conclusion

Many developing countries have a serious road accident problem. Fatality rates are high in comparison with those in developed countries and whilst in Europe and North America the situation is generally improving, many developing countries face a worsening situation. Apart from the humanitarian aspects of the problem, road accidents cost countries of Africa and Asia at least one per cent of their gross national product each year—sums that these countries can ill afford to lose. Compared with causes of death more commonly associated with the developing world, deaths from road accidents are by no means insignificant. Lack of medical facilities in these countries has been shown to be an important factor leading to high death rates.

In order to identify priorities for action, it is important that there is a clear understanding of the road accident problem and the likely effectiveness of road safety improvements. It is therefore a priority for countries to have an appropriate accident information system (such as TRL's MAAP) which can be used to identify accident patterns, the factors involved in road accidents and the location of hazardous sites. In order that an overall budget for, say, a five year action programme can be determined, it is essential that developing countries set up procedures for costing road accidents. This will also do much to ensure that the best use is made of any investment and that the most appropriate improvements are introduced in terms of the benefits that they will generate in relation to the cost of their implementation. Other basic requirements are for safety improvements to be coordinated by means of a National Road Safety Council (or the equivalent) and for a well trained safety team capable of implementing a wide-ranging programme of road safety improvements, which are preferably low cost.

Although developing countries may have made a late start in road safety, many are now beginning to take appropriate action to reduce road accidents and there are some encouraging signs for the future. For example, a survey of 23 African countries (Yerrell, 1991) suggested that nearly half were implementing a wide range of improvements. National aid agencies such as ODA and international lending agencies such as the World Bank are aware of the seriousness of the problem in developing countries and most loans for major highway or urban sector projects now have a road safety component built into them.

ODA is also to be applauded for the funding of TRL's long-term programme of research in developing countries which has done much to draw attention to this growing problem. This, in turn, has led to other promising developments. For example, at the second African Road Safety Congress (ECA, 1991), one of the key recommendations was for the strengthening of research centres at the national or sub-national level. The Sixth Conference of the Road Engineering Association of Asia and Australia dedicated a special workshop to the problem of road safety (REAAA, 1990). This year's REAAA Conference in Taiwan will also contain a special safety workshop.

Developing countries have accelerated their efforts to improve road safety in recent years. It is hoped that these trends will continue and that all countries will, through joint programmes of research and development and by sharing information, maintain an effective and scientific approach to reducing road accidents throughout the world.

Acknowledgements

The work in this chapter forms part of the programme of the Transport Research Laboratory and the paper is published by permission of the Chief Executive. The cooperation provided by all the countries participating in joint road safety research projects is gratefully acknowledged. The author is particularly grateful for the assistance given by the cooperating governments and organizations in Botswana, Egypt, Ghana, Indonesia, Jamaica, Pakistan, Thailand, Papua New Guinea and Zimbabwe. The author also wishes to acknowledge the contribution to this chapter provided by his colleagues and also the Engineering Division of the Overseas Development Administration for providing the funding for TRL's programmes of research on road accidents in developing countries.

References

Downing AJ (1985) Road accidents in Pakistan and the need for improvements in driver training and traffic law enforcement. In PTRC, *Developing Countries: Transport and Urban Development*. Proceedings of Seminar H, PTRC Summer Annual Meeting, University of Sussex, 15–18 July 1985, PTRC Education and Research Services, London
Downing AJ (1991a) Pedestrian safety in developing countries. In *The Vulnerable Road User: Proceedings of the International Conference on Traffic Safety*. McMillan India Ltd, New Delhi
Downing AJ (1991b) Driver training in Africa: the UN-ECA driving manual. In *Proceedings of the Second African Road Safety Congress*. Institute of Transport Economics, Oslo
Downing AJ, Sayer IA (1982) *A Preliminary Study of Children's Road Crossing Knowledge in Three Developing Countries*. TRRL Supplementary Report 771. Transport and Road Research Laboratory, Crowthorne
Downing CS (1987) The education of children in road safety. In Berfenstam R *The Healthy*

Community: Child Safety as Part of Health Promotion Activities. Stockholm
Economic Commission for Africa (1991) *Conference Recommendations: Proceedings of the Second African Road Safety Congress.* Institute of Economics, Oslo
Everest JT (1991) *Drinking and Driving.* Transport and Road Research Laboratory, Crowthorne
Fouracre PR, Jacobs GD (1976) *Comparative Accident Costs in Developing Countries.* TRRL Supplementary Report 206. Transport and Road Research Laboratory, Crowthorne
Gaber Gen MA, Yerrell JS (1983) Road safety research in Egypt. In *Proceedings of the International Association for Accidents and Traffic Medicine 9th International Conference, Mexico, September 1983.* IAATM, Mexico
Harral C, Faiz A (1988) *Road Deterioration in Developing Countries: Causes and Remedies.* World Bank, Washington DC
Hills BL, Elliott GJ (1986) *A Microcomputer Accident Analysis Package and its Use in Developing Countries.* Proceedings of the Indian Road Congress Road Safety Seminar, Srinigar
Jacobs GD (1975) *Road Accident Data Collection and Analysis in Developing Countries.* TRRL Laboratory Report 676. Transport and Road Research Laboratory, Crowthorne
Jacobs GD (1981) *A Preliminary Study of Road User Behaviour in Developing Countries.* TRRL Supplementary Report 646. Transport and Road Research Laboratory, Crowthorne
Jacobs GD (1986) Road accident fatality rates in developing countries: a reappraisal. In PTRC, *Developing Countries: Transport and Urban Development.* Proceedings of Seminar H, PTRC Summer Annual Meeting, University of Sussex, 15–18 July 1985, PTRC Education and Research Services, London, pp. 107–120
Jacobs GD, Bardsley MN (1977) *Road Accidents as a Cause of Death in Developing Countries.* TRRL Supplementary Report 277. Transport and Road Research Laboratory, Crowthorne
Jacobs GD, Cutting CA (1986) Further research on accident rates in developing countries. *Accident Analysis and Prevention, 18,* 119–127
Jacobs GD, Fouracre PR (1977) *Further Research on Road Accident Rates in Developing Countries.* TRRL Supplementary Report 270. Transport and Road Research Laboratory, Crowthorne
Jacobs GD, Hutchinson P (1973) *A Study of Accident Rates in Developing Countries.* TRRL Laboratory Report 546. Transport and Road Research Laboratory, Crowthorne
Leburu FM (1990) Training the children: Traffic education in Botswana. In *Proceedings of the International Conference for Road Safety and Accidents in Developing Countries.* Academy of Scientific Research and Technology, Cairo
Organisation for Economic Cooperation and Development (1974) *Research on Traffic Law Enforcement.* OECD, Paris
Organisation for Economic Cooperation and Development (1978) *Chairman's Report and Report of Sub Group 11 and Road Safety Education.* Transport and Road Research Laboratory, Crowthorne
Organisation for Economic Cooperation and Development (1979) *Traffic Safety in Residential Areas.* OECD, Paris
Organisation for Economic Cooperation and Development (1986) *Effectiveness of Road Safety Education Programmes.* OECD, Paris
Road Engineering Association of Asia and Australasia (1990) *Proceedings of the Sixth Conference,* March 1990. REAAA, Kuala Lumpur
Sabey BE, Staughton GG (1975) Interacting roles of road environment, vehicle and road-user in accidents. In *Proceedings of the International Association for Accident and*

Traffic Medicine 5th International Conference, London, September 1975. IAATM, London

Sandwith A (1980) *Traffic Safety in Zimbabwe*. Zimbabwe Traffic Safety Board, Harare

Sayer IA, Downing AJ (1981) *Driver Knowledge of Road Safety Factors in Three Developing Countries*. TRRL Supplementary Report 713. Transport and Road Research Laboratory, Crowthorne

Simmons V (1990) Alcohol and road traffic accidents. In *Proceedings of the First Caribbean Conference on Transportation and Traffic Planning*. Caribbean Epidemiology Centre, Trinidad

Spolander K (1977) *Trafikoevervakning*. National Road and Traffic Research Institute Rapport 139. NRTRI, Linkoeping (Sweden)

Transport and Road Research Laboratory (1990a). *Blood Alcohol Levels in Fatalities in Great Britain, 1988*. TRRL Leaflet LF 2017. Transport and Road Research Laboratory, Crowthorne

Transport and Road Research Laboratory (1990b) *A Guide for Drivers of Heavy Goods Vehicles*. Transport and Road Research Laboratory, Crowthorne

Transport and Road Research Laboratory (1991) *Towards Safer Roads in Developing Countries: a Guide for Planners and Engineers*. Transport and Road Research Laboratory, Crowthorne

World Bank (1990) Road safety: a lethal problem in the Third World. *The Urban Edge*, 14(5), special edition

Yerrell JS (1991) Road safety in Africa: background and overview. In *Proceedings of the Second African Road Safety Congress*. Institute of Transport Economics, Oslo

Yerrell JS (1992) Traffic accidents—a worldwide problem. *First International Seminar on Road User Behaviour*. Transport and Road Research Laboratory, Crowthorne

SECTION 3

THE WIDER PUBLIC HEALTH

12
Introduction

Tony Fletcher and Anthony J. McMichael

London School of Hygiene & Tropical Medicine, UK

This section addresses a number of intersecting themes: understanding the place of transport policy in the 'new public health' framework for analysing urban health issues; developing health concerns in the transport priority setting, for example in the framework of the healthy cities movement; and exploring the health promoting benefits of non-motorized transport, an antidote to dwelling too much on avoiding negative aspects of some transport choices.

Ashton reviews how the piecemeal urban development into sprawling cities dependent on car use has led to many adverse effects, expensive in both personal terms—the destruction of communities—and environmentally, with the excessive movement of essential goods in the globalized economy. This has its roots in the NIMBY ('Not In My Backyard') tradition of dealing with public health problems, of moving waste, pollution and slums to somewhere else. In response to these problems a new public health has emerged, based on more ecological principles: sustaining the environment which sustains you, and ideas of social justice. The principles of the Ottawa Charter for Health Promotion offer a way forward, with community participation lying at the centre of strategies for developing urban planning strategies. He concludes by underlining the important role played by non-governmental organizations in offering imaginative local solutions to the crisis of urban over-development.

Goldstein discusses ways forward to address the relative failure of health concerns in the setting of urban development agendas. Intersectoral collaborations need to be two-way, with the apparent disparities in health being communicated to planners, and the health sector appreciating and promoting the health opportunities offered by urban development strategies. The study of intra-urban health differences and their presentation in a form readily understood by decision-makers, requires an understanding of how these decision-makers currently perceive the situation. Finally, the widening of the basis of decision-making

Health at the Crossroads: Transport Policy and Urban Health.
Edited by Tony Fletcher and Anthony J. McMichael © 1997 John Wiley & Sons Ltd

to include more community participation would form an important part of the strategy to raise the profile of health.

Hillman identifies the disturbing trend of reducing fitness in the UK, both among adults and children (where habits of taking exercise are established). The growing recognition of the importance of fitness reflected in jogging, attending gyms and swimming, is not enough given the attendant risks of injury and the lack of sufficient facilities. Walking and cycling offer both an effective means of transport and a excellent source of regular exercise. The National Travel Survey has demonstrated that people in the UK walk and cycle much less than in the past, but given the low current level, there is great scope for increasing cycling and walking. Some success in this regard has been achieved in the Netherlands. However, people harbour genuine fears for their safety (or that of their children) on the roads. The risk for cyclists is somewhat exaggerated argues Hillman and in fact at a population level the gain in life years due to improved health far outweighs the risks of fatal accidents, even given the higher risks per kilometre cycled in the UK as compared to the Netherlands. The scope for increasing this relative advantage by improving the environment for cyclists is considerable. Hillman persuasively argues the case on health promotion grounds in addition to the other benefits to the urban environment of a modal shift from car use to cycling and walking.

13
Evaluating the wider impact on health and quality of life

John R. Ashton

North West Regional Health Authority, UK

The renaissance of public health over the past two decades began with a focus on the biomedical aspects of disease prevention, a preoccupation with individual risk factors and an emphasis on health education. Concern at victim blaming in the early 1980s led to the emergence of the concepts of health promotion which paved the way for a more appropriate balance to be struck between the individual and the collective and the agent, the host and the environment, in a reworking of the classical paradigm more suited to the contemporary health agenda.

What has emerged as the new public health is an understanding that health is fundamentally an ecological matter which is dependent on an optimal balance and relationship between populations and their environments. In this relationship, the precautionary principle *primum non nocere* long taught as part of the sound practice of clinical medicine acquires a new meaning or perhaps reinvokes an original one (Ashton and Seymour, 1988). In the new public health this principle finds itself in the company of another powerful and related principle well understood by people from so-called less-developed societies—the principle of reciprocal maintenance.

At the heart of this principle is the notion of looking after the things that look after us, be they our relationships, our bodies or the environment which sustains us and provides for us. It is perhaps increasingly understood as eco-sanity and it is one of the two fundamental challenges to human society as we approach the millennium; the other being social justice. It is in this context that the ideas behind the Ottawa Charter should be considered (Figure 13.1).

Here the central idea of the old public health, the sanitary idea, can be seen to have been deeply flawed. The sanitary idea was an idea of its times, very

Health at the Crossroads: Transport Policy and Urban Health.
Edited by Tony Fletcher and Anthony J. McMichael © 1997 John Wiley & Sons Ltd

| • Build policies which support health |
| • Create supportive environments |
| • Strengthen community action |
| • Develop personal skills |
| • Reorientate health services |

Figure 13.1   The elements of the Ottawa Charter for Health Promotion
Source: World Health Organization, Health and Welfare Canada, Canadian Public
Health Association (1986) *Ottawa Charter for Health Promotion.* World Health
Organization, Copenhagen.

mechanistic and imbued with images of 'man' conquering nature and of imposing
human will on natural phenomena and systems. The central theme was the belief
in the need to separate the miasmas associated with sewage, waste and pollution
from food, potable water and human habitation; it began with privies, paved
streets, and piped water supplies and finished with garden suburbs, new towns
and motorways. This approach has been very much in the 'NIMBY' (Not In My
Back Yard) tradition where, having removed wastes, pollution or slum-dwellers
to somewhere else they could be forgotten about. This has been an essentially
linear approach to the environment, to natural and social systems and the
resources which they represent (including those of family networks). It is an
approach which involves plundering and moving on, hardly a sound base for the
construction of a self-sustaining economy and one which is destined to build up
ecological debt for future generations when the limits to the carrying capacity of
natural and social systems are ignored. Interestingly, in at least one newly
developing country—Indonesia—which has high rates of growth, this issue is a
matter for hot debate and the official figures for economic growth are being
discounted by a significant proportion in an attempt to obtain a true perspective
on the relationship between development and sustainability.

The role of transport in this sorry tale, particularly the role of the motor car, has
been intimately bound up with urbanization and with efforts to deal with its
consequences. Other forms of modern transport are bound up with the move from
a local to a global economy as the world becomes one huge networked metropolis.

The urbanization issue has belatedly begun to receive serious attention.
According to Sir Donald Acheson, General Chairman of the technical discussions
at the 44th World Health Assembly in 1991 on the topic of 'Health for all in the
face of rapid urbanization': 'By the year 2000, a majority of the world's
population will live in large towns or cities. For most city dwellers the urban
setting will play a major part in determining their level of health. Moreover it is
becoming increasingly clear that the way in which we choose to organize and run
our cities will be critical to the future ecology of the planet itself. These essential
facts lie behind the recent emergence of a sense of crisis about the condition of the

world's cities and about the situation of the urban poor' (WHO, 1993). In Europe and North America where the urbanization experience began almost 200 years ago, the poor were living in appalling, insanitary conditions, crowding into urban slums and vulnerable to epidemic infectious disease. Governments seemed reluctant to introduce reforms and it fell to campaigning bodies such as the Health of Towns Associations in England to campaign for change (Ashton, 1992; Ashton and Ubido, 1991). The ensuing movement for sanitary reform was, as already inferred, very mechanistic albeit pursued with the best of intentions. The awfulness of the situation led visionaries such as William Morris to describe what health should be about for urban dwellers, 'At least I know this, that if a person is overworked in any degree they cannot enjoy the sort of health I am speaking of; nor if they are continually chained to one dull round of mechanical work, with no hope at the other end of it, nor if they live in continual sordid anxiety for their livelihood, nor if they are ill housed, nor if they are deprived of the natural beauty of the world, nor if they have no amusement to quicken the flow of their spirits from time to time; all these things, which touch more or less directly on their bodily condition, are born of the claim I make to live in good health' (Morris, 1884).

Musings such as these and those of others fed in to pioneers such as the town planner Ebenezer Howard who developed the first 'garden city' suburbs in the United Kingdom at the end of the last century as a technical solution to the slums (Hancock and Duhl, 1986). At first such developments were local, constrained by the transport technology of the day to the limits of tram and railway routes but the principle of integration in cities which had characterized the ancient Mediterranean cities, where people lived, worked and played in the same neighbourhood, had been breached and the functional city had arrived. This functional city which was embraced by town planners and public health reformers alike sought to divide cities up into functional zones for industry, residence and recreation. Their motives were laudable and very much in the sanitary tradition but their impact was hard to foresee. With the advent of the internal combustion engine, the ratchet apparently turned, the cities of the developed world began to thin out, urban sprawl, ribbon development, outer suburbs, new towns all came to be indivisible as the motor car democratized personal transport. However this fragmentation, functional division and the tyranny of mobility does not end with the city or county boundaries. According to David Morris 'We embrace the planetary economy with a fervour that borders on the religious' (Morris, 1990). Morris goes on to describe four principles which underpin the development of this global economy:

1. separation of producer from consumer with long distribution lines and transport implications;
2. dependence on other communities, regions and countries for essential goods and products in place of self-sufficiency;

3. fragmentation of production, distribution, consumption, residence, commerce and industry;
4. loss of community autonomy (often accompanied by increased responsibility for coping with the adverse consequences of the changes).

What has become of us?

As a child growing up in Liverpool I was free to wander and explore the city from quite an early age. In the holidays I would often go out all day with friends exploring on foot, bicycle or bus, and at secondary school I cycled the three miles each way daily for several years.

For today's children, all that has changed. The combination of at least three factors has rendered our cities unsafe and made today's parents anxious and wary. The creation and tolerance of an alienated and hostile underclass, the evacuation of city cores through slum clearance and the abandonment of our cities to cars and urban motorways to facilitate middle-class escape to safe havens, have together vandalized our urban heritage. Mayer Hillman argues cogently about the impact of the motor car on the quality of life in cities and identifies six consequences of our infatuation and lack of vision and control (Hillman, 1990):

1. traffic danger;
2. grief, suffering and anxiety;
3. loss of autonomy;
4. noise;
5. air pollution; and
6. lack of exercise.

In accepting this, and admitting our political bankruptcy, we are not only accepting the tragic medical consequences of physical and mental harm but we are failing to optimize what has occasionally been and what can be a pinnacle of civilization. Indeed the 'city' is literally, and should be, at the heart of 'civilization'.

At their best, cities can provide an external living space of immense stimulus and challenge. Len Duhl, one of the originators of the WHO *Healthy Cities* initiative talks of cities 'to grow people in' and there is a kind of Piagetian sense in which, as children grow and their sense of scale develops, they should be able to stretch and challenge themselves in a secure, supportive environment to enable them to discover themselves and become self-assured, confident adults—something which we increasingly recognize as being central to positive health behaviour and which underpins many of the social class differences in health status. At the other end of the age spectrum, there is a similar issue. As frailty restricts mobility and a sense of scale once more shrinks, we deserve an environment which maintains our autonomy, our options and our safety, but urban transport today is largely hostile to the elderly.

What is to be done?

One of the key issues identified in the *Healthy Cities* project has been the lack of vision (Ashton, 1988). People just do not allow themselves to entertain the lateral thoughts that are needed to develop effective approaches to creating healthy cities. Yet we have the methods. Trevor Hancock has described a methodology for running vision workshops for politicians and policy-makers, community groups and practitioners which actually works in creating a realistic agenda (Hancock, 1988). Tjeerd Deelstra has written extensively and eloquently on ecological approaches to urban planning in which we can move toward city management based on working *with* nature and natural systems, rather than on them, and work in ways which are self-sustaining (Deelstra, 1990). Moreover, the World Health Organization has generated a set of four practical principles derived from ecological science that should be followed in ecologically sound urban planning (WHO, 1988):

1. Civic design, agriculture and other human interventions should aim as far as possible at working with the natural topography and biological systems rather than mechanically imposing themselves on them.
2. Diversity and variety should be aimed at in the physical, social and economic structuring of communities. Land uses should be mixed where this does not create hazards. (Increasing the integration between work, residence and leisure should reduce the volume of traffic and its associated consequences).
3. Artificially created systems should be as closed as possible—human and solid waste should be recycled locally wherever possible, with a shift towards renewable sources of water, energy and raw materials.
4. There should be an optimal balance between populations and resources. Urban and population change needs to be related to the fragile state of natural systems and the environments that support them. There seem to be optimal sizes for cities above which many aspects of urban management including transport become much more complex.

Translating these into practice in a timescale of 10–20 years is becoming a global issue. Sadly many of the new megacities of the developing world are still slavishly following the Western model which has been shown to be such a disastrous cul-de-sac. Massive infrastructure investment continues to be made in transport systems which are road based, which benefit the few, add to international debt and are unsustainable. The alternatives based on integrated approaches to public transport, including walking and cycling have been well described by Mayer Hillman and to community organization by David Morris (Hillman, 1990; Morris, 1990).

Time is short, the challenge is great. The Scandinavian countries and the Netherlands are showing the way. However, there are signs of mobilization of which the highly successful conference on which this book is based is but one. The self-centred preoccupation with personal health-behaviour in the 1980s has led into the environmentalism of the 1990s, and even the British Government does not appear to be completely deaf to the lobbying organizations such as Friends of the Earth and the Cyclists Touring Club. However, as is often the case, the imagination and innovation has tended to come from the voluntary sector and from coalitions of groups including local authorities. Examples such as Sustrans' bold designs for a comprehensive country-wide network of cycleways linking the towns and cities, and specific initiatives such as the Trans-Pennine Trail from Hull to Liverpool with links to the coast which involves the cooperation of 30 local authorities together with the private sector and the Countryside Commission, shows what can be done. It would be nice if it had a proper place in national transport policy (Transpennine Trail Project, 1994).

References

Ashton J (1988) Esmedune 2000: vision or dream (a healthy Liverpool). In Ashton J (ed) *Healthy Cities: Concepts and Visions*. Department of Public Health (University of Liverpool), Liverpool

Ashton J (ed) (1992) *Healthy Cities*. Open University Press, Milton Keynes

Ashton J, Seymour H (1988) *The New Public Health*. Open University Press, Milton Keynes

Ashton J, Ubido J (1991) The healthy city and the ecological idea. *Social History of Medicine*, 4, 173–181

Deelstra T (1990) The ecological city. In Ashton J and Knight L (eds) *Proceedings of the First United Kingdom Healthy Cities Conference, Liverpool 28–30 March 1988*. Department of Public Health (University of Liverpool), Liverpool

Hancock T (1988) Healthy Toronto 2000: a vision of a healthy city. In Ashton J (ed) *Healthy Cities: Concepts and Visions*. Department of Public Health (University of Liverpool), Liverpool

Hancock T, Duhl LJ (1986) *Healthy Cities: Promoting Health in the Urban Context*. Working paper for the Healthy Cities Symposium, Portugal 1986. WHO, Copenhagen

Hillman M (1990) Transport and the healthy city. In Ashton J and Knight L (eds) *Proceedings of the First United Kingdom Healthy Cities Conference, Liverpool 28–30 March 1988*. Department of Public Health (University of Liverpool), Liverpool

Morris D (1990) Ecological economies and healthy cities. In Ashton J and Knight L (eds) *Proceedings of the First United Kingdom Healthy Cities Conference, Liverpool 28–30 March 1988*. Department of Public Health (University of Liverpool), Liverpool

Morris W (1884) quoted in the *Proceedings of the First United Kingdom Healthy Cities Conference, Liverpool 28–30 March 1988*. Department of Public Health, University of Liverpool 1990

Transpennine Trail Project (1994) *Transpennine Trail Annual Report 1993–94*. Barnsley Metropolitan Borough Council

World Health Organization (1988) *Ecological Models for Healthy Cities Planning*. WHO, Copenhagen

World Health Organization (1993) *The Urban Health Crisis: Strategies for Health for All in the Face of Rapid Urbanisation*. Report of the technical discussions at the 44th World Health Assembly, Geneva

14
Raising the profile of health in setting urban agendas

Gregory Goldstein

World Health Organization, Geneva, Switzerland

This chapter discusses how the profile of health in setting urban agendas—including the transport agenda—can be raised.

The WHO programme, *Healthy Cities*, spends enormous energy in efforts to place health on the urban agenda. In this work we have sought to ensure health and environment issues are addressed in municipal and national plans for development, by many key development sectors (industry, housing, local government, agriculture, transport etc.) (WHO, 1992a). This function is often termed intersectoral collaboration (ISC), or using an 'integrated approach'. In this chapter I will identify some major problems and issues about ISC, and then attempt to present solutions.

Out of all elements of primary health care, ISC may be the least successful. Although ISC has been an essential part of WHO's Primary Health Care policy—especially since 1978 and the Alma Ata Conference—a report to the UN Commission on Sustainable Development in 1994, by WHO (as Task Manager of Chapter 6 of Agenda 21), indicated that *health issues are frequently not being addressed in many countries in development planning in key sectors.* This apparent failure of ISC is surprising, given the importance that a majority of health planners attach to it. I will propose that one reason is the persistence of myths or false beliefs, such as the pervasive myth that good health is the result of medical and hospital services; furthermore there is a lack of understanding of the nature of health, and of the important influence of social and living conditions on health, sometimes by people within the health sector itself.

But we are starting to understand there may be a second major reason for the failure of ISC. As health sector workers, we have often blamed the housing sector, or the industry sector or local government, for ignoring health considerations in

Health at the Crossroads: Transport Policy and Urban Health.
Edited by Tony Fletcher and Anthony J. McMichael © 1997 John Wiley & Sons Ltd

their work. We may have overlooked a serious problem within the health sector itself. The health sector at present in most countries generally lacks the capacity to undertake studies or to collect data to measure or estimate the health impacts of development activities. Until it develops this capacity, its ability to participate in sustainable development planning or intersectoral work may be limited. Thus mortality and morbidity data is of interest to other development sectors, only to the extent that: firstly, some linkage can be established between the health problem being measured and the activities of the development sector. That is, the *health burden* of the development activities should be measured (in terms of death, disability etc.), with an estimation of the contribution that the various social and environmental factors are making to health problems; and secondly, there is identification made, and promotion given to various *health opportunities* presented by development programmes.

Thus urban development activities such as housing or industrial development have the potential to enhance health status of the population *if* health promotion and protection measures are undertaken in implementing the development; for example, in industrial development, occupational safety considerations and pollution control should be integral; or in housing development, basic environmental services and primary health care measures should be implemented with community participation.

In summary, the basis of intersectoral work on health and environment is measurement of and drawing attention to health impacts and health opportunities, using health statistics and epidemiological methods. In most countries, responsibility for health statistics and epidemiological work is wholly or partially divested in the Ministry of Health, with important contributions often coming from universities. However, at present capability is often lacking for the necessary health sector role. The above implies the health sector must undertake, in the case of many countries, two new roles:

1. an *information based role*, in which health impacts are monitored, involving measurement of health status and estimation of the contribution that various social and environmental factors are making to health problems, followed by an analysis of health requirements and opportunities in various development sectors that are significant for health; and
2. a *policy and advocacy role*, in which sector specific health policies for each development sector are formulated (for urban, rural, agriculture, local government, education, industry, labour (e.g. workplace health) etc., and are advocated by policy-makers in development planning. The WHO Commission on Health and Environment (WHO, 1992b), and Agenda 21, provide a clear illustration of what sector specific health policies look like.

Staff with expertise in environmental epidemiology and policy analysis are essential for this work. In the urban health arena, we are finding that the measurement of intra-urban differences is often a useful approach.

Armed with information and policies, the health sector will then have something to say to the other development sectors. Without these, which regrettably is often the case, it is not surprising that health and other sectors have little to say to each other.

In our Healthy Cities work, we have learned that ISC is enhanced by political support. *Mayors/municipalities* may commit themselves to a Healthy City process that will involve formulating and adopting a *municipal health plan*, which leads to work by many different agencies that are required to work together to prepare the plan. Developing solutions to problems on a community-wide basis requires the *partnership approach*, with partnerships of municipal government agencies (health, water, sanitation, housing, social welfare etc.), universities, NGOs, private companies and community organizations and groups.

In the area of transport, the above comments on the lack of ISC may apply. The health sector is forced to accept the health consequences of transport, in the sense that it provides hospital beds and services for victims. But the health sector does not, and in some cases cannot, accept that prevention of health consequences of transport are its responsibility, and that it has some responsibility to work with the transport sector to prevent adverse health impacts of transport. In most countries there is a serious deficit in the health sector's ability to conceptualize health problems in terms of their social and environmental causes; for example, deaths and injuries from traffic accidents, perhaps broken down into pedestrian and vehicle occupants categories. In reality, transport–health links are so much more than deaths and injuries, e.g. impacts of social isolation due to lack of access to transport, but even a basic analysis (limited to accident deaths and injuries) may be lacking.

I will now move on to my effort at solutions. I will discuss solutions under the two related headings, 'measurement of intra-urban differences', and 'development of a communications strategy'.

Measurement of intra-urban differences

One valuable analytic and promotional tool for ISC is measurement of intra-urban differences. Such studies (for example the excellent study by Stephens *et al.*, 1994, and other studies reported by the WHO Commission on Health and Environment Panel on Urbanization) have shown that localities within a city that have poor living conditions and deprivation of basic services have mortality and morbidity rates much higher, sometimes three-fold or more, than adjacent areas with good living conditions. The particular significance of differentials or differences in health, in my view, is that they are myth-shattering.

In particular, there are at least five serious myths that such studies help to shatter.

Myth 1. The first and perhaps the most important myth is that *health status is mainly related to activities that are undertaken by the health sector, and health professions such as medicine, nursing, pharmacy etc.*

These studies make it clear that conditions in the social and physical environment are the most important determinants, and *the effect of the health sector alone is limited.*

The lack of access to transport is part of a pattern of deprivation in low-income areas that has major and measurable health impacts. Moreover, this clarification by the studies is achieved in a convincing fashion that ordinary policy-makers and managers, without epidemiological training, can readily understand.

The studies make the point that not only is health status the result of development activities in the housing, industry, transport, agriculture and education sectors, but also that health development activities should be undertaken in collaboration with these sectors.

Myth 2.   Nothing can be done to correct health problems of the urban poor and prevention is of limited use; clearly, these studies indicate huge gains in health can be made by socio-economic development and improved living conditions; studies like these demonstrate that there are correctable weaknesses in local government in relation to basic services and requirements, that are at least partly responsible for the health problems (e.g. lack of water, lack of access to education, and transport).

Myth 3.   Wealthy communities are not interested in the conditions of the poor. If this is true, then why do such studies attract so much interest and promotion in the newspapers and other media? While it is naive to suppose that simple information alone can lead to reform in local government and elsewhere, public scrutiny of results like these creates space and opportunities for reformers to operate.

Myth 4.   Poor people suffer lack of services because they cannot pay for them. Many studies of this type show that poor people do pay—they pay relatively more for water than rich people, or that they may be paying considerable sums for private medical services. In relation to transport, studies by United Nations Commission on Human Settlements (UNCHS) refer to 20% of income of people being spent on transport.

Myth 5.   Poor people need to have more 'community participation' in the provision of basic environmental and health services. These studies reveal that commonly, poor people in cities currently are shouldering great and sometimes total responsibility for their basic needs in health, welfare, transport and employment creation. The concept of collective welfare provision is often a 'pipe-dream'.

In many cases local government may fail to offer any support to poor households, for example:

Water: may be collected from a river, ditch, or household well, or purchased from vendors and consumed without any testing for safety, or treatment by public health officers.

Housing: structures are erected by household members without professional assistance or consideration to health, safety or local government provisions, and not according to any plan for the site or area.

Transport: public transport with government subsidy may be available only in limited areas, and poor communities may bear the full cost of their privately run services.

I propose that city or district-wide systems are required in crowded urban areas, instead of this 'do-it-yourself' provision by each household. Systems administered by local government are required for water supply, sanitation, health care (including a referral system for hospital care), transport, education, and housing and land-use planning. To create these systems we need establishment of *partnerships* between community groups, community based organizations, NGOs, local institutions and municipal agencies.

Communications strategy

A communications strategy might be prepared at an early stage in planning of studies on health issues of transport, by which the study and results are to be presented to the decision-makers, in such a way that their significance for future action is evident.

Some important aspects of the strategy may be:

Who are involved

It is important to understand who are actually or potentially involved in taking action on the findings. Relevant actors in the health and environment arena in cities include various municipal and government agencies, individuals from community groups, university and training institutions, private sector companies, and so on.

Perception of the decision-makers

The perception of the decision-makers on the issue should be considered. There may be more than one decision-maker, and they may have different perceptions. For example, in one city a well-executed study showed poor health in low-income areas due in part to lack of municipal services for these areas. When the researchers discussed this finding with the authorities, it turned out they already knew about the health problems and the lack of services, but had not done anything about it because they thought the people in these areas were lazy and of poor personal character, and not deserving of their attention. The attitude to poor people was the foundation of the problem, and not, as the researchers had assumed, some combination of lack of knowledge, lack of technical ability, or lack of resources. A communications strategy might have been able to address this attitude/perception, and might, for example, have included getting more participation of the poor in government, ensuring they have a spokesperson on the decision-making bodies, making sure their point of view was expressed to improve understanding of their plight by decision-makers.

Tackle 'nothing can be done'

To counter the common perception that 'nothing can be done', consideration must be given to the possible range of actions by decision-makers in responding to the results. How can change be obtained incrementally? What is the first step? Consideration may be given to selection of the specific causal factors or environmental determinants over which the decision-maker feels he has some control, and can influence fairly quickly and with a modest commitment of resources, as opposed to trying to move on all factors.

Offer quantitative analysis

Another reason to try to separate out individual factors and related actions to address them is that it enables one to perform risk-based priority ranking of problems and influential factors. It seems a likely proposition that the case for change will be strengthened by sound quantitative analysis, by offering the opportunity for the decision-maker himself/herself to use science-based analysis as a basis for arguments with colleagues on municipal government issues.

Channels of communication

How can the involved decision-makers be reached, to discuss the above issues and background and findings of a study? Possible alternatives are: a personal interview with each one; a city consultation; a study tour; or recruitment of local communication experts to develop options.

Identification of possible motivations of decision-makers

Difficult and personally hazardous decisions may be needed by the decision-makers, for example, to devote some attention of their agency to the problems of low-income areas may be unpopular with their colleagues. Why should they take such a risk, apart from the fact that their government committed them to the principles of sustainable development?

In fact there are many examples of where people do take such risks, for reasons such as:

- A problem can be turned into an opportunity; for example, the use of results to get a grant for slum renewal from donors that can benefit not only slum

dwellers but improve the city as a whole.
- The decision-maker can show that benefits will offset initial costs (for example, the scheme may benefit the tourist industry).
- The decision-maker may personally benefit. Are there reasons such as to assist re-election? Do they feel compassion for the situation of low income-dwellers? Do they want to become an innovator or crusader? Do they want to expand their horizons, and to be part of a larger scene through national or international networking?
- The decision-maker may become interested in new reasons, such as the 'right argument', for example, contrary to the assumption of the educators, prostitutes in an AIDS education project that promoted condom use did not care about themselves getting AIDS and dying in 10 years. However, they were horrified to learn that their children could be infected, and were prepared to take action to avoid this.

Consideration should be given to recruitment of experts in the communication field to address in a systematic way the preparation of a communications strategy.

I would like to finish by emphasizing three mechanisms whereby health issues or information may influence urban decision-making, based on experiences of various WHO programmes:

1. By a widening of the basis of decision-making (by allowing inputs from community organizations, NGOs, the private sector, universities etc. into the decision-making about urban services, urban development and urban planning). A mechanism for participation is a 'city consultation' on the issue, whereby all stakeholders and above-listed institutions are allowed and encouraged to develop their proposals for action. (Urban programmes such as *Healthy Cities*, or UNCHS Sustainable Cities, or Urban Management Programme all use city consultations.) A city consultation is preceded by a period of data gathering and situation analysis that typically lasts 3–12 months.
   A related approach to participation is the organization of concerned persons. The organization of the AIDS lobby in the USA may provide a lesson. In the case of AIDS, we see that people affected by HIV and their friends and families work hard and effectively to mobilize resources and strengthen programmes to control the AIDS epidemic, and to improve services for patients. By comparison, transport-related health issues have a nearly non-existent profile. It is possible with some simple calculations to demonstrate that the number of people in any society whose lives have been damaged by road accidents is very large, and includes close relatives of victims, and those with persisting disabilities. All these people have a strong, albeit latent, motivation to do something about this issue, and doing something about transport safety may even improve their health by helping them to deal with their grief. Why is there no equivalent political lobby for transport safety? (Of course, there are countries or municipalities that are exceptions.) I suggest the

reason may be a simple one, a lack of leadership on the part of people such as ourselves.

2. Through what may be termed an appeal to 'enlightened self-interest', whereby the links between poor health and environmental conditions in one area or region, and various health and environmental threats that affect all city dwellers, are made evident by studies of the above type. Outbreaks of fearsome diseases such as cholera, meningitis and dengue, or air-pollution-related diseases, or traffic gridlock, threaten many cities, and may damage tourism and investment in urban development, and create alarm among all urban dwellers. Decision-makers can use the studies to show expenditures on improvements in health and environmental conditions—including transport services—are a wise investment.

3. Use of monitoring data as an implementation/education tool. Health and Welfare Canada has undertaken to inform people about health and environment and 'make all segments of society more aware of their actions and what they can do to improve and protect the environment'. Indicators are used to keep the public aware of progress in health and environmental protection, and efforts are made to publicize the monitoring data, some of which have become part of weather forecasts. Transport and health indices may be part of this monitoring.

References

Stephens C, Timaeus I, Akerman M et al. (1994) Environment and Health in Developing Countries: An Analysis of Intra-urban Differentials Using Existing Data. London School of Hygiene & Tropical Medicine, London

World Health Organization (1992a) Our Planet, Our Health. Commission on Health and Environment, Geneva

World Health Organization (1992b) Twenty Steps for Developing a Healthy City Project. WHO Regional Office for Europe, Copenhagen

15
Health promotion: the potential of non-motorized transport

Mayer Hillman

Policy Studies Institute, UK

Numerous epidemiological studies have revealed links between physical exercise and positive and negative health. Medical studies have established the physiological and psychological mechanisms accounting for them. People who exercise regularly—about 30 minutes a day and about three times a week—are fitter and less prone to illness, can perform everyday tasks with less stress and fatigue, have better physical control and sense of balance and are therefore less likely to fall.

Evidence of the benefits of exercise is now so universally accepted, and the literature on it so extensive, that neither is there space nor is it necessary to attempt to even summarize it here. Suffice it to say that exercise has a preventive role for many medical conditions, including heart disease (accounting for over a quarter of all deaths in England, that is a far higher proportion than in France or West Germany), stroke, osteoporosis (the risk of hip fracture has doubled in the last 25 years), asthma, some types of diabetes and some forms of cancer, loss of muscle mass, weakening of the immune system, and depression and anxiety.

In the circumstances, it is not surprising that exercise has been found to be associated with increased longevity. A major longitudinal survey of Harvard alumni recorded a 60% higher death rate from heart attacks among those who did not exercise at all compared with those who exercised either moderately or more intensively (Paffenbarger *et al.*, 1986) and, in this country, a similar study established that middle-aged men who engaged in moderate physical activity had a much reduced risk of heart attack compared with those who are inactive or those who were addicted to vigorous exercise (Morris *et al.*, 1990).

However, in common with the USA and other affluent countries, the fitness of the population of this country is decreasing: for instance, one in three adults is

Health at the Crossroads: Transport Policy and Urban Health.
Edited by Tony Fletcher and Anthony J. McMichael © 1997 John Wiley & Sons Ltd

overweight (Gregory *et al.*, 1990), partly owing to the increasingly sedentary nature of our lifestyles; three-quarters of the age group 35 to 64 are at risk of a heart attack (Working Group of the Coronary Prevention Group and British Heart Foundation, 1991); and seven in ten men and eight in ten women are below the age-appropriate activity level necessary to achieve a health benefit (Sports Council and Health Education Authority, 1992). The consequences of this for individuals are a lowering of the quality and length of life and, for society, the imposition of avoidable demands both on health and social services. Indeed, it would seem that some of the benefits of reduced morbidity and mortality that would otherwise have been gained from less smoking and better nutrition may be being lost because most people are taking insufficient exercise.

A related cause for concern is that some of the characteristics of lifestyle adopted during childhood are highly influential in the incidence of some diseases in later years—active adults are far more likely to have been active children. For the prevention of many diseases, childhood is the ideal time to instil appreciation of the benefits and practice of health-related patterns of activity, such as the habit of regular exercise (Coronary Prevention Group, 1992).

It is disquieting to note, therefore, that the physical condition of children is also at an all-time low, and declining, with low levels of sustained activity being recorded among both boys and girls (Armstrong, 1993). A major contributory factor to this is very likely to be the outcome of the growing restrictions imposed by parents on their children's independent travel—which almost by definition involves exercise—owing to fears about their safety outside the home (Hillman *et al.*, 1991), and their relatively poor condition is probably exacerbated by too much television viewing. In addition, pressures on the school curriculum are limiting the timetable for physical education. A study of secondary schools in 21 European countries has found that least time is spent on this in Britain (Armstrong and McManus, 1994).

Routes to fitness

Nevertheless, there is growing recognition among the public of the benefits to health of exercise, principally through the medium of education. But how can a public health strategy on physical fitness and active lifestyles featuring as a major element of an individual's daily life be promoted? To date, the focus of attention has been on sports and much discussion has been devoted to ways to motivate people and to make more appealing a routine which involves regular 'work outs' in gyms and health clubs, playing games such as tennis, squash, and badminton, or swimming, running and jogging.

The problem with most of these types of exercise is that they place high stress on hips, knees, ankles and Achilles tendons, and this would certainly be more apparent if they were adopted as a lifelong routine. In any case, most people who are initially attracted to such an exercise regime, where it entails an 'add-on' to their leisure schedule on a several times a week basis and therefore much self-discipline, have been found to be unlikely to maintain it year after year. Only the few highly motivated will do so. Moreover, for most sporting activities, there are not only the constraints of weather and time, but often costs of entry and problems of access and availability. In the case of team games, there is the additional problem of organizing for the mutual convenience of participants. For children, there is often for a range of reasons the requirement that they be escorted to and from their destination. Moreover, whilst games and physical education are appealing during the younger stage of childhood, other forms of leisure activity can prove more attractive as they grow older (Fox, 1994).

Swimming has been identified as a highly effective way of keeping fit as virtually all muscles are used in unstressed movements. However, it does not represent a realistic solution to propose other than for a very small proportion of the population who are attracted to and in a position to swim regularly during the whole year and throughout their lives, not least owing to the dearth of facilities: in Britain, there is only one public swimming bath for every 47 000 people. Indeed, on average, one sports centre caters for every 40 000 of the population (Central Statistical Office, 1994).

On the other hand, though not entirely ideal from the viewpoint of fitness as measured in terms of suppleness, strength and stamina, cycling and brisk walking are realistic means whereby the great majority of the population can keep fit. Both are forms of aerobic exercise which minimize the risk of muscle or ligament injury, and represent straightforward, cheap and much more widely available means of maintaining good health than sports. They can also provide a sense of achievement on longer journeys, particularly by cycle. In addition, their use rather than that of other means of transport also results in less damage to the health of other people otherwise stemming from the danger and anxiety generated by motorized vehicles and, of course, the adverse environmental effects especially from pollution and noise (Hillman and Cleary, 1992).

Cycling or walking can be used as a mode of travel by most people from childhood through to old age, and often tied in to the daily pattern of travel to school, to work, to leisure destinations and so on. By this means, they can have a functional role with less self-motivation required in order to adhere to what can otherwise develop into a boring routine. Walking, and more so cycling, can be especially advantageous for children for whom the world is considerably extended in the sense of the range of accessible destinations once their parents allow them to get around on their own.

Brisk walking on a regular basis has been found to provide sufficient stimulus to improve the fitness of young and old alike, including previously sedentary middle-aged men and women (Hardman et al., 1992; Stensel et al., 1994) and to delay the stage in life among the elderly where functional capacity falls below a quality threshold. It is also popular: walking, though not necessarily briskly, is the most preferred recreational activity (Central Statistical Office, 1994). Since it is weight-bearing, it contributes to maintaining bone density and therefore reducing the risk of osteoporosis. It can also provide wider opportunities for conversation on the street and thereby lower the incidence of social isolation. In the case of cycling, the benefits to health are greater. Some years ago, a study recorded a marked decrease in heart disease among all the cyclists examined, and a ten-fold decrease in its incidence among those over the age of 70 (Robertson, 1977). A study among factory workers concluded that regular cyclists enjoy a level of fitness equivalent to that of individuals ten years younger (Tuxworth *et al.*, 1986), and another found that those who cycled 60 miles a week from the age of 35 could add $2\frac{1}{2}$ years to their life expectancy (Paffenbarger *et al.*, 1986). A small additional consideration is that cycling is not weight-bearing and, as a result, people with some forms of arthritis find it easier to cycle than to walk.

Current patterns of travel in Britain and abroad

In spite of the considerable scope for enabling people to keep fit in this simple and routine way by using their feet more to get around, the current National Travel Survey (NTS) for Britain shows that only 3% of mileage is made on foot and less than 1% by bicycle. These represent marked reductions on those revealed in the equivalent survey for 1975/76. Indeed, the annual distance walked since then has fallen by 15% and that by cycle by 25% (GB Department of Transport, 1994).

The annual distance walked by children between the ages of 5 and 10 is in the region of 190 miles and, for those aged 11 to 15, 330 miles (GB Department of Transport, 1994). When these two figures are compared with those for the 1975/76 NTS, it reveals falls of 20% and 13% respectively. Equivalent figures for the annual distance cycled by the two age groups in the 1989/91 NTS are 20 miles and 12 miles for boys and girls respectively aged 5–10 years; and 198 and 46 miles for boys and girls respectively aged 11–15 years. For the younger age group, these figures represent falls of close on a third compared with the equivalent figures for 1975/76; and for the older age group, falls of about a sixth.

Some indication of the considerable scope for ambitious yet realistic targets on increasing fitness through the medium of increasing the extent of non-motorized travel in the course of the routine of daily life can be gained by looking at figures available from the Netherlands. At the beginning of the 1970s, the Dutch government decided to pay far more attention to the creation of safe cycle networks. As a consequence of this, there has been a dramatic increase not only in the proportion of journeys by cycle but also in cycle mileage: although mileage on foot in the Netherlands and in this country is fairly similar, cycle mileage there is 18 times higher (Centraal Bureau voor de Statistiek, 1994). Indeed, five times as many journeys there are made by cycle than by all forms of transport combined.

It is salutary to compare the figures for Dutch male and female teenagers aged 12–15 years with the equivalent figures for British male and female teenagers aged 11–15 years—precisely comparable age groups are not available in published figures. These show that male Dutch teenagers cover 9 times the distance on cycles than British male teenagers, and female Dutch teenagers cover 35 times the distance than their female counterparts here.

In the Netherlands, 29% of all journeys and 60% of school journeys are made by cycle compared with 2% and between 3 and 4% respectively here. And, it is not only a popular mode for children: a quarter of the journeys of women pensioners there are made in this way (Centraal Bureau voor de Statistiek, 1994).

Nor is the Netherlands the only country where cycle use is relatively high. Four in five households in Denmark have at least one adult bicycle and the average Dane—male and female—cycles about 1.5 kilometres each day and makes 18% of their journeys by bicycle (Denmark Ministry of Transport, 1993). Cycling also forms a fundamental part of children's lives there, with cycling being their predominant form of travel and less than 1 in 20 of the cycle trips of those aged between 6 and 15 are made with a parent (Denmark Ministry of Transport, 1993).

Disincentives to walking and cycling

Why then are the non-motorized modes not recognized as convenient and environmentally friendly means of travel in Britain and as ideal means of keeping fit? After all, few people are unable to walk and, in the case of cycling, low cycle ownership or ability to ride cannot be cited: there are about 15 to 18 million bicycles in the UK, and a survey has shown that 99% of men and 87% of women claim that they can cycle (Mintel, 1989). The PSI study, referred to earlier, found that over 90% of junior schoolchildren and 75% of young teenagers own a bicycle, and presumably can ride it (Hillman et al., 1991).

People are discouraged from walking for a variety of reasons. The principal problems established in surveys are difficulties in crossing the road owing to the danger and intimidation of the growing volume and speed of traffic, and its severance effects on activity that entails crossing main roads; cracked, uneven and narrow surfaces leading at times to injury from tripping and falling; pavements cluttered with street furniture, obstructed by parked vehicles, and often made unpleasant by litter, dog faeces, and other detritus. And, in many urban areas, fears of assault, especially on streets that are poorly lit and deserted are commonly cited. Most of these problems can be remedied by the diversion of small amounts of money relative to those currently invested in roads and public transport improvement.

The existence of these disincentives has of course disadvantaged groups in the population most dependent on walking, such as people with mobility handicaps for, paradoxically, in general, the more difficulty they have in getting about on foot, the more likely it is that they rely on walking as their main means of transport. The mobility of those on low incomes who cannot afford a car, and that of children in particular has suffered. Indeed, there is evidence that the restrictions on children's freedom to get about on their own, which their parents impose because of their fears about the dangers of traffic, are associated with harmful effects on children's physical, social and emotional development (Hillman, 1993a).

Other attitudinal surveys show that the low use of the bicycle is explained by a wide range of real and perceived concerns among current and prospective cyclists. One of these is the consequences of breathing air polluted by the harmful ingredients of the combustion of transport fuels. Much evidence exists on the link between air pollution and morbidity and mortality from bronchitis, asthma and lung disease (Whitelegg *et al.*, 1993). An important question to be answered is whether this pollution poses any greater risk to the health of cyclists than of other road users.

The evidence suggests that, insofar as face masks, if worn correctly, can filter out some of the more noxious gases, all road users, including pedestrians and motorists, should wear one as they breathe the same air polluted by the fumes discharged through motor vehicle exhausts. A recent study in Austria has shown that nitrogen dioxide and carbon monoxide from exhausts have more harmful effects on motorists than on cyclists (Knoflacher *et al.*, 1992). Clearly, the most effective approach to this problem is to reduce pollutants at source.

However, the prime deterrent to cycling in Britain lies in public perception of the risk of a road accident. Certainly the growth in the speed and volume of traffic over the last few decades has made roads less safe, particularly for cyclists. The statistics show that pedestrians and cyclists are vulnerable road users. Their accident rate is many times higher than that of car or bus users. These concerns have led consciously or otherwise to cycling rarely being included as a recommended form of exercise. Nevertheless, it could be argued that the dangers of cycling have been unduly influenced by exaggerated fears about the scale of risk entailed for the fatality rate is only one in every 25 million kilometres cycled, and that this rate should be compared first, with the much lower rate in the Netherlands where safe routes are commonplace for cyclists, and second and even more importantly with the fatality rate attributable to heart disease resulting from lack of exercise.

Life years lost versus life years gained

As road safety policy is almost invariably aimed at lowering road accidents, it is thought inadvisable to encourage the general public to take up cycling. As a consequence, the extent of the health benefits of this unique means of maintaining fitness, as well as the appropriateness of its primacy as a form of transport, have been poorly if at all appreciated. In turn, this has led to oversight of the means of promoting this 'public interest' mode and to considerable under-investment of resources for cycling which, compared with provision for motorized transport, is highly cost-effective. Special provision for cycling is remarkably cheap: the capital costs per kilometre for the new type of public transport systems currently under construction or being reviewed are between 100 and 600 times that for cycling provision. Indeed, the total cycle network proposed for London would cost the equivalent of two kilometres of the Leeds Supertram system or 400 metres of the Jubilee Line extension (Hillman, forthcoming).

Analysis aimed at relating the loss of 'life years' in cycle fatalities to the gain of 'life years' through improved fitness among regular cyclists, and thus their increased longevity, has important implications for the development of policy on cycling. It represents perhaps the most telling argument in this paper.

The loss of life expectancy among cyclists from road fatalities can be established from road accident and actuarial data. The increased longevity likely to be attributable to those engaging in exercise regimes several times a week compared with those leading relatively sedentary lives can be derived from studies in the UK and USA and special tabulations from the UK Office of Population Censuses and Surveys. Contrasting these figures shows that, even in the current hostile traffic environment, the benefits gained from regular cycling in terms of life years gained outweigh the loss of life years in cycling fatalities (British Medical Association, 1992). One calculation has shown the ratio to be around 20 to 1 (Hillman, 1993b), and that there is considerable scope for increasing this ratio through two interrelated means: first, the environment for cyclists can be made more user-friendly—as indeed is being attempted in some UK cities, following exemplary and highly successful initiatives in cities such as Freiburg, Groningen and Copenhagen, through the construction of safe and convenient pedestrian and cycle networks and the discouragement of car use; second, that improvement is very likely to release the considerable latent demand for cycling attributable to most road users' fears about the risks of injury in an accident involving a motor vehicle.

Conclusions

One of the most obvious and universally agreed elements of our lifestyles that is conducive to positive health is the adoption of a regime of physical exercise. The emphasis placed on encouraging people to take part in sports and some forms of recreation as the primary route to this end may be misplaced. Owing to a variety of limiting factors, including the paucity of facilities, difficulties of access and the time and expense involved in participation and, not least, self-motivation, only a very small proportion of the population is likely to do so regularly, several times a week, and throughout their lives.

By contrast, this chapter has outlined reasons why brisk walking and cycling are activities which can realistically feature as part of the routine of daily travel for most people, throughout the seasons, and from childhood through to old age. They have the potential for improving fitness in a way that, given proper provision for these modes, cannot be matched by any other comparable exercise regime. In the process, they can contribute significantly to reaching government health targets, for instance that of reducing mortality from heart disease by 30% by the year 2000 (GB Department of Health, 1992).

It would seem that the role of the two modes has been overlooked in public policy owing to their association with injurious impacts on health, especially in road accidents. However, these impacts are far more a reflection of the absence or inadequate quality of provision for them rather than something intrinsic to them. Evidence from such countries as the Netherlands and Denmark points to the scope for significant increases in the use of the bicycle in this country once sufficient investment in attractive environments is made for it. For instance, half of the journeys currently made by car in Britain are less than four miles in length—no more than a 15 to 20 minute cycle ride. And land use decisions and traffic management measures can strongly influence people's propensity to make their journeys on foot.

The necessary policy changes and the diversion of resources to that end are justified on social, environmental and, not least, economic grounds as well as those of health promotion. They would bring in their wake substantial benefits not only to the individuals whose use of the bicycle or walking is facilitated but also to society at large owing to the consequent reductions in road accidents among those not travelling by car or public transport and danger leading to restrictions on preferred patterns of travel, especially affecting children's independence; pollution leading to increased morbidity and mortality; noise, interrupting concentration and disturbing sleep; and congestion on traffic-filled streets causing severance and disrupting community life. They are justified too from the viewpoint of furthering the objectives of policies on equity, economy and energy conservation.

The speed with which these changes are made is dependent upon the extent of cultural shift in attitudes to motorized transport, particularly the car. There is much evidence that that shift is already taking place, with acknowledgement of the role of walking and cycling featuring increasingly in policy and policy-oriented documents, such as the recent Report by the Great Britain Royal Commission on Environmental Pollution (1994) which called for a quadrupling of the level of cycling by the year 2005.

As a means of furthering policy on health promotion as well as that on transport and the environment, it would appear to be very much in society's best interests that the current situation, with its environment so hostile to walking and cycling, is reversed, and that they be given pride of place in the transport hierarchy—that is going well beyond simply treating them as worthy of some consideration in the allocation of public resources.

References

Armstrong N (1993) Independent mobility and children's physical development. In Hillman M (ed) *Children, Transport and the Quality of Life*. Policy Studies Institute, London

Armstrong N, McManus A (1994) Children's fitness and physical activity: a challenge for physical education. *British Journal of Physical Education*, (Spring), 25

British Medical Association (1992) *Cycling: Towards Health and Safety*. Oxford University Press, London

Centraal Bureau voor de Statistiek (1994) *Mobility of the Dutch Population in 1993*. Voorburg/Heerlen, Netherlands

Central Statistical Office (1994) *Social Trends: Volume 24*. HMSO, London

Coronary Prevention Group (1992) *Prevention of Coronary Heart Diseases: Recommendations for National Governments*. Unpublished paper

Denmark Ministry of Transport (1993) *The Bicycle in Denmark: Present Use and Future Potential*. Denmark Ministry of Transport, Copenhagen

Fox K (1994) Understanding young people and their decisions about physical activity. *British Journal of Physical Education*, (Spring), 15–19

Great Britain Department of Health (1992) *The Health of the Nation: a Strategy for Health in England*. HMSO, London

Great Britain Department of Transport (1994) *Transport Statistics Report: National Travel Survey 1991/93*. HMSO, London

Great Britain Royal Commission on Environmental Pollution (1994) *Eighteenth Report: Transport and the Environment*. HMSO, London.

Gregory J, Foster K, Tyler H, Wiseman M (1990) *Dietary and Nutritional Survey of British Adults*. HMSO, London

Hardman AE, Jones PRM, Norgan NG, Hudson A (1992) Brisk walking improves endurance fitness without changing body fatness in previously sedentary women. *European Journal of Applied Physiology*, 65, 354–359

Hillman M (ed) (1993a) *Children, Transport and the Quality of Life*. Policy Studies Institute, London

Hillman M (1993b) Cycling and the promotion of health. *Policy Studies*, *14(2)*, 49–58

Hillman M (1994) Curbing car use: the dangers of exaggerating the future role of public transport. In *Transportation Planning Systems*, 2, no 4, 27.

Hillman M, Cleary J (1992) A prominent role for walking and cycling in future transport policy. In Roberts J *et al.* (eds) *Travel Sickness: The Need for a Sustainable Transport Policy for Britain*. Lawrence and Wishart, London

Hillman M, Adams J, Whitelegg J (1991) *One False Move: a Study of Children's Independent Mobility*. Policy Studies Institute, London

Knoflacher H, Macoun T, Wurz A (1992) Schadtstoffbelastung bei Verschiedenen Mobilitätsformen. Summary of paper supplied by Adrian Davis

Mintel (1989) *Bicycles*. Mintel International Group, London, September 1989

Morris JN, Clayton DG, Everitt MG *et al.* (1990) Exercise in leisure time: coronary attack and death rates. *British Heart Journal*, 63, 325–334

Paffenbarger RS, Hyde RT, Wing AL, Hseih CC (1986) Physical activity, all-cause mortality and longevity of college alumni. *New England Journal of Medicine*, *314*, 605–613

Robertson HK (1977) Heart disease in life-long cyclists. *British Medical Journal*, *2(6103)*, 1635–1636

Sports Council/Health Education Authority (1992) *Allied Dunbar National Fitness Survey: a Report on Activity Patterns and Fitness at all Levels*. HEA/Sports Council, London

Stensel DJ, Brooke-Wavell K, Hardman AE *et al.* (1994) The influence of a 1-year programme of brisk walking on endurance fitness and body composition in previously sedentary men aged 42–59 years. *European Journal of Applied Physiology*, 68, 531–537

Tuxworth W, Neville AM, White C, Jenkins C (1986) Health, fitness, physical activity and

morbidity of middle aged male factory workers. *British Journal of Industrial Medicine*, *43*, 733–753
Whitelegg J, Gatrell A, Naumann P (1993) *Traffic and Health*. Lancaster University, Lancaster
Working Group of The Coronary Prevention Group and The British Heart Foundation
(1991) An action plan for preventing coronary heart disease in primary care. *British Medical Journal*, *303*, 748–750

CITY CASE STUDIES

16
Introduction

Tony Fletcher and Anthony J. McMichael

London School of Hygiene & Tropical Medicine, UK

In this section, contrasting examples have been selected to illustrate a wide range of opportunities and obstacles, local achievements and larger scale problems where much remains to be done. Coming as they do from different backgrounds in town planning, environment departments, health and academic research, the emphasis of each example reflects both the position of the author and the specific location being considered.

Hass-Klau focuses on several specific examples of achievements in reducing car use in urban centres. In the town of Lüneberg, experience in implementing a car-free town centre underlines the importance of an integrated package including very frequent services between city centre and car parks, covering off-peak times, encouraging employers to provide public transport passes, facilities for cycle and pedestrian traffic and building political support for the changes. However, many people are still driving to the car parks just outside the car-free zone. One example of an experiment to reduce car dependence is to redesign residential areas to reduce the need for car ownership. Two examples of new car-free housing estates in Bremen and Amsterdam are presented. Connections to public transport and safe cycle networks need to be designed into it, but there is clearly a demand for such living conditions with people willing to pledge themselves not to own a car. As well as a cleaner, safer environment, people have more space for houses and gardens because of the reduced need to consign land to parking spaces.

Bunde, from Århus Municipal Council in Denmark, provides a good example of a systematic review and establishment of detailed target setting and establishing priority for different aspects of transport. These range from the general, such as overall transport volume, to very specific solutions to specific problems, such as improving safety at specific crossings. The different areas of concern identified were: overall volume; infrastructure provision; reduction of energy consumption; air pollution and noise; road safety; the barrier effect of dividing communities; and visual aspects. In each case, different levels of intervention are considered in

Health at the Crossroads: Transport Policy and Urban Health.
Edited by Tony Fletcher and Anthony J. McMichael © 1997 John Wiley & Sons Ltd

relation to planning, purchasing and public works, traffic management and information or education.

Kenworthy vividly describes the nightmare scenario of Bangkok's streets clogged by the very rapidly rising car ownership: people are clearly deterred from walking or cycling in the noisy, polluted and hazardous streets. Large Asian cities differ in many aspects of urban infrastructure from their Western counterparts, in particular higher urban density, high use of public transport, less road and less parking space per person. Bangkok, however, is unusual in having a higher car ownership and lower public transport provision (or use) than other Asian cities. Public transport, such as it is, is almost exclusively buses (stuck in traffic jams) which are not popular. In contrast to Singapore, there has as yet been a reluctance to control car growth by restrictive licensing or by providing alternative, attractive public transport. Public transport and cycling are ideally suited to such a densely populated area but have been poorly supported, in part because of Japanese pressure to develop their car and motorcycle export market in Thailand. The network of canals also provide an under-developed opportunity for more sustainable public transport. The percentage of urban land devoted to roads is lower than in most Western cities, a fact used by planners to justify road building, which would lead if successful to massive social disruption. The author contrasts policies based on demand management, using restrictions such as those successfully employed in Singapore, with the current policy of trying to increase road provision. Alternative policies are advocated, based on provision of mass rail transit, environments conducive to walking and cycling and planning to provide residential developments integrated with the public transport infrastructure.

Tiwari, presenting a detailed analysis of New Delhi, India, draws out some differences in road use compared to highly motorized countries. Firstly, the population of road users is highly heterogeneous, including significant proportions of animals and human drawn vehicles. Apart from a few cycle paths the Delhi master plan is more oriented to improving traffic flow in a city that already has a relatively high proportion of space devoted to roads (20% compared to 6% in Calcutta). Another feature of the master plan is an intention to develop mixed land use which should reduce commuting time. This, however, has not been successful because employment opportunities do not necessarily develop in tandem with the new residential developments. So, for example, people who have been relocated out of 'unauthorized settlements' with no sanitation provision, may have to travel long distances to find work. While the complex mix of users have to negotiate on the roads to keep moving, large accident risks evident in the increasing fatality risks and the high pollution levels are exacerbated by the constantly accelerating and decelerating motorized vehicles. The type of roads for different types of users vary in design. Models and theories developed for more homogeneous road use situations are of limited applicability, and conflict resolution at various levels of decision-making is advocated to represent the interest of this complex set of road users.

Greenbaum describes the development of transport infrastructure in the Boston area of the USA, a country which has arguably taken car dependency further than any other. It provides a fascinating insight into the difficulty of maintaining a momentum for policies which attempt to interrupt unrestrained car growth. Boston did, however, have its origins as a relatively compact urban area served by train and street cars. After the Second World War, the shift towards the car as the primary means of travel and the development of widely scattered communities continued unimpeded until the 1970s when awareness was growing of the adverse environmental impacts of exhaust pollution, and of the adverse social effects of fragmenting communities of urban highways. These concerns were of course underpinned by the increases of oil prices in the early 1970s. The plan for an expanded highway system was abandoned, car use was discouraged by, for example, banning the construction of any new parking spaces in downtown Boston, and laws requiring commuters to reduce travelling to work without taking fellow workers.

These initiatives had some impact but it was only short-lived. The benefits were not felt outside downtown Boston and the ride-sharing policy fell into disuse. The failure of these policies to achieve a substantial reduction in car dependency offers some positive lessons, including the importance of perceived health and social effects of transport to motivate people to support change, the central place in land use controls, the need to think wider than just protected urban cores, perceived sudden changes in price can have a strong deterrent effect, and, overwhelmingly, the personal freedom offered by the car is something that few in the USA would relinquish. A resurgence of interest in air pollution in the last few years has led to controls on emissions from vehicles, but there is intense opposition to transportation control measures.

Ferguson and McCarthy review transport policies in London, which have a particular administrative and political obstacle to their resolution since the abolition of the Greater London Council, from the sharing of transport policy development between individual London boroughs and central government. While the population of London has been falling, many people commute into London to work and car use is, as a consequence, predicted to rise. London has a very developed public transport infrastructure, with the provision of the underground network pivotal in shaping the expansion of London into the country areas to the north. However, recent under-investment in rail transport compared to (comparable) European countries has contributed to increased road congestion. While train use is tending to increase slowly there is a trend away from bus use and a long-term decline in cycle use. Some policy initiatives are outlined, including some improvements in bus services, cycle route provision and provision of facilities for the disabled. A number of proposals are presented and are currently under consideration, such as road pricing and establishing targets for air quality, road traffic reduction or modal shifts to walking and cycling.

17
Innovative urban transport planning—examples from Europe: car-free town centres and residential areas—utopia or reality?

Carmen Hass-Klau

Environmental and Transport Planning, UK

The message from the Continent has consistently been that environmentally friendly transport policies are vital to the creation of towns that are lively and pleasant to live in. Over the last 20 years, it has predominantly been the Netherlands, Switzerland and Germany that have implemented these transport policies. The continental package normally contains large-scale pedestrianization schemes in the town centres, traffic calming in residential areas, and a serious financial commitment by both the local authorities and the government in favour of public transport and cycling. Attempts have also been made to enforce planning restrictions against out-of-town shopping developments and to encourage the economic strengthening of town centre shopping, housing and other employment. This is in contrast to Britain which has invested little in public transport, privatized its bus industry and is planning to fragment and privatize the rail network. An important ingredient in the increased level of car-borne shopping has been the relaxation of planning regulations on suburban and edge-of-town retailing development, with the resulting wave of hypermarkets and shopping centres reducing the commercial potential in town centres.

The question one might ask, taking into account the contrast between Britain and the Continent, is whether the gap is widening between the two in terms of transport policies? In the conclusion I will try to offer an answer to this question. But first I will highlight two typical developments from the Continent, one

Health at the Crossroads: Transport Policy and Urban Health.
Edited by Tony Fletcher and Anthony J. McMichael © 1997 John Wiley & Sons Ltd

relating to the formation of a car-free town centre, and the other to progress towards car-free residential housing estates.

The making of a car-free town centre

As an example of a car-free town centre I have chosen a prosperous small town called Lüneburg, located about 50 km south-east of Hamburg. I have carried out research in Lüneburg for over three years. In 1994, it had 64 000 inhabitants and the wider hinterland includes some 250 000 inhabitants. Lüneburg could easily be compared with Chichester or Winchester or a number of other small county towns.

The town centre is of medieval and renaissance character and motor vehicle traffic has been a problem for some time. Car ownership is high, amounting to 510 cars per 1000 inhabitants. A comparison with Chichester and Winchester shows that the level of ownership in British county towns is about the same as in Germany.

A new transport strategy

As a result of the high level of motor vehicle traffic in Lüneburg and the daunting forecasts of further growth, the Town Council agreed in 1991 to implement a new transport policy strategy, with the objective of encouraging people to leave their cars at home, especially for short journeys, and to travel by public transport, cycle or on foot.

Local public transport

This strategy was planned to improve public transport considerably with more frequent bus services and better interchange facilities supplemented by collective taxis for evening services.

One of the first policies was to give public transport priority throughout the town by means of priority signals and bus lanes, but although the town was happy to pay for this, there was great reluctance to provide any additional subsidy to the bus operator. The bus company had operated previously as a private company with no subsidy at all from the city. However, the frequency in bus services could only be increased with the financial help of the town.

Every Saturday, and on weekdays before Christmas, a city bus service operates which is free of charge, delivers people every 15 minutes from the larger car parks to the town centre. In addition a stationary bus in the town centre is used as a left luggage office where shopping can be stored without payment.

A dial-a-ride taxi service picks people up at three locations in the town centre at off-peak times, from 20.30 and operates as late as 23.00 (Fridays and Saturdays at 23.00, 24.00 and 1.00). The taxi, which has to be ordered by telephone at least half an hour before the fixed times, delivers customers from the town centre to their front doors for the price of a bus fare plus an additional cost of DM1.50 (£0.60). The service covers not only the town but also the region.

Special family and 'environmental' travelcards were introduced in order to reduce the price of public transport, particularly for frequent use. Students have travelled free since October 1994.

'Jobtickets' have been implemented by the local bus company (KGV) and the Town Council. These tickets are available for council employees at a cost of DM35.00 (£15.75) per month and are intended to encourage people to travel to work by bus. It will be important for the bus company to persuade other employers to support the scheme.

Imagine how easy it would be to reduce traffic jams in many British towns if all local authorities committed to environmentally friendly transport policies provided such travel tickets for their employees instead of free car parking spaces.

Cycling

A comprehensive cycle plan was quickly adopted and an extensive cycle network has been built including segregated routes along roads, and generally cycle facilities have been improved. The overall aim is to increase cycling to the same level as in Münster where 34% of all trips within the town are made by bike.

Pedestrianization

Before 1993, Lüneburg already had a number of well-established pedestrianized streets (Figure 17.1). By 1993, as a first result of the implementation of the new transport policy plan, the area of pedestrianization had trebled. In some of these newly car-free streets, access has been provided for cyclists, public transport, taxis, residents and service vehicles. Commercial vehicles have access to the town centre between 18.00 and 11.00.

The closure of the town centre

The main change brought about was the closing of additional parts of the town centre to vehicular traffic in May 1993.

During the weeks leading up to May there was an increased publicity campaign to draw people's attention to the changes in the transport system.

Despite the publicity it was expected that initially these road closures would bring complete traffic chaos to the town centre. Eighty police officers were on patrol on the first day to enforce the new regulations and a strong police presence was maintained for the first week. However, these concerns turned out to be ill-founded. Observations tended to confirm the view that congestion and chaos was less than had originally been feared. During the first days a steady stream of motorists tried to enter the restricted areas of the town centre and were politely redirected by police to alternative routes. A few car drivers attempted to enter the town centre via the cycle lanes, driving happily along with two wheels on the pavements!

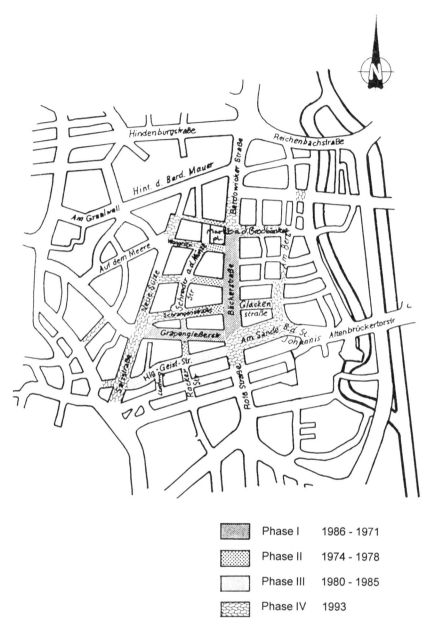

	Phase I	1986 - 1971
	Phase II	1974 - 1978
	Phase III	1980 - 1985
	Phase IV	1993

Figure 17.1   Phases of pedestrianization in Lüneburg

Pedestrians also took time to become used to the new environment. As traffic lights were still working on those streets which were now closed to general traffic, the majority of pedestrians were still waiting for a green light despite no cars: behaviour unlikely to be observed in Britain.

It was, however, difficult for the traders to accept these changes. Only one month after the town centre was closed to car traffic, traders complained about a fall in turnover. These complaints escalated into a large political campaign against the town centre closure by some of the traders and the local press just before the local election. Instead of accepting the transport policy changes, which had been agreed by an overwhelming political majority, the changes were criticized unmercifully by a vocal minority. It seems they may in part have been those people who could have gained from a political change in the Land election which was due in spring 1994. After the election, which did not bring any political change, the accusations and complaints about the town centre closure virtually ceased.

Most of the town centre streets which were closed to traffic in May 1993 have now been redesigned. The change in appearance of the same street can be stunning, as may be seen when comparing Figure 17.2 with Figure 17.3.

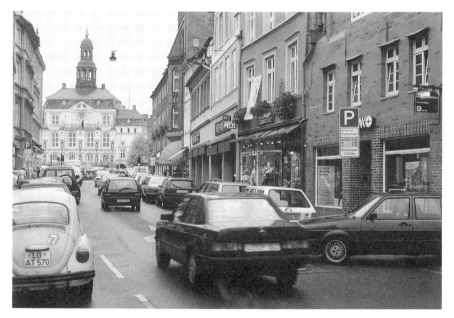

Figure 17.2   Town centre street before traffic was removed

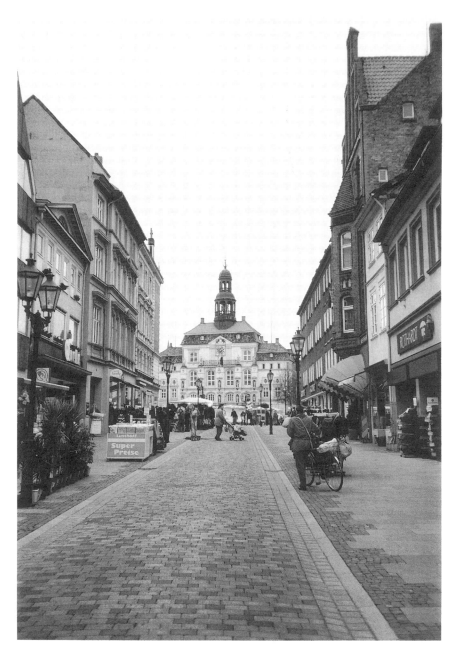

Figure 17.3   The same street as in Figure 17.2 but pedestrianized and redesigned

The effects on traffic

Three years after the new transport policies were put in place, one can already see a number of the intended effects. According to traffic counts shown in Table 17.1, there has been a significant decline over 1991–94 in the number of cars on the inner ring roads and the roads leading to the town centre.

The same counts indicate a large increase in cyclists (59%) and pedestrians (48%). The figures for bus travel are misleading because the weather was much better during the two surveys in 1994 than in 1991. Hence a number of people who took the bus in 1991 cycled or walked in 1994. Despite this, according to the public transport operator, overall bus travel was higher in 1994 than three years before.

Car ownership in Lüneburg slightly increased by 1% in the time period which already indicates a slowing down in the growth rate. This can be contrasted with the region as a whole, where there was an increase of about 9%.

Another very important effect of the transport policy has been the reduction in personal injuries from accidents by 13.5% from 422 to 365 in one year (1993/94).

The second example of new transport policies on the Continent goes one step further from the car-free town centre schemes which have been achieved by a small number of local authorities, to car-free housing estates.

This may be the beginning of a significant policy change and could have dramatic effects in terms of land use planning if implemented on a large scale. So far there have been only a few such projects in Germany and the Netherlands.

Car-free housing estates

Bremen-Hollerland

The best-known car-free housing estate in Germany is located in Bremen, a city of about 500 000 inhabitants. Its local authority is well known for its environmental approach to transport and urban design. Its large city centre is virtually car-free.

The planned car-free housing estate is situated in the north-east of the city and

Table 17.1 Change in traffic flows on inner ring road and roads leading to the town centre

Mode	Absolute			Modal split (%)	
	1991	1994	Change (%)	1991	1994
Cars	106 002	90 597	− 14.5	81.0	73.3
Motorbikes	1 720	1 889	9.8	1.3	1.5
Bus	7 095	6 490	− 8.5	5.4	5.2
Bicycles	7 905	12 541	58.7	6.1	10.2
Pedestrians	8 136	12 067	48.3	6.2	9.8
Total				100.0	100.0

Source: Pez (1994).

is close to a nature reserve and other recreational sites. The size of the land area on which the car-free housing will be constructed is 2.6 hectares (ha).

Design. In total 1000 housing units are planned, of which only 210 will be car-free. The houses themselves will be two to three storeys high. Figure 17.4 shows the outline of the estate but the exact design has not been finalized. Some of the buildings will be constructed according to ecological principles, including the use of construction material which can be recycled.

Transport. There is no through road in the housing estate but it has easy access to an excellent cycle network. Additional cycle facilities are planned in the estate to promote cycling further. A newly constructed tram line (No. 4—Bremen to Lilienthal) will connect the housing estate with the city centre. It will be the first new tram line built in Bremen for decades.

Pledge of car freedom by the residents and car parking facilities. The most interesting aspect of this housing estate will be that residents have to commit themselves not to own a car. Of the people so far interested who want either to buy or rent, 75% do not have a car. About 30 car parking spaces will be available for visitors and 12–15 spaces for car sharing. It is assumed that one car will be shared between 10–15 users.

Advantages. The houses which will be rented and sold are advertised with the following advantages: living will be less noisy and housing will be cheaper because normally for the same housing units 200 parking spaces would be needed using about 7000 square metres. There will be better air, no accidents and energy savings.

Interests. Regular meetings have been held since the early planning stages between the potential residents and the planning department, and information leaflets have been written and distributed. Originally 342 households were interested. This has been reduced to 152 of which 37 would like to buy either a house or a flat, and another 37 have not yet decided whether to buy or rent. The reason for the decline in interest is that the cost of the housing, despite the saving in car parking spaces, is rather high.

Stages of the construction programme. The planning process has now been completed. The construction of housing will begin in autumn 1995 and it is assumed that the first houses will be available in 1996.

Amsterdam

As in Bremen, Amsterdam's city centre allows little private car access. About 70% of people living in Amsterdam do not own a car. Westerpark quarter, an inner

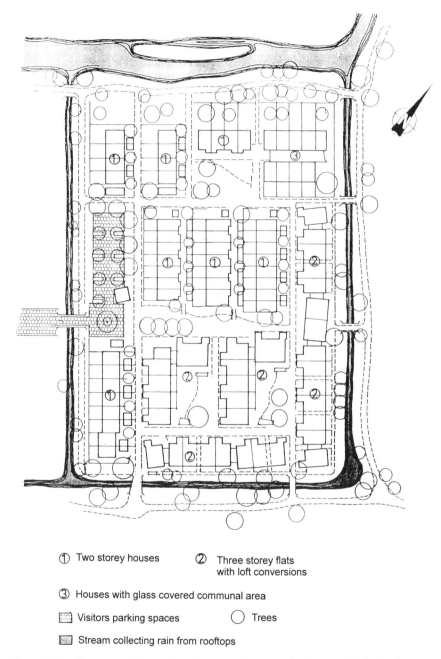

① Two storey houses ② Three storey flats
with loft conversions

③ Houses with glass covered communal area

▨ Visitors parking spaces ○ Trees

▨ Stream collecting rain from rooftops

Figure 17.4 Proposed design of car-free housing estate in Bremen-Hollerland

city area to the west of the city centre, will be the first car-free settlement in the Netherlands. The size of the area is small, only 6 ha, and the 600 apartments will be four to nine storeys high; about half will be owner occupied and half social housing.

Planning started in November 1992 and construction began in mid-1995. The flats will be built by different housing cooperatives which are all non-profit organizations. Flats will be of different sizes and the cost for the owner occupied housing will be about the same as for similar flats in Amsterdam. Only one car parking space for three apartments is planned in Westerpark (a maximum of 180 parking spaces in all). A car hire company will locate itself close to the car-free area.

When the District of Westerpark advertised their new car-free apartments in the local newspaper, about 4000 people responded in seven days and during the same month another 2000 expressed interest either in buying or renting.

Other car-free housing estates

There are a number of other planned car-free housing estates, for instance in Berlin where a pressure group promotes car-free living. About 1000 households or roughly 2500 people were committed to this idea. There is one potential project, in Lichterfelde Süd in West Berlin. In Dortmund, a small housing estate is planned by the City Council containing only 100–150 housing units.

In München-Neuriem about 2200 apartments are proposed close to two underground stations and the Munich exhibition centre. If the plans come to fruition, it would be the largest car-free area so far, but the firm behind this scheme has not yet been able to convince the Council to give permission.

Conclusion

This chapter has described two developments in Europe: a car-free town centre and examples of car-free housing estates. Both issues, although consistent in being the next logical step to complement previously established transport policies, are still not as common on the Continent as they should be.

One of the most important lessons one can learn from Lüneburg is that if a Town Council decides to implement major changes, momentum has to be established by doing it quickly, with conviction and with style. In addition, money has to be available to do it well. A slow and cautious pace does not in practice lead to consensus, but on the contrary gives the critics endless opportunities to prevent anything happening at all.

Lüneburg can be seen as a model for a number of German towns. Whether it can act as a model for Britain is more questionable; not only is the financial commitment which is necessary to change a town significantly more difficult to achieve in Britain, but there are a number of other factors which make it easier in the Netherlands or in Germany to change towns. For instance, they have significantly greater political freedom as a local authority.

The lesson from the car-free housing estates is that even small projects like the one in Amsterdam and Bremen take a very long time to come to fruition. There is always interest from a number of people who are willing to buy a property without access to a car parking space. However, the psychological situation in Continental Europe is different from Britain, where car ownership appears to be a central concern for property owners. The transport policies over the last 20 years in Germany and the Netherlands makes such experiments possible. These housing estates are only the start of a movement which seems set to continue on a much larger scale in future years.

Coming back to Britain, certainly there has been a change in the overall policy approach by the local authorities and the British government, and an acceptance that unrestrained car use cannot be sustained. Even so, Britain and the Continent are drifting apart, not in theory but in practice because major elements of a 'car orientated' transport policy have to be pursued in Britain, simply because there are no alternatives, and land use trends have already been set. How can one ask people to use the car less if public transport either does not exist or is in a poor state, expensive and unreliable? How can one ask people to cycle if facilities are lacking? It is here where experiences on the Continent offer people real alternatives. There is another important difference: although funds for environmentally friendly transport policies are lacking on the Continent too, far more is still being spent there than in Britain.

Experts who are trying to change people's transport habits know that it is still very difficult to change attitudes and behaviour in favour of an environmentally friendly transport policy even after most of these facilities are in place and despite the greater environmental awareness of the population on the Continent. What chance does Britain have to catch up with the Continent if the pace of change is not speeded up dramatically, or does Britain wish to remain a car-orientated society?

Further reading

Billinger H (1994) Car-free residential area in Munich, Neu Riem: concepts and legal provision for a new residential area in Munich without private cars. In *Environmental Issues: Proceedings of the 22nd European Transport Forum*, University of Warwick, 12–16 September 1994 (pp. 207–218). PTRC Education and Research Services, London

Pez P (1994) *Auswirkungen der Innerstädtischen Verkehrsberuhigung in Lüneburg eine Zwischenbilanz: Verkehrswissenschaftliche Arbeiten 8*. Universität Lüneburg, Lüneburg

Reutter U (1993) Autofreie Haushalte in Neubaugebieten—Machbarkeitsstudie. In *Monatsbericht*. Institut für Landes—und Stadtentwicklungsforschung des Landes Nordrhein, Westfalen

A more detailed report on Lüneburg has been published by ETP and is available under the title *Lüneburg: The making of a car-free town centre* (1994) from the author.

18
Transport and environmental quality in Århus, Denmark: targets and priority areas of action

Jørgen Bunde

Århus Council, Denmark

Environmental problems have been receiving increased attention, in Denmark and in other countries.

The World Commission on Environment and Development proposed in *Our Common Future* (World Commission on Environment and Development, 1987) that all future environmental efforts be based on the concept of sustainable development. Sustainable development meets the needs of the present generation without compromising the ability of future generations to meet their own needs. The Commission emphasizes that world economic growth can only occur within the limits set by nature and that the benefits of economic growth and the efforts to solve environmental problems should be shared in an equitable manner globally, nationally and locally.

In 1990 the European Commission published the *Green Paper on the urban environment*, (Commission of the European Communities, 1990) which emphasizes the problems of cities with high levels of pollution and noise caused by road traffic, large distances resulting from the growth of mass consumption and increased motor vehicle use, and large transport facilities that disfigure Europe's cities and contribute significantly to global pollution. One of the solutions the

This chapter Copyright © 1997 the Municipality of Århus. Reproduced by permssion. Compiled from *Transport and Environment Quality* (1993), published by funds provided by the Spatial Planning Department, Ministry of Environment, Denmark, and *Traffic & Miljø* (1994). For further information please contact: Office of the City Engineer, Municipality of Århus, Orla Lehmanns Allé 3, Postboks 539, DK-8100 Århus, Denmark.

Health at the Crossroads: Transport Policy and Urban Health.
Edited by Tony Fletcher and Anthony J. McMichael published 1997 John Wiley & Sons Ltd

Green Paper proposes is to promote more functional diversity in cities. Land use and transport planning should be integrated and transport should be managed, based on environmental considerations.

Denmark's goals

As a follow-up to the Brundtland report, the Government of Denmark published an action plan for environment and development in 1988 (Denmark Government State Information Service, 1988) describing how the Government's efforts to achieve sustainable development could be carried out within the various ministerial areas.

Since developments in the transport sector are decisive for both economic growth and environmental quality, it is important to integrate the solutions to environmental problems into the decisions on the expansion of the future transport system.

The Government of Denmark therefore published a special transport action plan (Denmark Ministry of Traffic, 1990) for environment and development in 1990. This plan analyses the environmental problems and energy consumption of the transport sector, sets targets for energy consumption, air quality and noise levels until the year 2030 and describes several priority areas of action at the national and local levels.

At the same time, the Road Safety Commission (Ministry of Justice) published a report in 1988 (Denmark Ministry of Justice, 1988) that analysed the general state of road safety in Denmark, proposed a series of targets for the efforts to promote road safety until the year 2000 and presented action plans for realizing the targets both at the national and local levels.

Work on transport and environmental quality initiated in Århus

In May 1991, the Municipality of Århus accepted an invitation from the Ministry of Environment and Energy to cooperate with the Ministry and four other municipalities in Denmark on transport and environmental quality. The aim was to survey the environmental impact of transport in these municipalities and to investigate the local opportunities to improve this. One of the starting-points for the survey was the Ministry's published guidelines on transport and environmental quality (Denmark Ministry of Environment, 1992). The cooperative group also aimed to produce a strategy for administering a transport and environmental quality-related state fund, with an allocation of 150 million Danish crowns for 1992–95, to support the implementation of the local action plans.

As part of the cooperation with the Ministry of Environment and Energy, the Århus Municipal Council decided to make transport and environmental quality a special planning focus and to implement a special planning project on this topic in connection with the scheduled revision of the municipal plan. In spring 1992, the Municipal Council therefore published a planning report intended to promote debate on the long-term environmental impact of transport. The report later resulted in the final action plan for traffic and the environment (Municipality of Århus, 1994).

The results of the special focus on planning for transport and environmental quality are presented in the form of a set of targets and priority areas of action for the Municipality's future activities in transport and the environment.

The chapter on targets and priority areas of action was prepared in the form of a proposal for the guidelines of the municipal plan on transport and environmental quality. It includes proposals for the municipality's overall guidelines, targets and strategies for future efforts to reduce the environmental impact of transport, and thereby creates the basis for setting priorities in administration and investment in roads, and for the extension and revision of the municipal sector plan on roads.

Targets and priority areas of action

The municipality of Århus has identified how it can influence the environment in which transport is carried out, in a broad sense. In each of the following eight areas, targets and priority areas have been established in planning, public works, traffic management and information/education.

1. Volume of transport   5. Noise
2. Infrastructure   6. Road safety
3. Energy consumption   7. Its barrier effect
4. Air pollution   8. Visual environment

Some examples of the targets and policy proposals are summarized below.

Based on the national targets for improving the environment, local targets and priority areas of action are proposed in the following areas: planning; public works and purchasing; traffic management; and information and education.

The volume of transport

The target of the Municipality of Århus is to reduce the total volume of transport within the Municipality and thus to reduce the environmental burden of transport. The Municipality especially aims to improve the total environment in the city centre by rerouting traffic. The interests of all the users of the city centre will be considered in this restructuring, including residents, shoppers, visitors, the people who work in the city centre and those who are employed to drive in the city centre.

Planning

The Municipality will attempt to reduce the volume of transport through appropriate transport and land use planning, with the aim of conserving energy and reducing carbon dioxide emissions from transport. A comprehensive policy on the location of dwellings, workplaces, shopping centres and institutions will be implemented to attempt to reduce the transport distances as much as possible, so that the setting for most transport is within each local community. A transport model for the city centre that can describe the pattern of personal and freight transport will be prepared to assess the opportunities for, and impact of, shifting the distribution of transport between the various modes and means of transport and the distribution of road traffic on the road network.

An initiative is already underway between Århus sporveje (public transport authority) and the Office of the City Engineer to investigate the potential of using modern technology to manage, give priority to and provide information on city and regional bus routes in urban traffic. This initiative will continue with the aim of improving the efficiency of mass transport and thereby encouraging a shift from individual transport to mass transport. Realizing this potential will also improve air quality, reduce noise and improve road safety.

As part of the planning proposals being prepared for land currently used by the repair yards of the Danish State Railways, alternative options for establishing a common transport terminal for city and regional buses, taxis and trains will be explored. The route network and user pattern of public transport will be analysed with the aim of determining the future routes for public transport in the city centre and assessing the financial and environmental impact of using various sizes of bus or electrified public transport (trams). The opportunities to improve the accessibility and efficiency of taxi transport in the city centre, and especially in the most congested part of the city centre, will be investigated in cooperation between the Municipality's Taxi Commission, the police in Århus, Århus public transport authority and the Office of the City Engineer.

The Municipality of Århus is encouraging the Ministry of Transport and the Ministry of Environment and Energy to cooperate in planning and implementing pilot projects in the city centre, and especially in the most congested part, with the aim of improving the overall environment there, including pilot projects to develop new modes and means of transport and new ways to organize transport services.

Traffic management

Road traffic will be rerouted in the city centre, subject to fiscal limitations, with the aim of:

1. improving the overall environment in the city centre by restricting car traffic and giving higher priority to public transport and bicycle transport;
2. creating large, coherent squares and pedestrian areas; and
3. restructuring parking areas.

Parking in the city centre will be restructured in such a way that street parking is eliminated and replaced by large parking facilities on the outskirts of the city centre. A parking information system will be developed that can direct motorists to available parking spaces when they enter the city. This should reduce the total number of motorists seeking parking, and improve the ease of access, efficiency and stopping conditions for transport related to errands in the city centre, including taxi traffic.

Information and education

A general educational campaign will be conducted on the impact of road traffic on environmental quality, including the need to reduce the volume of motor vehicle transport. Such a campaign will also provide education on: the problems of air pollution and the potential to reduce them through a more considered use of vehicles and more energy-efficient and smooth operation of vehicles; the noise pollution caused by motor vehicle traffic and the potential to reduce the nuisance from noise; and the importance of the pattern of car traffic on road safety and the reinforcement or reduction of the barrier effect. These kinds of educational campaigns play an important role in relation to meeting all the specific targets including those for air pollution, noise, accidents and energy consumption.

Infrastructure

The infrastructure target of the Municipality of Århus is to modernize the overall transport infrastructure with the aim of creating rapid and efficient transport connections in the Municipality and improving the environment on and along the roads. This will be achieved by changing and extending the road network, so that car traffic can be shifted from more environmentally sensitive stretches of road to ones that are more environmentally robust. The transport networks for public transport and bicycle transport will be simultaneously given higher priority.

The opportunities to establish a more extensive network of bicycle routes in the most congested part of the city centre will be investigated with the aim of shifting personal transport to bicycles. This network will be specially designed to provide rapid and safe routes around the city centre and will be based, in part, on the potential provided by the overall rerouting of road traffic in the most congested part of the city centre. An increase in bicycle transport in the long term will improve air quality, reduce noise levels, conserve energy, promote road safety, reduce the barrier effect and make it possible to improve the visual environment.

In connection with the annual revision of the restriction of routes for vehicles carrying hazardous goods, the Municipality's Division of Technical Services is currently cooperating with the police in assessing whether sufficient attention is being paid to the environmental considerations mentioned in the municipal plan for transport and environmental quality.

When the main road network around the existing urban area is completed, some of the existing main road network within the motorway in Jylland on Viborgvej, Silkeborgvej, Skanderborgvej and Grenåvej can be renovated, for example, by using traffic calming schemes on through roads. With the aim of eliminating through traffic in large, residential areas and concentrating the traffic on main roads and highways, traffic calming schemes will continue to be implemented, including creating culs-de-sac, speed bumps, traffic signals and signs. This will improve air quality, reduce noise levels, enhance road safety (routes to and from school) and reduce the barrier effect.

Energy consumption

The energy conservation target of the Municipality of Århus is to help to reduce energy consumption in accordance with the targets of the transport action plan for environment and development of the Government of Denmark.

The Municipality will attempt to reduce energy consumption in the transport sector through integrated transport and land use planning, and analysis will be undertaken of the Municipality's total energy consumption through transport. Energy efficiency will be taken into consideration in the purchase of new vehicles for municipal use.

Air pollution

The target of the Municipality of Århus on air pollution from road traffic is to help to reduce air pollution in accordance with the targets of the transport action plan for environment and development of the Government of Denmark. In particular, the Municipality of Århus will try to reduce the general emission of carbon dioxide, nitrogen oxides and hydrocarbons and to reduce the concentration of nitrogen dioxide and carbon monoxide in the streets of the central district.

Local plans that affect transport will have a separate report on the present and projected air quality. The stretches of road designated as especially critical in the survey of environmental conditions will be investigated further with the aim of improving air quality. The use of modern technology to manage and give priority to mass transport, especially through signal-controlled intersections, was described earlier. A report will be prepared outlining the practical and economic impact of requiring that goods be distributed in the city centre using vehicles with a maximum gross weight of no more than five tonnes.

Reduced emissions will be a consideration in the purchase of new buses for Århus sporveje (public transport authority).

With the aim of reducing air pollution along the roads in Århus by ensuring a smoother flow of traffic, the speed limits on the municipal road network will be assessed and revised in cooperation between the Office of the City Engineer and the police. The planned rerouting of road traffic away from the city centre, which aims, among other things, at reducing air pollution there, will be carried out as fast as available funds allow. An attempt will be made to reroute heavy vehicles to roads on which the air quality is not crucial.

Noise

The target of the Municipality of Århus on noise from road traffic for the next five years is to reduce the number of dwellings subjected to a noise level from traffic exceeding 65 dB(A) by 2.5% per year.

Planning

The zoning limit values intended to ensure an acceptable level of noise from such sources as road traffic will continue to be used in the planning of new residential areas and the renovation or changed zoning of existing residential areas. Local plans that affect transport will have a separate report on the present and projected noise level. Future urban zones for noise-sensitive purposes will be located at a distance from roads so that the noise level from road traffic does not exceed 55 dB(A). The already-initiated registration activity will be continued, especially with the aim of determining the exact number of dwellings subjected to excessive noise, their type, location and noise level and possible measures to reduce the noise level.

Public works and purchasing

The Municipality of Århus will ensure compliance with the municipal guide-lines on noise, which state that new municipal roads must be constructed such that the noise level in the outdoor areas of dwellings adjacent to the new road does not exceed 55 dB(A) or, if this is not possible for technical and financial reasons, then 30 dB(A) indoors. For significant renovation of existing roads, a maximum noise level of 60 dB(A) outdoors or 30 dB(A) indoors must be ensured.

The Municipality of Århus will recommend to the state and Århus County that the same standards are used in the construction of state or county highways.

The Municipality will attempt to reduce the noise level for the dwellings most subjected to noise along municipal roads through sound baffles or façade insulation, to ensure an acceptable indoor noise level. An attempt will be made to create a special fund for matching-funds financing of noise-reducing measures by the Municipality of Århus and the owners of the noise-impacted dwellings as part of the municipal road plan. The extent of any municipal subsidy will depend on the priorities determined in the annual budgeting process.

Reduced noise emissions will be a consideration in the purchase of new buses for Århus public transport authority.

Traffic management

With the aim of reducing noise levels along the roads, the speed limits on the municipal road network will be assessed and revised in cooperation between the Office of the City Engineer and the police. An attempt will be made to reroute road traffic to fewer, larger arteries by traffic-control measures, which will calm traffic in more and larger local residential districts and eliminate the annoying fast-moving through traffic. An attempt will be made to reroute heavy vehicles to roads on which the noise level is not crucial. The planned rerouting of road traffic away from the city centre, which aims, among other things, at reducing the noise level there, will be carried out as fast as the available funds allow.

Road safety

The target of the Municipality of Århus on improving road safety for the years 1991–96 is to reduce the number of deaths and injuries from road traffic as proposed in the action plan of the Road Safety Commission by 5% per year (cumulative, with 1990 as the base year). The Municipality of Århus intends to contribute to reaching this target by its current efforts, corresponding to the most cost-effective municipal measures proposed in the Commission's report, as follows.

Planning

The ongoing work of improving road safety in the integrated planning of future transport facilities and land use will be continued. Local plans that significantly affect transport will include a separate report on the present and projected road safety conditions.

The Traffic Safety Committee of the Århus Municipal Council created a special working group in spring 1992 with technicians from the school system and the Office of the City Engineer. The group's task is to survey the safety problems of schoolchildren on their way to and from school and, based on this, to make proposals for the priority areas of action to improve road safety. This work is continuing and is expected to be completed in autumn 1993.

In 1992, the Office of the City Engineer cooperated with the Traffic Safety Division of the National Road Directorate in beginning to analyse the stretches of road and intersections among Århus's roads and paths that account for the most accidents. The causes of the road accidents are being analysed, and proposals will be made on how to reduce this number. The already initiated work of planning traffic calming schemes in the city centre, and especially the area around the central railway station, will be continued.

A study will be initiated of the potential to establish a more extensive network of bicycle routes in the densest part of the city centre, especially because of the opportunities created by the rerouting of road traffic there.

Public works

To alleviate the strain on the existing road network, the overall road network will continue to be expanded with motorways, main roads to the harbour and the city centre and roads to serve commercial areas as fast as available funds permit.

Based on, among other things, the priority areas of action determined using the results of the ongoing analysis of the pattern of road accidents, attempts will be made to integrate efforts to improve safety in the areas with many road accidents into the public works programmes of the next few years. Special attention will be paid to projects that can make intersections safer for bicyclists. The public works budget of the municipal road sector will be allocated special funds to improve safety and environmental quality. The priorities for these projects must be determined within the fiscal limits imposed by the Århus Municipal Council.

With the aim of eliminating through traffic in large residential areas and concentrating the traffic on main roads and highways, traffic calming schemes will continue to be implemented, including creating culs-de-sac, speed bumps, traffic signals and signs. Road traffic will be rerouted in the city centre with the aim of calming traffic in the most congested part, including restricting car traffic, giving higher priority to reducing the travel time of mass transport, creating large, coherent squares and pedestrian areas and restructuring parking areas.

Traffic management

With the aim of reducing the speed of road traffic and ensuring a more smooth and even flow of road traffic, the speed limits on the municipal road network will be assessed and revised in cooperation between the Office of the City Engineer and the police. The travel time by bus will be reduced by establishing streets on which buses will be given high priority or through giving buses special lanes on other streets, signal synchronization, etc., as fast as the available funds allow.

Information and education

A general educational campaign will be conducted on the impact of road traffic on environmental quality, including the increasing risk of road accidents at higher speed. On one day all young drivers-to-be are invited to drive at a testing track. Annual road safety campaigns are conducted in connection with the first days of school. A campaign will be conducted to promote the increased use of bicycles as part of daily transport and to inform the public about the safety aspects of bicycling. A campaign will be conducted to inform the public about the risks associated with jumping red lights. In cooperation with the municipal Department of Social Services, the education of elderly people on road safety problems associated with their role as pedestrians will be expanded.

The barrier effect

The target of the Municipality of Århus in reducing the barrier effect of road traffic is therefore to attempt to reduce the volume and speed of traffic on stretches of road where many pedestrians and bicyclists need to cross the street more safely and securely or where it is necessary to create passages for wild animals.

In coordination with the ongoing analysis of schoolchildren's routes to school, it will be determined where pedestrians and bicyclists have a special need to cross large traffic arteries in Århus and currently have problems doing so.

The ongoing rerouting of road traffic around residential areas will be continued, especially with the aim of reducing the amount of through traffic and reducing speed in general.

The planned rerouting of road traffic away from the city centre, which aims, among other things, at reducing the barrier effect there, will be carried out as fast as available funds allow.

The visual environment

The target of the Municipality of Århus in improving the quality of the visual environment is to create beautiful and harmonious street spaces, with special consideration for their use as areas for walking and bicycling and as residential areas. Creating more interesting and attractive street environments in the city centre will be emphasized, to maintain the area as the commercial and cultural centre of Århus. The Municipality will attempt to convert public street spaces in cooperation with and with co-financing from the adjacent property owners. The significance of the visual environment in promoting road safety will be emphasized in the creation and improvement of visual environments.

References

Commission of the European Communities (1990) *Green Paper on the Urban Environment: Communication from the Commission to the Council and Parliament, Brussels, 27 June 1990*. OOPEC, Brussels

Denmark Government State Information Service (1988) *The Government's Action Plan on Environment and Development*. DGSIS, Copenhagen

Denmark Ministry of Environment, National Agency for Physical Planning (1992) *Transport and environment in municipal planning*. Ministry of Environment, Copenhagen

Denmark Ministry of Justice Road Safety Commission (1988) *Action Plan on Road Safety*. Ministry of Justice, Copenhagen

Denmark Ministry of Traffic (1990) *The Government's Action Plan for Environment and Development*. Ministry of Transport, Copenhagen

Municipality of Århus (1994) *Traffic and Environment, Municipal Plan 1993–2005*. Municipality of Århus, Århus, Denmark

World Commission on Environment and Development (1987) *Our Common Future*. United Nations and the International Association

19
Automobile dependence in Bangkok: an international comparison with implications for planning policies and air pollution

Jeffrey R. Kenworthy

Institute for Science & Technology Policy, Murdoch University, Australia

Any discussion of automobile dependence today will usually involve some reference to Los Angeles. As an archetype for cities that have tried to build their transport systems almost totally around freeways and failed, it is almost unparalleled. However, the Asian region is rapidly developing its own archetype of urban traffic dysfunction and air pollution: the Bangkok metropolitan region.

Interestingly, an historical coincidence underlies the similarities between Los Angeles and Bangkok today. In 1781 the Spanish Governor of California, Felipe de Neve, established the community that we know today as Los Angeles or 'the City of Angels'. In 1782, in an almost prophetic leap that would seal a strange connection between the two places, King Rama I of Thailand established a new capital for his country, the original name of which means 'the Great City of the Angels.'

Whether we want to read any more into this coincidence depends a little on our penchant for intrigue. But for those who once knew Bangkok as the Venice of the East with its serpentine river and network of canals, the unfortunate reality is that it is fast becoming the Los Angeles of the East. Most canals have been paved over with congested roads. Elevated freeways and spaghetti junctions punctuate the urban landscape. The air is heavily laden with automotive air and noise emissions. And in true Los Angelino style, there are plans to turn the Chao Phraya River into a floating freeway. Bangkok presently adds about 600 new cars

Health at the Crossroads: Transport Policy and Urban Health.
Edited by Tony Fletcher and Anthony J. McMichael © 1997 John Wiley & Sons Ltd

daily to the traffic stream, which equates to an extra 3 km of bumper-to-bumper traffic. At this rate, in less than four years enough cars will be added to fill the entire road system with one lane of traffic.

Bangkok's traffic predicament and severe air pollution raise some interesting questions about how a city can descend into such chaos and what factors underlie the situation. Importantly, they raise questions about what policies and strategies are best for relieving the situation, irrespective of the present political likelihood of implementing them. An effective way of providing the perspectives needed to answer these questions is to compare Bangkok to other cities around the world, especially other Asian cities in the region.

This chapter provides a detailed comparison of Bangkok's land use and transport system characteristics with cities in North America, Europe and Australia and in particular, other Asian cities such as Kuala Lumpur, Jakarta, Manila, Seoul, Surabaya, Singapore, Hong Kong and Tokyo. The data on the developing Asian cities other than Bangkok are taken from Barter *et al.* (1994) and Bangkok data come from Poboon *et al.* (1994). This paper also briefly summarizes the air pollution situation in Bangkok, with some reference to health impacts. Areas of planning policy that need attention are highlighted, suggesting a suite of policies that are likely to improve the present transport and air pollution situation in Bangkok.

Land use patterns

One of the most important factors in determining a city's level of car use and the viability of public transport, walking and cycling is urban density (Newman and Kenworthy, 1989). Higher densities, and the mixed land uses associated with them, shorten the length of trips by all modes, make walking and cycling possible for more trips and create sufficient concentrations of activities for an effective, frequent public transport service. Figure 19.1 depicts the relationship between urban density, energy use per capita and the percentage of workers using public transport across a global sample of cities. Higher urban densities, particularly those characteristic of Asian cities such as Tokyo, have much lower energy use per capita for transport and much higher use of public transport for work trips.

Figure 19.2 provides average urban densities for cities in the USA, Australia, Europe and a selection of Asian cities. The Bangkok Metropolitan Area with 6 million people living at 162 persons per hectare (ha) is clearly a densely settled city in an international context, and is a little above average for an Asian city. Within Bangkok, the inner zone of 3 million people has a density of 257 persons per ha (virtually the same as Manhattan and central Paris), the middle zone of 2 million people is settled at 138 per ha and the outer zone of 1 million people has 74 persons per ha, which is still some five times denser than the average metropolitan area in the USA and Australia (Poboon *et al.*, 1994). Bangkok therefore fulfils one of the chief criteria for minimizing automobile dependence.

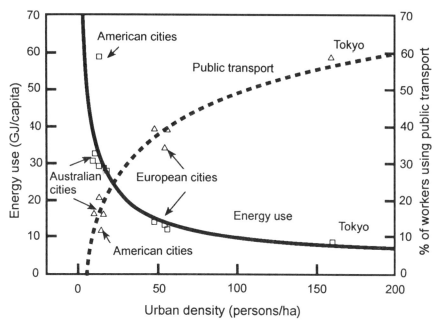

Figure 19.1 Urban density, energy use and public transport for the journey-to-work in a global sample of cities. □, energy use; △, percentage of workers using public transport

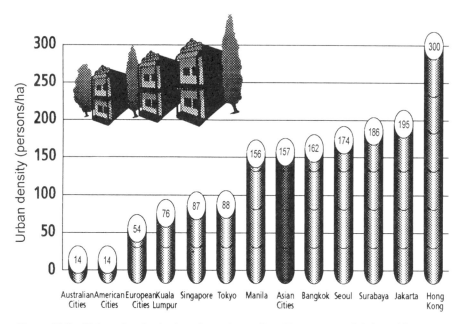

Figure 19.2 Urban density in American, Australian, European and Asian cities

Provision for the automobile

Another key factor in automobile dependence is how well the automobile is catered for in basic infrastructure. The length of road per person and the amount of parking in the Central Business District (CBD) are indicative of this factor. Figure 19.3 summarizes the length of road per person in cities and shows that the Asian cities are extremely low in this factor (0.7 metres per person compared to as high as 8.7 in Australian cities). Bangkok is about average for an Asian city but this relatively low road provision only partly helps to explain the congested traffic, as shown later. Figure 19.4 provides the number of parking spaces per 1000 jobs and shows that Bangkok with 338 exceeds the average Australian city and is only a little less than the average US city with 380. By contrast, Singapore, Tokyo and Hong Kong average a mere 67 spaces per 1000 CBD jobs.

Vehicle ownership

Vehicle ownership varies considerably in cities around the world as shown in Figure 19.5. US and Australian cities are clear leaders in car ownership but they have very low motorcycle ownership (95% of the combined car and motorcycle ownership is cars). At the other end of the spectrum Hong Kong has only 47 vehicles per 1000 people, and again these are mainly cars (91%). Bangkok is the highest of the Asian cities in total vehicle ownership (296 per 1000 people) and is only a little behind the European average of 341. However, only 56% are cars in Bangkok, unlike in European cities with 96% cars. Motorbikes are popular in

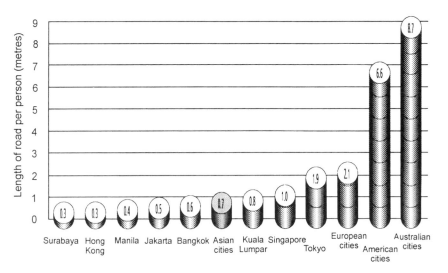

Figure 19.3   Length of road per person in American, Australian, European and Asian cities

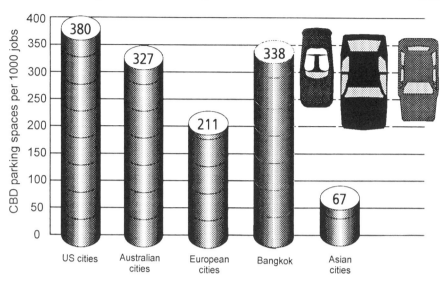

Figure 19.4   Parking spaces in the CBD in Bangkok compared to American, Australian, European and other Asian cities (Singapore, Tokyo and Hong Kong)

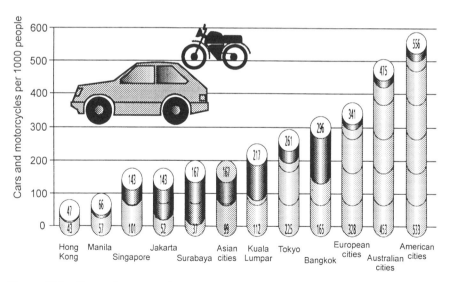

Figure 19.5   Car and motorcycle ownership in American, Australian, European and Asian cities. Note Asian cities are for 1990, the others for 1980

Bangkok and other Asian cities such as Jakarta and Surabaya where they dominate vehicle ownership. They are cheaper, smaller and easier to park, and can cut a path through congested streets and negotiate the narrow streets of the urban kampongs. They are, however, responsible for a very significant amount of pollution, especially suspended particulate matter.

Bangkok is very much higher in total vehicle ownership than the average Asian city (296 per 1000 people compared to 167). It has double the level of much wealthier Singapore which has only 143 vehicles per 1000, and is even higher than Tokyo with 261 vehicles per 1000 people (although Tokyo's ownership is 86% cars).

Figure 19.6 shows the paradox associated with such high levels of vehicle ownership in Bangkok by comparing national purchasing power per capita in various nations in 1990. For example, Thailand had only 29% of the purchasing power of Hong Kong, but Bangkok in 1990 had some six times more vehicles per capita. Similarly, Bangkok's car ownership is 63% higher than Singapore, but Thailand's purchasing power is only one-third that of Singapore. Wealth levels alone are clearly not the only determinants of vehicle ownership. This is considered further in the paper.

What kind of transport patterns are associated with these basic land use and transport features?

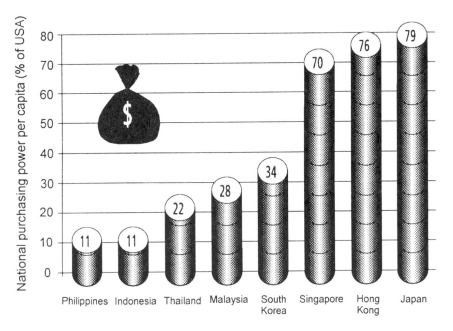

Figure 19.6   National purchasing power per capita (1990) in Asian countries compared to the USA

Transport patterns

Private transport

Figure 19.7 provides the total vehicle kilometres of travel per person in the various cities. As expected, the US and Australian cities are clear leaders (9747 and 7090 km respectively), followed by the European cities with much lower levels (3959 km). Bangkok, however, is heavily motorized for its physical characteristics, being 74% higher in vehicle use than the average Asian city. It has almost the same level of private vehicle use as in Tokyo, which based on national figures in 1990, had 3.5 times more purchasing power than Bangkok. Again, there are clearly more factors than wealth at work in urban automobile dependence. In Bangkok, 51% of all trips are by private means, compared to an overall average for Asian cities of 33%, with Manila as low as 21%.

Public transport

Figure 19.8 shows that the use of public transport expressed as transit's share of total annual passenger kilometres, is very low in US and Australian cities (4% and 8% respectively), while in Europe it is 25%. The Asian cities in this graph are Singapore, Tokyo and Hong Kong which have 64% of all passenger travel by public transport and which today are heavily dependent on rail-based transit. By comparison, Bangkok, with its gridlocked bus-only transit system, has only half this level of public transport use. Although this is quite high in an international

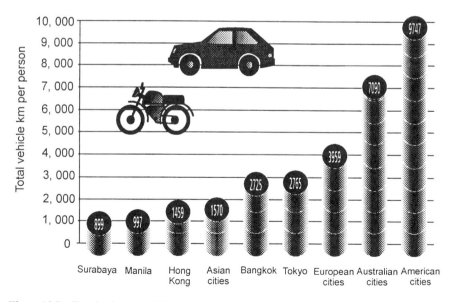

Figure 19.7 Total private vehicle travel in American, Australian, European and Asian cities

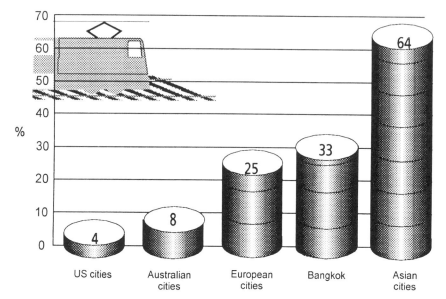

Figure 19.8   The proportion of total annual passenger travel by public transport in Bangkok, compared to American, Australian, European and other Asian cities (Singapore, Tokyo and Hong Kong)

sense, it is too low for a city of Bangkok's type with low road provision and a dense urban fabric unsuited to accommodating automobiles.

With respect to public transport's share of all trips, Bangkok does moderately well with its basic bus system and other collective modes (33% compared to an average for Asian cities of 35%). Nevertheless, Manila and Seoul have much higher levels of public transport (49% and 65% of all trips). Figure 19.9 shows the proportion of motorized work trips on public transport, for an even larger sample of cities. This is very revealing as it shows that for those trips undertaken in the peak when road space is at a premium, Bangkok has rather low use of public transport (only 31% compared to an average for the Asian cities of 55% and more particularly, between 62% and 89% in Tokyo, Singapore, Manila and Hong Kong).

Non-motorized modes

Figure 19.10 shows the use of walking and cycling for the journey to work in cities around the world and reveals that US and Australian cities with their low densities, heavily zoned land uses and long trips have only 5% of workers walking or cycling; European and Asian cities have 21% and 25% respectively, while Bangkok is very low with only 10%. Figure 19.11 shows that, as a percentage of all daily trips, walking and cycling in Bangkok is about as low as it gets in Asian

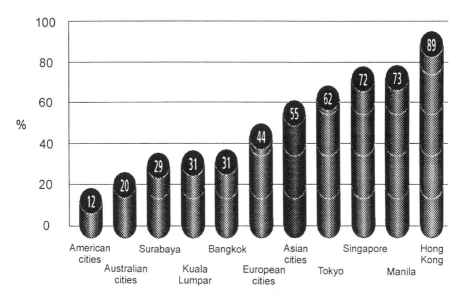

Figure 19.9   The proportion of motorized works trips on public transport in American, Australian, European and Asian cities

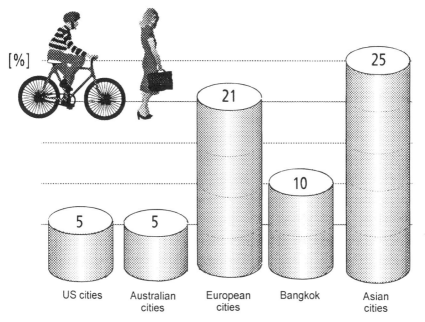

Figure 19.10   The proportion of workers using walking and cycling for the journey to work in Bangkok compared to American, Australian, European and other Asian cities (Singapore, Tokyo and Hong Kong)

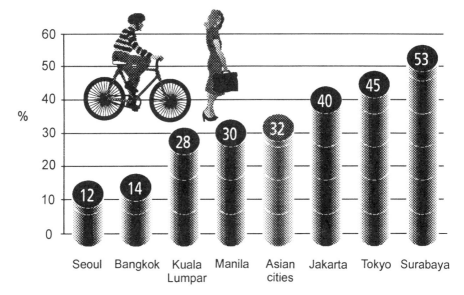

Figure 19.11   The proportion of all daily trips by non-motorized modes in Asian cities

cities (14%, or less than half the Asian city average of 32%). Tokyo on the other hand has a massive 45% of all trips by foot and bicycle, exceeded in this sample only by Surabaya with 53%.

Implications of the international comparisons

What are the implications for Bangkok of these comparisons in the land use and transport patterns of cities across the globe?

Vehicle ownership

Bangkok clearly has a burgeoning vehicle population which is higher than expected if wealth were the only factor involved. It can be argued that the absence of a real public transport alternative and the serious problems associated with walking and cycling are helping to fuel exponential growth in vehicles, especially since 1980 (Poboon *et al.*, 1994). There is also nothing in government policy which would help to curtail the trend. On the contrary, close ties with Japanese car and motorcycle manufacturers, financial aid from Japan and other financial institutions for road projects, plus low tariffs and other government charges associated with vehicle ownership, suggest that high vehicle growth will continue (Kenworthy, 1994; Mallet, 1994).

Singapore's experience highlights Bangkok's need to establish some policy constraints on motor vehicles. The suppression of vehicle ownership in Singapore compared to Bangkok can be seen in Figure 19.5. Singapore's tough economic and physical planning disincentives against cars and its excellent public transport explain this picture, especially in the light of the city's economic capacity to purchase cars, as depicted in Figure 19.6 (Kenworthy *et al.*, 1994). Singapore's policies include all-day (07.30–18.30) restrictions and high charges for vehicles entering the CBD, and the Certificate of Entitlement (COE) system which requires purchase of the right simply to buy a car (costs depend on vehicle size and the time that the vehicle will be operated but range from S$28 150 for a weekend only car, through to S$63 000 for big cars (*The Straits Times*, 17 December 1993).

Public transport

Bangkok's dense urban fabric, combined with intensively mixed land use throughout a major part of the city, makes it a potentially ideal environment for public transport and particularly walking and cycling. This is especially true because of the linear nature of the city where residential areas and commercial/retail strips are densely built up along road corridors. This is well-suited to a fixed route, segregated transit system, whereas currently buses attempting to ply these corridors find themselves at a standstill with other traffic. Public transport use in Bangkok is correspondingly low for an Asian city because only occasionally do buses operate on effective bus lanes (in particular contraflow lanes). In addition, the crowded, mostly non-air-conditioned buses are unable to provide an acceptable transport alternative for the growing middle class who are fuelling the demand for car travel. The Asian cities which do have high levels of public transport use are those that have effective rail systems and have been able to capture middle-class travellers on attractive, air-conditioned fast trains (e.g. Hong Kong and Singapore).

An effective rail-based public transport system would appear to be a priority for Bangkok if public transport is ever to compete with private cars.

Walking and cycling

Bangkok's level of walking and cycling is atypically low for an Asian urban environment. Much of this appears to be related to the hostile nature of the pedestrian environment and the absence of bike lanes or other facilities. Most main roads have poor footpaths and where they have been widened and perhaps planted with trees to relieve the hot climate, there is so much noise and fumes that walking is an ordeal.

The residential roads on which most of Bangkok is built are narrow, and those that connect them with major roads are particularly crowded with traffic and speeding motor bikes. Their narrowness, combined with the high walls which surround the houses, creates a very unattractive environment for pedestrians and cyclists, and there is almost nowhere to walk or cycle safely. For trips to the shopping areas on main roads or to catch buses, many people use hired motorcycles. If priority were given to improving pedestrian environments and facilities for walking and creating a shaded cycleway system, people would naturally choose non-motorized modes for short trips because they are the most convenient modes in dense environments with fine-grained mixed land uses. Tokyo strongly demonstrates this point.

Waterways

Water transport is an attractive, fast way to travel in Bangkok. It provides passengers with relief from the hot climate and separation from the fumes and noise of the roads. However, many canals have been filled in for roads and even the river is the focus of an attempt to build a floating freeway. Water transport's present contribution to passenger transport is thus very low, but with more and better boats, improved jetties and effective feeder services, waterway transport could be built up.

Paratransit

Bangkok's tuk-tuks, silor-leks and hired motorcycles currently fill an important transport niche and offer cheap fares. Their overall contribution to daily trips is very small when compared to buses and other modes, but could be improved by using them as formal feeder services to bus stops, piers and railway stations, and through improved shelters and government regulation to maintain vehicle standards and safety.

Roads

The big issue in Bangkok is roads. The majority of capital investment in transport goes into large road projects (Poboon and Kenworthy, 1995), and the dominant perception of the root of Bangkok's traffic problems is that there simply are not enough roads. Much is made of the fact that Bangkok has only 11% of its urbanized area devoted to roads whereas other cities have upwards of 20% (Tanaboriboon, 1993).

As shown in Figure 19.3, however, Bangkok is not atypical for an Asian city in the length of roads it provides per person. Indeed, Jakarta, Manila, Hong Kong and Surabaya provide less. To compare Bangkok's road area with that of other cities is difficult due to data availability problems. However, it is worth doing because this parameter incorporates road widths. Figure 19.12 draws together data on a number of cities and shows that Bangkok is not so unusually low (e.g. Paris, Hong Kong and Munich are almost identical to Bangkok in this factor).

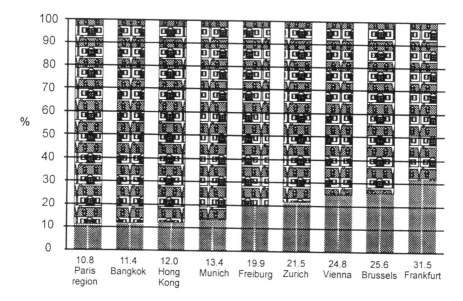

10.8   11.4   12.0   13.4   19.9   21.5   24.8   25.6   31.5
Paris   Bangkok   Hong   Munich   Freiburg Zurich   Vienna   Brussels Frankfurt
region   Kong

Figure 19.12   The percentage of urbanized land in Bangkok occupied by roads compared to a selection of global cities

The crux of the issue is that cities which have a low proportion of urbanized land under roads, also have extremely good public transport services, in particular, very good rail systems. They also have high levels of walking and cycling because of better infrastructure provision and environments more conducive to these modes. The important policy conclusion to be drawn from this is that Bangkok is not suffering so much from a lack of road space, as from a poorly developed transit system and a very low level of walking and cycling.

There is another very important point to stress here that is related to Bangkok's tightly woven urban fabric, which like many other Asian cities has not been built for the automobile. Non-motorized modes, especially waterway transport, were the basis of Bangkok's early development, followed by trams and buses. It is only since about 1980 that vehicle ownership and thus congestion have got out of control (Poboon *et al.*, 1994). It is certainly possible to try to accommodate Bangkok's growth in vehicles with an aggressive road building programme, but not without tearing apart the urban fabric.

Figure 19.13 estimates the results of trying to expand Bangkok's proportion of urban land devoted to roads from its present 11% up to 20%. Based on present average population and job densities, the new roads would displace the equivalent of a city the size of Chiang Mai. Resettling these people and employment enterprises at densities typical of the outer zone of Bangkok would require new land equivalent to 10% of Bangkok's present urbanized area.

equals....

Existing road space	3 844 ha	
Extra land needed for roads	2 888 ha	Lat Prao District
Displaced residents	469 000	City
Displaced jobs	145 800	of
Total activities displaced	615 100	Chiang Mai
Land required to resettle	14 598 ha	10% of BMA

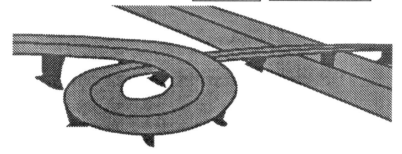

Figure 19.13   The implications of increasing the percentage of urbanized land under roads in Bangkok to 20%

Moreover, because they would be in automobile-dependent areas distant from public transport, they would themselves generate huge new volumes of traffic.

Air pollution

The transport patterns discussed in the previous sections are at least partly responsible for Bangkok's severe air pollution problem. Other important factors include climatic influences, less stringent motor vehicle standards and poor maintenance, especially of diesel fuelled trucks, buses and other vehicles. Although Bangkok does not presently experience photochemical smog (surface ozone) as in Los Angeles, it suffers from extremely high levels of suspended particulate matter (SPM) and high levels of carbon monoxide (CO) and lead (Pb). Boontherawara *et al.* (1994) report that SPM would have to come down by 84.9%, CO by 47.4% and Pb by 13.0% to reach proposed ambient air quality standards. Other emissions from transport such as nitrogen oxides (NO_x) and hydrocarbons (HC) are also a problem and Boontherawara *et al.* (1994) claim, based on WHO data, that all the major transport-related air pollutants in Bangkok are above the threshold considered harmful for human health.

General health impacts

Some general findings give an indication of the intensity of health impacts in Bangkok from traffic and associated air pollution. There is very high exposure to air pollution of a large proportion of Bangkok people as they negotiate the public environments of the city in non-air-conditioned buses or cars, in tuk-tuks and other forms of paratransit, on motorcycles and just walking along streets.

1. In 1990, over 1 million Bangkok residents received treatment for respiratory infections associated directly with air pollution (Magistad, 1991).
2. Particulate matter constitutes 'a serious threat to public health' and could lead to 1400 deaths per year (Mallet, 1992, quoted in Sayeg, 1992).
3. Bangkok's lung cancer rate is reportedly three times higher than elsewhere in Thailand (Magistad, 1991). (Differences in cigarette smoking, however, may partly account for this.)
4. A study of traffic exposed policemen versus non-traffic exposed policeman of the same age found that the incidence of respiratory health problems, as measured by a range of indicators, was higher in the traffic exposed group (Aekplakorn et al., 1991).
5. Transport is reportedly responsible for over one million cases of nervous disorders and anxieties from the strain and frustration of sitting in stalled traffic. Noise pollution from traffic is also another impact of concern (Sayeg, 1992).
6. Lead has been estimated to cause several hundred thousand cases of hypertension each year, up to 400 deaths, and possible, but as yet unproven, impacts on unborn foetuses (US Agency for International Development, 1990). One report suggests reduction of the IQ of an average Bangkok child by four points by the age of seven (Poboon and Kenworthy, 1995). Lead levels in some newborn babies are two to five times higher than those considered dangerous in the USA (Magistad, 1991). Food sold by the roadside is common in Bangkok and exacerbates lead intake.

Tackling air pollution

One of the most comprehensive studies to investigate the implications for transport policy of Bangkok's burgeoning air pollution comes from Boontherawara et al. (1994). The study, a direct result of the growing number and severity of transport-related health problems in Bangkok, attempted to model the transport and emissions impacts of a combination of three traffic scenarios and three technology scenarios for the year 2000 compared to 1994.

Traffic scenarios

1. Do nothing (1994 road network, no mass rapid transit);
2. Do as committed (more roads, mass rapid transit systems, truck terminals); or
3. Demand management (do as committed scenario, plus increased fuel prices, busways, bus signal priority in inner area, increase quality and quantity of buses, school bus system, traffic restraint projects).

Technology scenarios

1. Base case technology
2. Reasonable technology
3. Best technology

Two key results of the study were that:

1. Only the demand management scenario results in fewer total vehicle kilometres in the year 2000 than in 1994 (4.08 million compared to 4.38 million or a 7% reduction). The do-nothing approach entails a 15% increase, and the do-as-committed scenario, a 13% increase. The do-nothing approach maintains the automobile orientation of Bangkok but pushes new traffic away from gridlocked inner areas to middle and outer areas where some road capacity exists. The do-as-committed approach increases private vehicle travel by providing new roads, but replaces a considerable amount of existing car travel with use of the new mass transit systems.
2. In order to reduce SPM, CO and HC emissions to internationally acceptable standards, the only effective way for Bangkok is a demand management approach to transport planning in conjunction with the introduction of at least reasonable vehicle technology. That is, relying on technology *alone* is not enough for the desired overall improvement in air quality, though in conjunction with new transport projects, especially mass rapid transit, and transport demand management measures, air quality could be significantly improved.

Policy conclusions

This analysis suggests a range of essential policies which Bangkok needs to consider in order to begin resolving its desperate traffic situation and air pollution. These policies—discussed in detail in Poboon *et al.* (1994), Poboon and Kenworthy (1995), Kenworthy *et al.* (1994) and Barter *et al.* (1994)—can be summarized as follows.

Restraints on cars

This requires an economic approach in the form of increased vehicle taxes, registration duty and fuel tax and perhaps even a Singapore-style COE for car ownership. It also requires physical restraint and control of the level of CBD parking. Designating particular parts of inner Bangkok as pedestrian and public transport priority zones and at least some full-scale pedestrianization in central Bangkok would be appropriate.

Public transport development

To make restraints on private transport politically feasible, public transport would need to improve greatly. An absolute first priority is the establishment of a high quality mass rapid transit system, notwithstanding the enormous technical, institutional and political obstacles. Buses need to be given effective, enforceable priority in the traffic system in the form of bus-only lanes and bus-actuated signal priority, as well as improved waiting time, greater and more reliable transfers and improved vehicle quality. Waterway transport and paratransit modes need to be greatly improved.

Walking and cycling environments

In addition to pedestrianization in central locations, there needs to be a comprehensive programme to improve walking and cycling environments at a local and regional level. Shaded routes, continuity of footpaths and cycling routes, separation from dangerous traffic, noise abatement and bike facilities at destinations all need to be considered. If Tokyo can achieve 45% of daily trips on foot and bicycle, Bangkok must set its sights on more than its present 14%.

Transit-oriented, mixed use, development

Although much of Bangkok is already ideally suited to mass transit, there are enormous numbers of high-density apartments and dispersed townhouse and condominium developments being built with huge parking facilities and without any thought for public transport. In Europe and North America automobile dependence is being reduced through urban village style developments located around rail stations. These are high-density, mixed land use areas with minimal parking, with pedestrianized or traffic-calmed environments to encourage walking and cycling for local trips (Newman *et al.*, 1992). In Singapore and Hong Kong, it is an accepted model of urban development to focus a majority of new residential and commercial areas around stations on their mass rapid transit systems (Kenworthy *et al.*, 1994).

Institutional reform

Bangkok's quest to build a rail system has so far been thwarted by the plethora of agencies responsible for transport planning and implementation causing overlapping and conflicting mandates. There should be many fewer agencies, each with a clear-cut function, and overseen by a single coordinating committee with the authority for recommending decision-making to the government.

Adoption of stringent air emissions standards

Bangkok's current emissions standards for vehicles need to be strengthened to enforce the adoption of the best technology available for all types of vehicles. This would greatly enhance the positive impacts of other transport policies designed to minimize private travel.

A final word

Bangkok today is increasingly being referred to as the Los Angeles of the East. Although its present problems can be analysed and understood in a technical way using the data in this chapter, its problems extend deeper, as do those of Los Angeles. The transport and air pollution problems in these two cities stem from a lack of effective public planning for the 'common good' over many years.

Los Angeles has attempted to function almost totally on automobiles and has been reluctant to develop a public transport system of any significance or to control land use and car travel. The notion has been that if individuals are allowed to maximize their private good then the sum of these decisions will be a good city. This has not happened and Los Angeles is now one of the most problematic environments in the Western world. Bangkok too runs the risk of allowing itself to be plundered by private interests associated with road transport systems. Unless public planning for the common good can gain a foothold, as is now emerging in Los Angeles with the development of an extensive rail system, integration of some development around stations, and land use controls to minimize new travel, there is little hope that any of the policies outlined here can be implemented.

Acknowledgements

The illustrations in this chapter were drawn by Felix Laube, a PhD student in the Institute of Science & Technology Policy at Murdoch University. The research by PhD students Chamlong Poboon and Paul Barter in developing the data on Bangkok and Asian cities in newly industrializing countries is gratefully acknowledged. The data in this chapter on the less developed Asian cities represent the best available to date from studies and government sources.

References

Aekplakorn W, Metadilogkul O, Sawanpanyalert P, Rugronnayuth K (1991) *Comparison of Respiratory Health Between Traffic and Non-Traffic Policemen.* National Epidemiological Board, Thailand
Barter P, Kenworthy J, Poboon C, Newman P (1994) *The Challenge of Southeast Asia's*

Rapid Motorisation: Kuala Lumpur, Jakarta, Surabaya and Manila in an International Perspective. (Unpublished paper presented to Asian Studies Association of Australia Biennial Conference, 'Environment, State and Society in Asia: The Legacy of the Twentieth Century'; 13–16 July 1994, Asia Research Centre, Murdoch University, Perth)

Boontherawara N, Paisarnutpong O, Panich S *et al.* (1994) Traffic crisis and air pollution in Bangkok. *TEI Quarterly Environment Journal,* 2, 4–37

Kenworthy J (1994) Exit to Eden or highway to hell? *The Australian, (5 December 1994),* 9

Kenworthy J, Barter P, Newman P, Poboon C (1994) *Resisting Automobile Dependence in Booming Economies: A Case Study of Singapore, Tokyo and Hong Kong Within a Global Sample of Cities.* (Unpublished paper presented to Asian Studies Association of Australia Biennial Conference, 'Environment, State and Society in Asia: The Legacy of the Twentieth Century'; 13–16 July 1994, Asia Research Centre, Murdoch University, Perth)

Magistad MK (1991) Bangkok's progress marked by health hazards. *The Washington Post: Health Magazine Supplement, (7 May 1991),* 13

Mallet V (1992) Third World city, First World smog. *The Financial Times, (25 March 1992),* 11

Mallet V (1994) Thailand in driver's seat of Asia's accelerating car industry. *The Australian, (10 November 1994),* 39

Newman P, Kenworthy J (1989) *Cities and Automobile Dependence: An International Sourcebook.* Gower Publishing, Aldershot

Newman P, Kenworthy J, Robinson L (1992) *Winning back the Cities.* Australian Consumers Association/Pluto Press, Sydney

Panich S (1994) *Bangkok and its air pollution.* (Unpublished paper presented to the International Institute for Energy Conservation (IIEC) Workshop, 1–2 November, Sukhothai Hotel, Bangkok)

Poboon C, Kenworthy J, Newman P, Barter P (1994) *Bangkok: Anatomy of a Traffic Disaster.* (Unpublished paper presented to Asian Studies Association of Australia Biennial Conference, 'Environment, State and Society in Asia: The Legacy of the Twentieth Century'; 13–16 July, 1994, Asia Research Centre, Murdoch University, Perth)

Poboon C, Kenworthy J (1995) *Bangkok: Towards a Sustainable Traffic Solution.* (Unpublished paper presented to Urban Habitat Conference, Delft, 15–17 February)

Sayeg P (1992) *Assessment of Transportation Growth in Asia and its Effects on Energy Use, the Environment, and Traffic Congestion: Case Study of Bangkok, Thailand.* International Institute for Energy Conservation, Washington DC

Tanaboriboon Y (1993) Bangkok traffic. *Journal of International Association of Traffic and Safety Sciences,* 17, 14–23

United States Agency for International Development (1990) *Ranking Environmental Health Risks in Bangkok, Thailand: Volume 1.* USAID, Washington DC

20
Issues in planning for heterogeneous traffic: the case study of Delhi

Geetam Tiwari

Indian Institute of Technology, New Delhi, India

The Delhi metropolitan area is spread over 1483 square kilometres with an average population density of 5540 persons per square kilometre. The total population of Delhi is 8.2 million and the average annual growth rate is 4.5%. General trends of transport, socio-economic demographic patterns and travel characteristics are comparable to many other cities, especially in the low-income less motorized countries. These trends can be analysed at a disaggregated level to understand the close link between the transport system, socio-economic patterns and travel characteristics.

Transport system

Delhi has a road-based transport system. Commuter rail caters for a very small commuting population from the surrounding towns. Following the Delhi master plan, approximately 20% of the land area is devoted to the road network, compared to 6% in Calcutta and 17% in Madras (Table 20.1). The road network is used by at least seven categories of motorized and non-motorized modes. Delhi has the highest vehicle population—three times the average of Bombay, Calcutta and Madras. However, the percentage of two-wheelers is comparable to other metropolitan cities in India.

The variation in static dynamic and operating characteristics of these modes is given in Table 20.2. Vehicles ranging in width from 0.60 m to 2.6 m, and capable of maximum speeds ranging from 15 kmph to 100 kmph, share the same road space. Non-motorized vehicles (NMV) and motorized two-wheelers have freedom of lateral movement along with forward movement, thus interfering with the queues

Health at the Crossroads: Transport Policy and Urban Health.
Edited by Tony Fletcher and Anthony J. McMichael © 1997 John Wiley & Sons Ltd

Table 20.1 Transport infrastructure in selected metropolitan cities in India

City	Road length (km)	City area (km²)	Road length per 1000 population	Road length per 100 km²	Transport area as % of city area
Delhi	1595	446.3	0.28	357.38	21
Calcutta	840	568.0	0.09	147.68	6.4
Bombay	1423	438.0	0.17	233.83	NA
Madras	1670	572.0	0.39	291.96	17.0

NA: Not available.
Source: Central Institute of Road Transport (1988).

Table 20.2 Vehicle characteristics

Mode	Length (metres)	Breadth (metres)	Maximum speed (km/h)	Average occupancy	Fuel efficiency (km/l)
Car	2.5	1.5	100	2.4	10.9
TSR	2.5	1.3	45	1.8	20
Motorcycle	1.75	0.75	80	1.7	44.4
Bicycle	1.75	0.6	20	1.2	–
Bus	12	2.6	80	47	4.3
Cycle Rickshaw	2.0	1.3	15	2.5	–
Pedestrian	0.6	0.6	5		

TSR: Three-wheeler scooter rickshaw.
Source: Tata Energy Research Institute (1993) and manufacturers' publications.

of other motorized vehicles (Raghavachari and Badrinath, 1991). The occupants of these vehicles are vulnerable to impacts from motorized vehicles (MV). They are also exposed to the exhaust fumes of the MVs for longer time periods because of their slow speeds.

At present, the transport infrastructure of Delhi does not provide specific facilities for NMVs. The Delhi master plan prepared in 1961, and revised in 1971 and 1981, includes the provision of cycling tracks in some areas of Delhi. The tracks have not been planned as an integral part of the road network, i.e. they are discontinuous and have not been integrated at junctions. They have low utilization at places where they are partly implemented and, therefore, no further attempts were made to implement the complete network. Dedicated facilities for NMVs exist at some bridges and flyovers as a result of traffic management strategies conceived and planned by the Delhi traffic police.

In general, the road infrastructure in Delhi does not have any special provisions to meet the varying demands of different modes. Engineering design standards used in Delhi are similar to the recommended standards for homogeneous traffic (Indian Roads Congress, 1990).

Socio-economic patterns

Socio-economic characteristics coupled with land use patterns influence the travel demand (number of trips and mode choice). Vehicle ownership by different income groups reveals the role that each category of vehicle plays in providing mobility to different income groups (Table 20.3). Choice of mode depends on vehicle ownership and income level. The combined effect of land use patterns and the socio-economic status of people is reflected in distance to workplace and travel time to workplace (Table 20.4). A large percentage of low income people travel longer distances and spend 30–60 minutes on one-way travel. The majority of middle income and high income people have lower trip

Table 20.3   Personal vehicle ownership pattern

Household monthly income (Rs)	Percentage of households with		
	Cycle only	MTW only	Car only
<1000	37	12	–
1001–2500	13	39	1
2501–5000	11	53	10
>5000	2	64	35
All	13	45	15

MTW: Motorized two-wheeler.
Source: Central Institute of Road Transport (1988).

Table 20.4   Home–work distance distribution for various income households in Delhi

Household monthly income (Rs)	Percentage of households at			
	<3 km	4–10 km	11–20 km	> 20 km
<500	16.2	41.9	38.7	3.2
501–1000	21.2	37.9	34.2	6.7
1001–1500	16.5	43.2	30.0	10.3
1501–2500	22.1	39.3	31.4	7.2
2501–3500	17.7	44.0	31.3	7.0
3501–5000	19.5	37.3	32.0	11.2
>5000	19.6	39.1	31.2	10.1
Not stated	27.7	33.7	31.7	6.9

Source: Central Road Research Institute (1992).

times and travel distance than the average values for the whole population. Since the number of people in the lower income group is much greater than in the high income group, and the trend is not likely to change in the foreseeable future, the importance of NMVs in providing mobility to a large section of the population will not diminish.

One objective in land use distribution and density patterns as envisaged in the Delhi masterplan has been to contain the average trip length. A total of 23 commercial district centres have been planned along the periphery of the city. Rising land prices are another important factor which have contributed to the growth of mixed land use patterns and higher densities. In the past decade, a large number of single family dwelling units have been converted to multi-storeyed flats, and space has been rented to and bought by commercial and institutional organizations by outbidding the residential occupants. Mixed land use patterns have been successful in curbing the number and lengths of primarily non-work-related trips by motorized modes. The number of trips per household for different purposes remains constant, regardless of whether a person is living in the 'inner area', which has a heavy concentration of employment and commercial activities, or the 'outer areas' where new developments have been planned.

Despite these efforts to promote mixed land use planning, the presence and growth of 'unauthorized settlements' and pavement dwellings defy the masterplan. Nearly 40% of Delhi's population lives in these units with a minimal supply of drinking water, sewage disposal and electricity. A large number of people living in these units are employed in the informal sector, providing various kinds of services at low wages. In the mid 1970s, there was a conscious effort to move these people to the outer areas of the city where the new developments had been planned. However, due to lack of employment opportunities, people living in these areas have to commute long distances across the city in search of employment. NMV traffic in the outer areas is much higher, compared to the middle and central areas in Delhi. Unlike the traffic in highly motorized countries (HMCs), NMVs are present in significant numbers on the arterial roads and intercity highways which are designed for the fast-moving, uninterrupted flow of motorized vehicles.

The presence of an active informal sector introduces a high degree of heterogeneity in the socio-economic and land use system. These people are out of the formal housing market, and are incapable of making direct payments for minimal urban amenities. However, they are an integral part of the urban landscape, providing a variety of services at low wages, at locations where there is high demand for these services. Hawkers, pavement shops, cycle and motor vehicle part repair shops are viewed as unauthorized developments along the road, reducing the capacity of the planned network. However, since the market demands these services, they continue to exist and grow along the arterial roads as well.

The impact of heterogeneity

Flow patterns

The traffic flow observed on the network is the result of continuous interaction between the various modes (transport system) and demands of people in different income groups. This involves several levels of equilibrium flows. Each level has different requirements for efficient and safe movement. An ideal solution would be to provide a separate infrastructure for each flow pattern. On the other hand, the presence of all levels on the same infrastructure results in the trade-off of benefits between levels. For example, motorized vehicles cannot have uninterrupted flows because of the presence of NMVs. On the other hand, NMV occupants are exposed to higher risks of traffic crashes because of high-speed motorized vehicles.

The different flows not only have different, but often, conflicting requirements. Buses need frequent stops to pick up and drop passengers; however, private cars need uninterrupted movement. Motorized vehicles need clear pavements and roads, while bicyclists and pedestrians need shaded trees along the pavement to protect them from the summer sun.

The heterogeneous traffic flow is described as 'chaotic' by people used to measuring homogeneous traffic, because vehicles do not follow car-following logic. The variation in vehicle sizes and their acceleration permits them to advance through the roadway network by weaving through available gaps. This results in high conflict (as per the standard definition of conflict, Fazio and Tiwari, 1995) and reduced flow rates if measured in terms of vehicles per hour. Journey speeds of cars and other motorized vehicles are also affected by this. In Delhi, the speed of cars in central areas ranges from 10 to 15 kmph, and 25 to 40 kmph on arterial streets. Frequent braking and acceleration (75% on Delhi roads compared to 30% in the USA), reduces journey speeds and adversely affects the fuel consumption and emissions because the present motorized vehicles are not designed to operate in mixed traffic conditions.

Public health risks

The adverse effects of heterogeneous traffic flowing on an infrastructure designed to cater for the needs of motorized vehicles only is reflected in increasing air pollution and a phenomenal increase in traffic crashes. The World Health Organization (WHO) has classified Delhi as one of the ten most polluted cities in the world along with Mexico City, Seoul and Beijing. An estimated 1300 million tonnes of pollutants were emitted by the vehicles in Delhi in 1992, which is almost 50% more than in 1987 (CPCB, 1993). Estimation of eight-hourly average concentrations of different pollutants due to vehicular emissions alone on five major corridors in Delhi (Table 20.5) was found to exceed the ambient standards laid down by the Central Pollution Control Board (TERI, 1993).

Table 20.5 Estimated maximum ground level concentration of various pollutants due to vehicular emissions only on selected corridors in Delhi ($\mu g/m^3$)

Corridor	CO	HC	NO_x	SO_2	TSP	Pb
Minto Road	*5231*	*1962*	*252*	27	3	*3.5*
L.B. Road	*8500*	*2515*	*503*	42	4.5	*5.5*
M.G. Road	3923	*1308*	604	90	16	*2.5*
G.T. Road	*5281*	*3018*	101	28	3	*3*
Shahdra Mathura Road	1408	352	*352*	52	9.6	1

Note: 1. The values correspond to wind velocity of 2.1 m/s.
2. The italic values exceed the Indian standards for ambient air quality.
CO, carbon monoxide; HC, hydrocarbon; NO_x, nitrogen oxides; SO_2, sulphur dioxide; TSP, total suspended particulate; Pb, lead.
Source: Tata Energy Research Institute (1993).

Despite low vehicle ownership rates compared to HMCs, the number of crashes and fatalities has been rising in Delhi. In 1993, the city of Delhi had approximately 1900 reported traffic fatalities; more than double the total of all the other major Indian cities combined (*Indian Express*, 1994). This reflects the high proportion of both MVs and NMVs on Delhi roads. Most traffic fatalities involve collision between MVs and NMVs (Table 20.6). NMV users constitute 54% of the fatalities. The majority of crashes occur on straight stretches on divided roads (Tiwari, 1993). Buses and trucks are involved in more than 50% of the fatal crashes.

Issues for discussion

Consideration of total system

Traffic flow is the result of continuous interaction between socio-economic patterns and available transport technologies. The variations in transport modes and the volume and direction of travel are a reflection of the hierarchical structure of society and land use patterns. Therefore, the problems of traffic flow must be analysed in the context of social environment.

Conflicting requirements

1. Users of different transport modes have conflicting requirements. Motorized vehicles need clear roads for uninterrupted traffic flow, whereas bicyclists and pedestrians need shady trees, kiosks for drinks, food and bicycle repair shops etc. at shorter distances.
2. Motorized vehicles are designed to operate at much higher speeds for better fuel economy and emission levels than those recommended from the safety point of view for the NMV occupants and pedestrians.

Table 20.6   Distribution of road traffic fatalities in Delhi

Victims	Struck by									
	Pedes-trian	Bicycle	MTW	TSR	Car	Bus	Truck	Other	Unknown	Total (%)
Pedestrian	–	–	29	19	35	154	99	22	110	468 (42)
Bicycle	–	1	6	1	6	39	50	13	18	134 (12)
MTW	2	2	15	1	20	88	67	30	27	252 (23)
TSR	–	–	–	4	1	13	8	2	1	29 (3)
Car	–	–	–	–	3	3	8	3	–	17 (1)
Bus	2	–	1	–	–	47	10	47	–	107 (107)
Truck	–	–	–	–	1	4	15	11	–	31 (3)
Other	–	–	–	1	3	12	29	12	5	62 (5)
Unknown	–	–	–	1	–	2	–	1	10	14 (1)
Total	4	3	51	27	69	362	286	141	171	1114
(%)	(0.3)	(0.3)	(4)	(2)	(6)	(32)	(26)	(13)	(16)	(100)

MTW: Motorized two-wheelers; TSR: three-wheeler scooter rickshaw.
Source: Mohan and Bawa (1985).

Conflict resolution implies trade-offs

The requirements of any one particular group are met at the cost of others. If the infrastructure design encourages high speed, occupants of NMVs are exposed to higher risks. Mixed traffic flows have frequent braking and acceleration, reduction in average speeds and fuel efficiency of motorized vehicles. However, it provides higher mobility to a larger section of the population who cannot afford automobiles.

Transport planning needs to incorporate heterogeneity

The present methodologies for traffic planning and evaluation reflect the need and biases of one class of road users. Consequently, the present traffic infrastructure leads to suboptimal performance of various modes. A solution to the problems of heterogeneous traffic lies in recognizing the presence of heterogeneity in the socio-economic and transport environment. Planning and evaluation method-ologies based on this premise can lead to sustainable solutions.

References

Central Institute of Road Transport (1988) *Transportation in Eleven Cities*. Report submitted to the Ministry of Surface Transport, New Delhi, India
Central Pollution Control Board (1993) *Pollution Statistics of Delhi*. CPCB, Delhi, India
Central Road Research Institute (1992) *Development of Traffic and Transport Flow Data Base for Road System in Delhi Urban Area*. CRRI, Delhi, India
Fazio J, Tiwari G (1995) Nonmotorised-motorised Traffic Accidents and Conflicts on Delhi Streets. Presented at the 74th Annual Meeting of the Transportation Research Board, Washington, DC, USA

Indian Express (1994) Newspaper article, Saturday 26 February, Better Policing Urged. New Delhi, India

Indian Institute of Petroleum (1985) *State of Art Report on Vehicle Emissions.* Dehradun, India

Indian Roads Congress (1990) Guidelines for Capacity of Urban Roads in Plain Areas. *Journal of Indian Roads Congress,* paper no. 105

Mohan D, Bawa P (1985) An analysis of road traffic fatalities in Delhi, India. *Accident Analysis and Prevention, 17(1),* 33–45

Raghavachari S, Badrinath K M (1991) Accident Causative Factors Under Mixed Traffic Conditions. A case study of Hyderabad city. International Conference on Traffic Safety, New Delhi, India

Tata Energy Research Institute (1993) *Impact of Road Transportation Systems on Energy and Environment: An Analysis of Metropolitan Cities of India.* Final report submitted to Ministry of Urban Development, Government of India

Tiwari G (1993) Pedestrians and Bicycle Crashes in Delhi. Second World Conference on Injury Control, Atlanta, USA

21
Shaping transport and health policy: a case study in the Boston Metropolitan Area, Massachusetts, USA

Daniel S. Greenbaum

Health Effects Institute, Cambridge, Massachusetts, USA

The Greater Boston Metropolitan Area comprises the eastern portion of the State of Massachusetts, bordering on the Atlantic Ocean in the north-eastern United States. The region covers 1400 square miles (3600 square kilometres) and includes approximately 2.9 million inhabitants, centred around the city of Boston, Massachusetts (population 600 000). The region is one of the ten largest metropolitan areas in the United States.

One of the oldest urban areas in the United States, the region developed until the mid-1940s in a compact fashion, with development clustered around a concentrated urban core in Boston and immediately surrounding communities, and largely delimited by the extent of rail and street car transportation lines.

Following the Second World War, increased prosperity, the desire to provide individual homes for returning servicemen, and the low price of petrol, contributed to the development of a series of national and state government policies which dramatically reshaped the patterns of development in the region. Extensive construction by the state and federal governments of high-speed, radial and circumferential highways, and government-subsidized loans for new single-family homes, accelerated the development of widespread, largely unplanned development throughout the metropolitan area, which for the first time was independent of the rail and other public transportation infrastructure which had previously been the major constraint on sprawl.

This rapid development had several consequences. Car travel grew exponentially, resulting by the mid-1960s in substantial traffic congestion, in particular on

Health at the Crossroads: Transport Policy and Urban Health.
Edited by Tony Fletcher and Anthony J. McMichael © 1997 John Wiley & Sons Ltd

routes to and from jobs in the urban core. Communities throughout the region began, somewhat belatedly, to develop and strengthen land use plans and controls, but these efforts were hindered by land use control authority which was widely scattered (there are 101 individual cities and towns, with the only overarching planning organization—the Metropolitan Area Planning Council—being an advisory one). As use of the private car expanded, use of rail and other transportation declined, causing privately owned transportation services to close, reduce service, or be taken over by public authorities; public transportation services to require ever-increasing public subsidies to continue to operate; and in general a reduced investment in maintaining and upgrading these services. Thus, the Greater Boston public transportation system, the first of its kind in the United States, and one of the most extensive for the population served, was in serious decline.

The 1970s: changing priorities and policies

In the late 1960s and 1970s, several factors combined to alter these trends dramatically. First, the growing congestion reached a level of intense public and political concern, and calls from the business community and many political leaders raised pressure for reducing congestion through major investments in completing the radial and circumferential highway system. Specifically, there were proposals to build a new circumferential route through the urban core and extend the radial routes into the core.

At the same time, the 1970s ushered in an increased national and regional awareness of the environment and public health, with the passage in 1970 of national, and corresponding state, legislation such as the National Environmental Policy Act (which required a comprehensive analysis of the environmental and health effects of new highways and other transportation infrastructure before they were built), and the National Clean Air Act (which required the establishment of national health-based standards for air pollutants such as carbon monoxide and ozone, and required each metropolitan area in the country which violated these standards to implement plans to reduce pollution to acceptable levels).

In Boston, environmental concerns took two forms. First, there was growing concern among urban planners and citizens that the disruption and dislocation caused by new highway construction in the urban core would destroy neighbourhoods, harm the health and well-being of urban residents (many of whom were poor), and undermine the fabric of urban life by making it easier for wealthier residents to build homes far outside the city, and drive in to work. Second, there was also recognition among political leaders and citizens that the region regularly exceeded national, health-based standards for carbon monoxide (which comes largely from cars), and ground-level ozone (which is created by the mixture and transformation of emissions from a variety of sources, including cars).

A third factor which changed in the 1970s was the cost and availability of petrol as motor fuel. As a result of the world oil embargo in 1973, and the second round of embargo in 1978–79, the price of a gallon of petrol rose from under 30 cents per gallon, to over $1.20. These prices, while still low by international standards, represented a greater than fourfold increase over only six years. When combined with the occurrence of actual fuel shortages, these changes had a tremendous impact on public perception of transport options and solutions.

The result of these three factors was an intense public debate about the right transport policies to pursue to address congestion, environmental, and health concerns. Coalitions of urban citizens and regional environmentalist and health advocates argued strongly for stopping new highway construction, and reinvesting in public transport. Suburban citizens and businesses argued for continuing the road construction programmes and cautioned that stopping such programmes would choke off economic investment and well-being in the urban core. After a tumultuous debate (Lupo *et al.*, 1971) the region chose not to continue the traditional approach of building more highways but rather to implement a series of transport policies which sought to reverse the 25-year trend towards relying solely on the single-occupant car for urban and regional transport. These policies included:

1. **1970**: The then Governor of the State of Massachusetts, Mr Francis Sargent, after an extensive and public debate, announced that the state would abandon plans to complete the radial and circumferential highway system into and around Boston. In its place, the state would invest hundreds of millions of dollars in extending and upgrading the metropolitan rapid transit system, as well as in improved bus service, bicycle paths, and other alternatives to the car.
2. **1975**: As one part of its response to the National Clean Air Act, the Massachusetts Department of Environmental Protection imposed parking freezes on all commercial parking facilities in downtown Boston, the adjoining city of Cambridge, and the nearby Logan International Airport. These freezes, which did not allow the construction of any new commercial spaces unless they were accompanied by a reduction elsewhere in the freeze area, were intended to limit car-related development in the urban core and to cause a rise in the price of parking, which in turn would make the use of public transport more attractive economically, encourage drivers to shift to multiple occupant vehicles, and reduce air pollutant emissions from cars.
3. **1979**: In response to the second oil embargo, the State of Massachusetts promulgated a detailed and comprehensive ride-sharing rule, requiring all companies throughout the Greater Boston region which employed 100 or more individuals to develop and implement proactive programmes and incentives to increase substantially the percentage of their employees who came to work in other than single-occupancy vehicles.

In addition to these measures, throughout the 1970s a number of measures were implemented on the national level to increase fuel efficiency and reduce emissions of pollutants from new cars. The average fuel efficiency of the new car fleet nearly doubled during this period, and the average emissions from each vehicle were reduced by over 80%.

The results: some success, substantial problems remain

The immediate results of these policies, when combined with the underlying economic factors brought on by the oil embargo, were positive. The vehicle miles travelled into and out of the urban core slowed their rapid increase and in the late 1970s actually declined slightly (Falbel, personal communication, 1995). In large measure because of the substantial investment in new and improved rapid transit, the percentage of commuting employees travelling to the urban core in other than single-passenger cars continued to exceed 50% which, while lower than much of the rest of the world, is higher than most other metropolitan areas in the United States. Entirely new commuting services, such as a commuter boat service from south of Boston, were initiated and prospered.

For several years in the early 1980s, employers actively pursued their ride-sharing programmes, reporting their progress annually to the state Department of Environmental Protection, and offering their employees car-pooling incentives, opportunities to join low-cost vanpools, and subsidized passes for the metropolitan transit system. As a result of these and other measures to reduce air pollution, the number of days on which the Greater Boston area exceeded national air quality standards began to decline (Massachusetts Department of Environmental Protection, 1982).

At the same time, the 1980s saw a substantial increase in the development and redevelopment of Boston itself, seeming to confirm the arguments of those who advocated these policies that it was possible to have economic development without depending solely on the car for transportation.

These positive results were, however, overshadowed in the mid-1980s by a series of trends which undermined their effectiveness, and ultimately have led to a worsening of some of the original problems.

First, since most of these policies were aimed at reducing car travel into and out of the urban core, they did little or nothing to reduce, and may have caused an increase in, development along the circumferential highways ringing the metropolitan area. During the period 1970–90, for example, while employment in the urban core grew by 100 000 jobs, employment grew in the surrounding suburbs by over 400 000 (Falbel, personal communication, 1995). There were few constraints on this development, land costs were lower, and parking was not expensive to build, and provided free to employees and shoppers.

Second, the price rises in petrol of the 1970s stopped, as the turmoil on world oil markets subsided. Though prices stayed generally at their 1979 levels in absolute terms, in real dollar terms (adjusted for inflation), the cost of petrol began to decline. By the early 1990s, the inflation-adjusted price of petrol had declined to a level equal to, or slightly below the levels in 1973. This, along with stability of supplies, effectively eliminated the economic incentive which had driven much of the gain in the early 1980s.

Third, some of the policies, such as the parking freezes and ride-sharing rules, were complicated to implement and enforce, and sophisticated developers and businesses began to exploit what were originally considered narrow exceptions in the rules. Thus, over 9000 new parking spaces were added in Boston during the 'freeze' in the 1980s and businesses soon abandoned their efforts to implement the ride-sharing rule, in the face of diminishing public concern about energy prices and supplies, and diminished attention from the state agencies charged with enforcing the rules.

Finally, but by no means least importantly, the Massachusetts economy grew very rapidly in the period 1983–87, due to a number of positive economic factors nationally and regionally. Personal incomes rose substantially, and the ability to own a home, and purchase a first or additional vehicle, rose proportionately (Metropolitan Area Planning Council, 1989).

Lessons to be learned

While it may be tempting for those elsewhere in the world, where petrol prices are substantially higher and car ownership substantially lower, to write off this experience in the United States as not relevant to their own situation and experience, there are several lessons to learn from this case which would argue that that is not so.

Lesson 1. Urban health and social well-being considerations can be a significant contributor to shaping transport policy, though it is unlikely that they are sufficient in and of themselves.

There is no question that the concerns over urban air quality and general welfare were a factor in building the alliance of strong political support which led to the striking reversal in transport policy in the Greater Boston area in the 1970s. It is not clear, however, that they would have had as much impact in the absence of the other major motivating factor, the world oil crises of 1973, and 1978–79.

Lesson 2. Transport policy cannot effectively address problems of congestion and health impacts unless accompanied by a strong and effective programme of regional land use management and control.

Despite several strong and potentially effective transport policy decisions designed to reduce congestion and improve public health, the absence of any long-term, regional, land use strategy meant that when economic growth began to occur, it occurred along the same decentralized patterns as had growth prior to the transport decisions, soon voiding any positive benefits from the original policy decisions. In addition, to the extent that land use controls were adopted (e.g. the parking freezes), their effectiveness was limited by their complexity and the lack of sustained support for implementing them.

Lesson 3. Transport and land use policies, if focused primarily on addressing issues of congestion and health in the urban core, can inadvertently hasten the development of land use patterns that significantly worsen regional congestion and health problems.

The Greater Boston transport policies focused almost entirely on reducing congestion into and out of the urban core. During the period of their implementation, traffic and congestion in suburban and fringe areas grew substantially faster than travel to and from the core, in part hastened by the fact that the adopted policies increased the cost of developing facilities in the core and made the outer areas comparatively more attractive.

Lesson 4. The price of transportation (e.g. fuel costs, parking, etc.) can be an effective deterrent to rapidly increasing traffic and associated health effects, but that effectiveness may be due more to perceived changes in that price, rather than to the absolute level.

The dramatic increase in fuel prices in the United States in the 1970s was the single most effective factor in altering travel behaviour, improving fuel efficiency, and reducing, albeit temporarily, congestion. Since the early 1980s, however, and despite the fact that absolute prices have remained stable, rising personal incomes, and continued inflation of other items, have all but negated this powerful original price incentive. As a variety of new 'pricing' policies are considered for transport policy (e.g. congestion pricing, 'pay at the pump', emissions fees) it is important that the perception of the level of such prices over the long term, and not just the initial rise in prices, be factored into their design and implementation.

Lesson 5. The personal freedom offered by the car is intensely attractive, and once land use patterns which assume the availability of that personal freedom begin to emerge, it is very difficult to gain the support to alter or contain them to address issues of urban health and congestion.

The land use patterns put in place in the 1950s and 1960s in the United States were developed largely independent of existing public transportation infrastructure. Once those patterns, which assume widespread trip origins and widespread trip destinations, were in place, the development of policies to reverse them, in the absence of stringent new land use controls and extensive new investment in circumferential transit infrastructure, was nearly impossible. For those countries which are only now beginning to experience these land use changes (through increased vehicle ownership and rising personal incomes), this may be the most important lesson to be learned from the Massachusetts experience.

Postscript: transport and urban health policy in the 1990s

In the late 1980s, as congestion again grew, and air pollution rose, renewed public concern about air pollution and public health led to calls for action, and the enactment, in 1990, of sweeping new amendments to the National Clean Air Act. Those amendments include a number of measures to reduce air pollution from mobile sources, including new vehicle emissions standards, requirements for cleaner fuels, and a series of transportation control measures which the most seriously polluted metropolitan areas in the country are expected to implement. While the improvements in vehicle technology and fuels are moving forward, the transportation control measures have encountered intense opposition throughout the United States and, at the time of writing, are being reassessed. In the absence of other motivating factors to address travel behaviour (for example, a world oil crisis), it is unlikely that any significantly greater changes in behaviour will occur in the 1990s than in the 1970s. While there will be improvements in air pollution due to technology improvements, it is likely that these improvements will be, as they were between 1970 and 1990, offset by continuing increases in the vehicle miles travelled throughout the United States.

References

Falbel SM (1989) *The Demographics of Commuting in Greater Boston.* Massachusetts Executive Office of Transportation and Construction, Boston (Massachusetts)
Lupo A, Colcord F, Fowler EP (1971) *Rites of Way: The Politics of Transportation in Boston and the US City.* Little, Brown, Boston
Massachusetts Department of Environmental Protection (1982) *Reasonable Further Progress; Implementation of the Clean Air Act in Massachusetts.* MDEP, Boston
Metropolitan Area Planning Council (1989) *MetroPlan 2000: A Regional Plan for Metropolitan Boston.* MAPC, Boston

22
Transport in London and the implications for health

Jake Ferguson and Mark McCarthy

Camden and Islington Health Authority, London, UK

London is situated at the heart of the South East of England and covers an area of approximately 610 square miles. It is divided into 33 administrative boroughs of which 13 (including the City of London) lie in the Inner London Region and 20 in the Outer London Region. Together they make up Greater London which is bounded by the Green Belt.

This chapter describes the development of transport in London and the problems that London's increasing traffic volume poses for the health of its 6.3 million residents.

Transport networks

The history of travel in London

In the nineteenth century London was a rapidly expanding economic and industrial centre and had a transport system to match, with the world's first steam underground (1863) and the first electric tube railway (1890). The Underground became fully electric by 1907.

In 1820 London's population stood at just 1.5 million. Most journeys were by foot. Horse-drawn stage coaches served the outer districts, and only Hackney carriages were allowed to operate in the busy centre. Outward development of London was primarily along the main roads and the River Thames. The introduction of electric trams and motor buses meant people could cover longer distances with greater ease, promoting outward development and urban expansion. This allowed poorer people to live further out and encouraged speculative building near the new railways and Underground stations.

Public transport continued to develop in the first half of the twentieth century

Health at the Crossroads: Transport Policy and Urban Health.
Edited by Tony Fletcher and Anthony J. McMichael © 1997 John Wiley & Sons Ltd

but slowed thereafter. In 1948, buses made 4000 million journeys a year, falling in 1988–89 to 1200 million per year, as use of London's roads by cars and commercial vehicles increased. In 1846 Parliament decreed that no main line railways could enter the central area, so underground railways were built to join main line termini. Between the years 1907–40, the Underground was extended out into the countryside, and in the west buses fed the services it offered. The Underground continued to grow into the suburbs and improved in the centre with the introduction of the Victoria Line. The Jubilee Line Extension currently under construction will link the main line termini King's Cross, St Pancras, Euston and Victoria to Canary Wharf in the Docklands development.

After the Second World War the Green Belt restricted London's natural growth outwards, but urbanization continued beyond the Green Belt, increasing commuting distance. Cars became the dominant form of transport for non-central trips in London in the 1950s and 1960s. Motorways attracted large numbers of radial commuters, increasing commuter traffic further, with limited park-and-ride facilities outside the centre. Today, commuters are the cause of most private car traffic in the city (Figure 22.1)

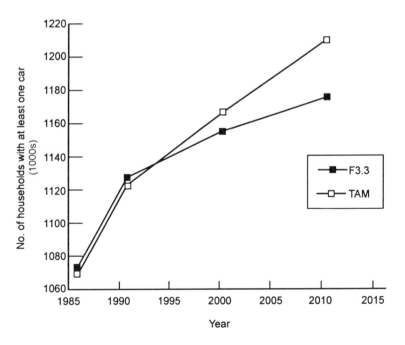

Figure 22.1   Increase in car ownership: Greater London. Source: MVA Consultancy, 1994

Travel surveys

The London Area Transport Survey

The London Area Transport Survey (LATS) (London Research Centre, 1994) was conducted in 1991 by the UK Department of Transport in partnership with the London Research Centre (which acted on behalf of the London boroughs). The data were collected in a number of different ways including a household survey and a roadside interview survey. The area studied was the area within the M25 London Orbital Motorway (and parts of two London boroughs that extend outside this motorway).

Weekday travel in Inner London is dominated by the car and walking. In Outer London the car is the most popular, with fewer people on foot. The number of people using public transport, that is the London Bus, the Underground and British Rail, is greater in Inner London in relation to other modes of transport than it is in Outer London. The use of taxis and pedal cycles is similarly greater in Inner London. The bus has seen a decline in use, from 1502 million bus passengers annually in 1970, to 1112 million passengers in 1993—a decrease of over 25%. Underground passengers remain relatively stable, 775 million in 1991 and 750 million in 1994.

The London Area Transport Survey (LATS) suggests that the number of people cycling in London has declined by 30% since 1981, although on London's central streets there has been a proliferation of cycle couriers. Cycling is more popular amongst men than women. On a typical day, 3% of males over the age of 5 travel by bicycle, compared with just 1% of females. In London there are approximately 12 million bicycles in present ownership. However, only 1 in 10 are used on any given weekday.

Most journeys involve some walking, and although the LATS study did not include journeys of less than 200 metres or two minutes in duration, Londoners make over 4 million trips where walking is the only form of transport. Women make approximately 14% more journeys on foot than men.

The Transport Prediction Model 'F3.3'

The MVA Consultancy prepares predictions of future London travel for the Government Office for London using complex computer models. The F3.3 model is the latest, revised in 1994, and uses demographic data from the 1991 Office of Population Censuses and Surveys (OPCS) survey. Forecasts of demographic changes are provided by the London Research Centre with car ownership changes from the Department of Transport forecasts. The forecasts also include employment changes and changes to public transport and highways over future years.

The forecasts are divided by the time of day (morning, inter and evening peaks) and divided by region using the GLC boundary as the outer cordon, an Inner London boundary and a central cordon.

The use of the car in London and the rest of Britain is predicted to continue to increase on its present levels. The total number of car/light goods vehicle trips made wholly or partly within the Greater London area on an average weekday in 1991 was estimated at over 8 million trips undertaken between 07.00–19.00. By 2001, the number of person/light goods vehicle trips made will have increased by 13% and to 24% by the year 2011 (Figure 22.2).

The number of inbound cars crossing the outer cordon between 07.00–19.00 is predicted to increase 26% by the year 2011—a further 209 000 vehicles entering Greater London. This trend reflects increased commuting by car/light goods vehicle from outside the Greater London area.

In Greater London, the number of households with cars is predicted to increase into the next century. By the year 2011, there will be an estimated 4% more households with one car and 58% more households with two or more cars, from 1991 figures.

Public transport passenger trips in Greater London are predicted to increase by 0.4% and 5.7% for the years 2001 and 2011 respectively. During the morning peak period (07.00–10.00) in Central London, British Rail are predicted to see an increase of 5.4% and 29.5% in passenger travel from 1991 in the years 2001 and 2011 (these increases are related to future plans to expand rail services entering London, for example, Cross Rail and the Thameslink). The Underground will also see an overall increase in the number of passengers of 9.5% to 2001

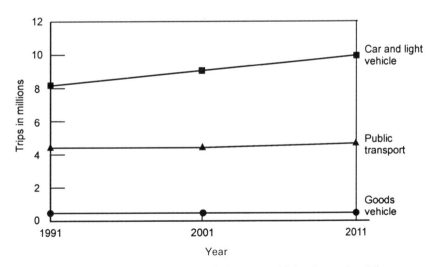

Figure 22.2 Predictions of the numbers of highway vehicle trips and public transport trips made wholly or partly in Greater London between 07.00–19.00 on an average weekday. Source: MVA Consultancy, 1994

over 1991 levels, but this will fall after the turn of the century to 5.3% over 1991 levels.

Bus passenger travel, which must compete with the car for city road space, is predicted to see a decline with 10.4% fewer passengers in 2001 and to 2011 an 18.4% decline from 1991 levels.

The forecast average speeds across London are predicted to decrease further, with an average speed in Central London over the three hour peak of just under 10 miles per hour.

It is of note that the F3.3 model does not predict the number of pedestrians or cyclists using Londons walkways and roads.

Accident patterns

This section describes the accident trends and patterns in Greater London using data provided by the London Research Centre's Accident Analysis Unit (LAAU). Casualty (injury and death) figures are often used to describe the degree of danger on London's roads, but they are not a true indicator of road safety.

In 1993, 45 801 road traffic casualties were reported in Greater London. There has been a downward trend in total casualties over the last 10 years, although casualties injured in cars account for about half of all casualties, and are not decreasing (Figure 22.3). However, this information must be examined carefully, since it provides no data on the numbers of users of each type of transport.

Age is an important determinant of mode of travel. For instance, people over sixty are much more likely to travel by public service vehicle than by motorbike. This is reflected in the casualty data. The largest percentage of casualties on pedal cycles, motorbikes, car drivers and car passengers is in the 25–59 age category. However, on public service vehicles approximately the same number of those over 60 are injured or killed as those in the 25–59 age group.

Children under 16 years make up 12% of all casualties. About 19% are injured going to or from school. Fifty-one per cent are injured as pedestrians, 29% as car occupants and 13% as cyclists.

In 1993, 58% of all casualties were male and 42% female. As pedestrians, there were 26% more male casualties than female (5588 compared with 4106). As cyclists, there were 74% more male casualties and as car drivers and passengers there were slightly more female car casualties (11 338 compared with 10 486) reflected, in part, by the larger percentage of car passenger casualties (64% female).

Casualty rates

Although they are not a true indicator of danger, the casualty rates by mode of transport allow comparisons to be made. Table 22.1 suggests that travelling by two-wheeled vehicles has the highest casualty rates—thirty times higher than

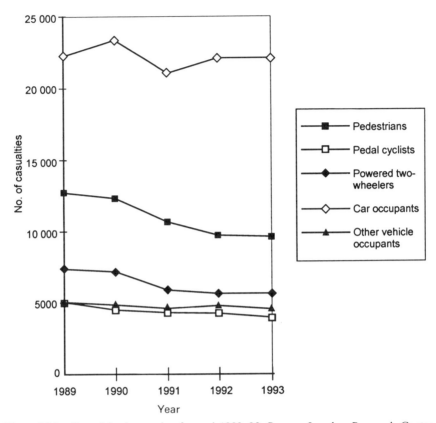

Figure 22.3   Casualties by mode of travel 1989–93. Source: London Research Centre, Annual Report, 1993

casualty rates per journey by car. Travelling by pedal cycle has the second highest casualty rates. For the number of passenger journeys, travelling by foot has equal casualty rates to that of a car. Bus, rail and air travel have the lowest casualty rates.

Air and noise pollution in London

Air pollution levels

In 1991 107 sites in the UK exceeded the EC Guide Value for nitrogen dioxide. Out of the 20 sites with the highest concentrations 17 are in London. (Bell, 1993)

Nitrogen dioxide (NO_2), one of the most dangerous air pollutants, has reached unprecedented levels in the UK, especially in London. Research conducted by the

Table 22.1 Passenger casualty rates (per 100 million killed and seriously injured)by mode of travel for Great Britain

Mode	Passenger kilometres	Passenger journeys	Passenger hours
Car	4.5	55	190
Van	2.4	30	75
TWMV	150.0	1600	4500
Pedal cycle	85.0	230	1200
Foot	55.0	55	225
Bus or coach	1.6	13	40
Rail	0.4	9	15
Water	4.6	170	90
Air	0.04	70	20

Source: GB Department of Transport (1994c).
TWMV, two-wheeled motor vehicle.
1992 rates except air and rail: average rates 1975–92; bus or coach: average rate 1988/9–1992/3; water: average rate 1983–92.

Warren Spring Laboratory (Campbell *et al.*, 1992) showed that in December 1991 the hourly average concentration of nitrogen dioxide in London exceeded 400 ppb in some areas which proved to be more than double the World Health Organization (WHO) guidelines (210 ppb) and the highest ever recorded in the UK since records began in 1976.

Air pollution in London is monitored on behalf of the London Borough Authorities (LBA) and the Association of London Boroughs (ALA) (which have now merged to become the Association of London Government) by the South East Institute of Public Health (SEIPH). Few boroughs use continuous automatic monitors. The government has its own sites in London. Its results are kept separate from those of the local authorities. At present the Department of the Environment has six automatic stations and one integrated site with Bexley Local Authority. It intends to have 80 similar sites by the year 1997. Many monitoring techniques do not meet EC guidelines. There is a great need for standardization across all the survey sites.

Noise pollution

A survey carried out in 1990 across England and Wales suggested that road transport produced noise outside 92% of the sample of houses, with aircraft noise at 62% of the sites (GB Royal Commission on Environmental Pollution, 1994).

Evidence from environmental health officers in London suggest that noise from traffic may be a contributory factor to stress-related illnesses. The main airports of London, Heathrow, Gatwick and Stansted generate noise as well as air pollution. Large numbers of people reside in the hundreds of square kilometres affected by the noise.

Borough policies

Road safety plans

The London boroughs have both shared and individual responsibility for road transport. The government is responsible for the strategic trunk road network and the local authorities the rest. Road safety is primarily the responsibility of the local authorities.

In 1987 the Secretary of State for Transport announced a target to reduce accident casualties by one-third on the baseline figure (the average over five years 1981–85) by the year 2000 (Figure 22.4). Local authorities were required to draw up road safety plans which outline their individual targets and strategies—usually a mixture of traffic calming measures, education, traffic enforcement and publicity. These road safety plans play an essential part in linking the different areas of road safety (health, education and engineering) together. The Traffic

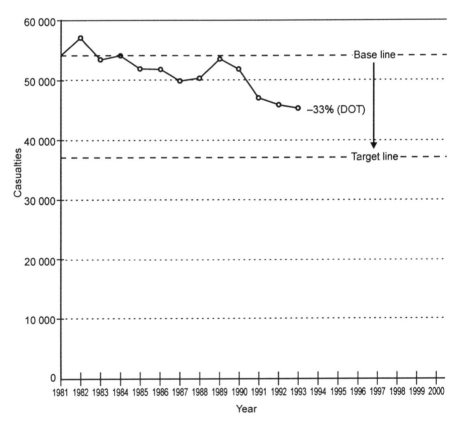

Figure 22.4   Greater London: all casualties

Director for London advises local authorities as to their plan of action but has no authority to enforce implementation of the proposed action, or to ensure that schemes are developed.

How well are these plans actually going? From the aspect of accident reduction a recent road safety briefing by the Department of Transport (GB Department of Transport, 1994a) indicated that a '. . . considerable further reduction in casualties will be required for the remainder of the period to the year 2000 if London's target is to be met. In effect, total casualties in Greater London will need to be reduced by an average of 2.5% per year until the millennium. This is double the progress made in recent years.'

Transport policies and development plans

Transport schemes and developments are funded by the government and local authorities. The long-term development strategies of local authorities are outlined in what are known as Unitary Development Plans (UDPs). These form a general policy framework around which more specific plans, such as the Transport Policies and Programmes (TPPs), are based. Both the UDPs and TPPs require central government funding in the form of Transport Supplementary Grants (TSGs), which are the route via which road schemes costing more than £2 million are funded. Whereas the UDPs are subject to public consultation, TPPs are not, although they do have to conform to the strategy laid out in the UDP.

While central government, represented by the Highways Agency, is responsible for the strategic trunk road network, boroughs generally act as their agents locally. This means that they have responsibility for monitoring safety on trunk roads, suggesting modifications, and supervising any work that results.

Government policy in London

> You have your own company, your own temperature control, your own music—and you don't have to put up with dreadful human beings sitting alongside you. (Stephen Norris, Transport Minister for London)

Public transport in London has no overall coordinating body linking all the public transport modes and thus lacks policies and programmes to develop them. On the other hand, the Department of Transport has many subdivisions that look after individual aspects of transport, for example, a rail division and a transport policies division. It encourages the interaction between transport operatives and local authorities but does not feel the need for a transport strategy document specific to London.

'Priorities for London', a Government Office for London briefing, outlines some of the government's 'achievements' (Bowmor, 1994):

1. Bus and rail privatization.
2. Central Line (Underground), Thames and Chiltern Line, and Kent Link

(British Rail) modernizations.
3. Appointment of a Traffic Director for London.
4. Local Authority safety schemes.

However, the government is still continuing to develop the road network in and around London.

Investment in public transport

Britain as a whole has not had a good history of public transport investment. Figure 22.5 shows the UK at the bottom of the table in rail infrastructure investment in 1989–91 per capita.

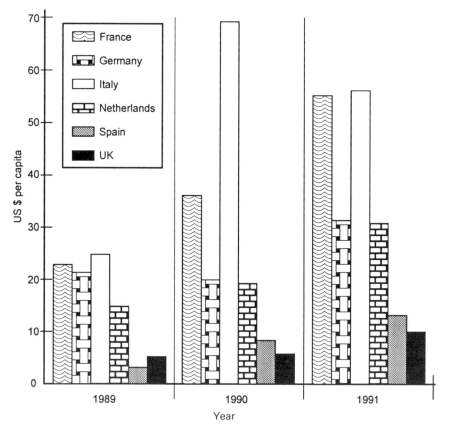

Figure 22.5   Investment in rail infrastructure in the EC: the UK left behind. Per capita spending for 1990 and 1991 calculated using 1989 as base. Expressed as US $ per head. Source: Great Britain Department of Transport, 1991; OECD, 1991

Investment in rail track entering London is likely to reduce the need to travel by car. Investment in rail in the South East area (including London) has been increasing since 1985/86, but the total investment is not comparable to investment in road infrastructure as the latter excludes private investment in motor vehicles.

New transport measures in London

The following are examples of the many existing schemes to improve road safety, road congestion and the general road environment, some at a London-wide level, and others implemented by local authorities and organizations such as London Transport.

London Bus Priority Network

Over 3.7 million people use buses in London every day, despite their poor reliability and slow speeds caused mainly by traffic congestion and inconsiderate or illegal parking. The London Bus Priority Network, to be completed by the year 2000, has been devised to tackle these problems on almost 500 miles of roads, containing 70% of the worst bus 'trouble spots'. It has been drawn up by the London boroughs through the Association of London Borough Engineers and Surveyors (ALBES) in conjunction with London Transport and the Department of Transport. It aims to introduce bus priority and traffic management measures along main corridors and key arteries so that there is '. . . at least an average 25% peak period and 15% inter peak period reduction in overall bus journey time'.

Priority Red Routes

According to the Network Plan Executive Summary (Traffic Director for London, 1993), congestion in London is estimated to cost around £10 000 million a year. The Priority (Red) Route Network (Red Routes), which should be fully operational in 1997, aims to remove the danger posed by illegally parked vehicles and to improve the flow of traffic. The scheme, which will cost £100 million to implement, to be funded by the Traffic Director for London, should pay for itself in terms of journey times and accident reduction, if properly enforced, within six months.

The scheme pays particular attention to improving access to those with disabilities by making special parking provision and improving footway mobility. Buses and coaches are likely to benefit from the effect of reduced congestion. Pedestrians may benefit from the reduction in the numbers of parked cars and also improvement of present crossing facilities. However, the increased speed of traffic may have a negative effect on the overall danger posed by busy main roads.

There was initial scepticism about the Red Route schemes, with many groups and associations insisting that the negative effects of the routes (encouraging more traffic, for example) outweigh the positive effects. Unfortunately the pilot scheme introduced in 1991 on the busy A1 at Archway was too small an area to provide any substantial analysis of the benefit.

London Cycle Network

In July 1994, a bid was submitted by Kingston upon Thames on behalf of all the 33 London boroughs for financial support of the London Cycle Network comprising 1300 km of routes and costing £36 million over five years. Its aim is to make cycling in London safer and will coincide with the other new road measures such as the Bus Priority Network. It is estimated to result in a 25% reduction in cycle accidents. The greatest potential for cycling is on local journeys, as over 70% of all commuting trips in London are under 10 km. It was announced in December 1994 that the cycle network would receive £3 million in government capital for its first year (1995/96) which amounts to over 1% of the forecast investment in roads in 1993/94 (GB Department of Transport, 1994b).

New measures to improve mobility for the disabled and elderly

At the forefront of current measures to provide better transport services for the disabled is the Low Floor Bus. All new buses are required to meet its specifications. There are currently 68 of these buses in service in the Outer London areas over five different routes. Unfortunately, due to the length of the Low Floor Bus (40 ft), services are not yet available in central London. The Low Floor Bus has experienced a few problems from cars parked at bus stops, requiring the use of the bus ramp which adds delay to the service. However, surveys carried out by the Transport Research Laboratory (TRL) on similar bus schemes in Europe suggest that the service may prove quicker than the standard bus. The Midicar, a smaller version of the Low Floor Bus, is soon to be introduced.

Other services for the less mobile include 150 Dial-a-ride buses in six regions across London and the Taxi Card scheme which enables disabled passengers to travel at a reduced fare.

The main problem for improving services for the disabled is the lack of legislation that commits transport industries to provide sufficient access to their carriages.

Road pricing

Road pricing as a means of reducing traffic congestion has been a consideration for London's problems. The government has conducted lengthy research into the efficacy of such programmes in London, which has proved inconclusive, and there is a need for further research into the subject. The methods of road pricing are varied and their effects uncertain. One of its major drawbacks is that congestion and expensive parking in central London does not seem to deter motorists from travelling by car at present so it is possible that motorists will readily accept road charges (pricing)—especially if they consider there to be no alternative methods of travel.

Strategies for London's transport and health

London Planning Advisory Committee (LPAC) strategy

The LPAC strategy (LPAC, 1994) has three main elements: to reduce the amount of travel; to restrain traffic, especially the car; and to improve public transport.

Modes of transport that improve health and the environment, e.g. walking and cycling, must be promoted and a modal shift to public transport should reduce the need for the number of trips made by car. LPAC 'opposes any net increase in the strategic highway capacity available to the car' except that which is required for the regeneration of East London. Part of this regeneration involves LPAC's proposal that there should be an international station at Stratford as an access point to the Channel Tunnel Rail Link.

Its recommendations to the government include:

1. Establishing traffic targets across the whole of London, in particular the outer London town centres, the major radials and the M25 and introducing transport policies to achieve them.
2. Improving air quality monitoring London-wide, and extending the targets to encompass more air pollutants.
3. Greater consideration of the impact of noise pollution of rail and air services.

Its recommendations to local boroughs include:

1. Reducing the need to travel by developing near existing and new public transport nodes, setting traffic targets and promoting public transport.
2. Introducing more parking restrictions and reallocating road space.
3. Promoting greener alternatives to the car including local boroughs' own transport fleet.
4. Reviewing existing UDP's and TPP's with an aim to stabilizing, then reducing traffic levels and their environmental impact.

The government itself has begun advising the motoring population, through the media when traffic pollution levels in London reach unacceptable levels, but is not planning actually to restrain traffic in such instances.

The Royal Commission's recommendations

The Eighteenth Report of the Royal Commission on Environmental Pollution: Transport and the Environment (GB Royal Commission on Environmental Pollution, 1994), follows a similar line as LPAC in that sustainable development is at the heart of its national strategy. 'To ensure that an effective transport policy at all levels of government is integrated with land use policy and gives priority to minimizing the need for transport and increasing the proportions of trips by environmentally less damaging modes.'

The strategy reiterates the need for a body to take an overview of transport problems and work closely with land use planners at a strategic and regional level. It recommends that in London, there should be a Passenger Transport Authority that broadly covers the area bound by the M25 with increased powers, especially over bus services, and be responsible for strategic planning; also that the present system of funding, the Transport Supplementary Grants (TSGs), be less restrictive (currently expenditure is only continued to highways and traffic regulation). It suggests TSGs should encompass environmental objectives and that the trunk road network be passed to local authority control so that land use policies can be facilitated. At a government level the Commission suggest that there is an overall restructuring in the Department of Transport to meet the requirements of a fundamentally different approach to transport policy.

Further important recommendations include one that 'all significant applications for planning permission should contain analysis of the transport implications, including pedestrian, cycling and public transport access'. The Commission's traffic targets for London propose a reduction in the numbers of journeys undertaken by car from 50% to 45% by 2000 and 35% by 2020. Its proposals for cycle use involve an increase of 10% of all urban journeys by 2005 and suggest that local authorities set up safe pedestrian networks, particularly for children travelling to and from school.

Commentary—the implications for London's health

Accidents and exercise

Accidents cause widespread suffering and incur huge costs in financial terms to the health system. Accidents are one of the major causes of premature deaths especially among children and teenagers. Nationally, motor vehicle traffic accidents make up about 60% of all accidents.

It is evident that the government's accident targets for London are unlikely to be met with respect to the largest casualty group of slight injuries. A strategic, London-wide view of traffic reduction measures is required and a greater emphasis on investigating pedestrianization in central areas.

Continuing improvements to access on public service vehicles are needed, such as the Low Floor Bus. Rail and bus services, as part of their policy programmes, should ensure that the less mobile are welcomed rather than seen as a problem group that must be 'catered for'.

Roads act as barriers to the small-scale day-to-day movements within communities, discouraging access to vital services such as hospitals, social services and also recreational establishments. It is the least mobile and vulnerable, i.e. the elderly, the disabled and children who are most affected by this phenomenon. Planning must encompass this principle and support methods of travel such as cycling and walking as links into existing and planned public transport nodes.

Motor vehicles are responsible for approximately 51% of nitrogen dioxide and 87% of carbon monoxide pollution in the air over London (Bell, 1993) along with other airborne particulates. The number of cars on London's roads is forecast to double by 2025. This will place a huge strain on the environment. Air pollution episodes similar to that in 1991 may become more commonplace, requiring regular 'pre-storm' warnings announced on national and regional television. The United Nations Economic and Social Council in 1990 published a report which concluded that '. . . immediate abatement and control action should be taken to reduce the severe impact of air pollution on human health . . . this action should not be delayed for additional studies' (United Nations, 1990).

References

Bell S (1993) *Capital Killer II: Still fuming over London's Traffic Pollution.* London Boroughs Association, London

Bowmor A (1994) *Transport in London: an overview.* Internal document for information produced by Government Office for London

Campbell GW, Cox J, Downing CEH, Stedman JR, Stevenson K (1992) *A survey of nitrogen dioxide concentrations in the United Kingdom using diffusion tubes: July to December 1991.* Warren Spring Laboratory, UK

Great Britain Department of Transport (1991) *Transport Statistics Great Britain 1991 C 11 + 3.15.* HMSO, London. Evidence taken from Steer Davies Gleave (1992) *Financing Public Transport: How does Britain compare?*

Great Britain Department of Transport (1994a) *Internal Road Safety briefing, 9 December 1994.* HMSO, London

Great Britain Department of Transport (1994b) *Transport Statistics London 1994.* HMSO, London

Great Britain Department of Transport (1994c) *Transport Statistics Great Britain 1994.* HMSO, London

Great Britain Royal Commission on Environmental Pollution (1994) *Eighteenth Report. Transport and the Environment.* HMSO, London.

London Accident Analysis Unit (1994) *Casualty Reduction Targets in Greater London: A Review of Existing and Possible Future Casualty Reduction Target Groups.* London Research Centre, HMSO, London

LPAC (London Planning Advisory Committee) (1994) *Advice on Strategic Planning Guidance for London.* ADV 26

London Research Centre (1994) *Travel in London: London Area Transport Survey 1991.* HMSO, London

MVA Consultancy (1994) *London Transportation Studies: Technical Note 246–F3.3: Planning data (Revised June 1994) and Technical Note 256–F3.3: Validation–Comparison with observed data and previous forecasts (October 1994).* MVA Consultancy on behalf of Department of Transport

OECD (1991) *National Accounts*, Volume 1, Paris (Population, exchange rates). Evidence taken from Steer Davies Gleave (1992) *Financing Public Transport: How does Britain compare?*

Steer Davies Gleave (1992) *Financing Public Transport: How does Britain compare?* Steer Davies Gleave for The Bow Group, Centre for Local Economic Strategies, Euro Tunnel, Railway Industry Association and Transport 2000
Traffic Director for London (1993) *Network Plan: Executive Summary.* Traffic Director for London, March 1993
United Nations (1990) *Impact on Human Health of Air Pollution in Europe.* UN, Geneva

SECTION 5

TRANSPORT POLICIES

23
Introduction

Tony Fletcher and Anthony J. McMichael

London School of Hygiene & Tropical Medicine, UK

This section takes us into the heartland of policy formulation. What, really, are society's priorities? Is public health important? Is there a role for market-based controls, via an economics attuned to human needs and environmental impacts?

Goodwin leads us through a linear argument: transport emissions affect health; emissions have increased as transport policy has stimulated traffic growth; now policy-makers are acquiring a 'new realism' and a realization that there is insufficient space for more roads; this facilitates consideration of the health impacts of excess and inappropriate urban traffic. Health concerns may not have driven the evolution of transport policy, but they are now well placed to contribute to a rational convergence of social interests.

Button captures the dilemma within an economic framework: how to maximize the net contribution of cars to society. He explores market-based management and pricing options. Despite common misperceptions, he argues, economists are interested in natural and social resource management—so, since we live in a market economy, we must ask what markets can achieve. Button explores some controversial issues: assigning property rights to 'commons' (such as the air); introducing road pricing (via privatization?) to control the negative environmental externalities of inefficient traffic; and the 'polluter pays' principle. He argues that these are *instruments* of policy attainment, of making markets responsive to social ends; full internalization of environmental and health burdens within the market is not possible.

Walter and colleagues' view of public health concerns important emergent criteria for sustainable transport policy. The traditional engineer's road-building approach has failed; there are new opportunities for economic incentives and controls. However, since people dislike paying more without getting more, it is crucial to lay bare the environmental and public health costs that are currently neglected by our myopic markets. Their paper summarizes various expert assessments of impact and costs in relation to air pollution, noise, accidents,

Health at the Crossroads: Transport Policy and Urban Health.
Edited by Tony Fletcher and Anthony J. McMichael © 1997 John Wiley & Sons Ltd

global warming and traffic congestion, and it concludes that we must embrace interdisciplinary discussion and solution of these macro-problems.

Whitelegg proposes, with persuasive examples, that the case for an alternative vision of the future of transport has never been stronger. Various transport crises have emerged around Europe, and a range of economic and social absurdities are apparent. He argues that health concerns are now prominent ('non-sustainable transport policies represent a large-scale experiment with people's lives'), as we begin to re-think cities as human habitat, as social structures. He cites compelling examples of Sustainable Cities Good Practice from the Netherlands and Germany, and urges involvement of public health professionals.

In a broadly integrative overview, Steensberg re-examines the role of scientific knowledge in social decision-making, and the political, social and ethical dimensions of formulating and implementing public policies. He concludes that sustainable transport policies are increasingly being adopted by governments, but that, through human frailties, their implementation is still lagging. Steensberg reminds us that 'sustainability' is a tall order, extending beyond local environments to wider issues of global warming and husbanding resources. Transport reform must be part of the solution.

24
Are transport policies driven by health concerns?

Philip B. Goodwin

ESRC Transport Studies Unit, University of Oxford, UK

Although this chapter is not concerned primarily with road safety, some mention of safety is important to set a context.

In 1896 at Crystal Palace, Mrs Bridget Driscoll became the first person to be killed by a car in Britain. At her inquest, the coroner said that he hoped such an event would never happen again. Now, road traffic accidents injure about 13 million people per year, worldwide, and kill over half a million. Although the word 'accident' hints that the phenomenon is often thought of as substantially outside human control, nevertheless safety considerations have mostly been afforded a very high profile in transport policy. A large part of traffic law, policing and design standards is essentially concerned with the regulation of speed and behaviour for safety objectives.

But for most of the current generation of transport policy, the central approach to other aspects of health has been summed up by a telling quotation from the UK Ministry of Transport in 1979 (requoted by Green (1994)):

> the effects of pollution by motor vehicles can be summarised: there is no evidence that this type of pollution has any adverse effect on health.

Clearly, as long as this was the accepted view, then health considerations could not be expected to play a substantial part in transport policy discussions. Health was, simply, irrelevant.

Aspects of transport policy which cause problems for health

However, in retrospect the health aspects of transport policy cannot be dismissed so lightly. Three propositions are argued here: first, transport emissions do have an effect on health; second, the magnitude of those effects is dominated by the

Health at the Crossroads: Transport Policy and Urban Health.
Edited by Tony Fletcher and Anthony J. McMichael © 1997 John Wiley & Sons Ltd

growth and pervasiveness of the total volume of traffic; third, transport policy has broadly acted to increase that growth.

Transport emissions do have an effect on health

Papers in the recent Ashden Trust report, summarized by Read (1994), review the evidence, and the following quotations are broadly representative:

Dr Claire Holman: 'Urban concentrations of nitrogen dioxide and carbon monoxide exceed international health guidelines in many areas with heavy traffic ... Motorists and car passengers ... are exposed to the highest concentrations.'

Dr Sarah Walters: 'There is now a wealth of published evidence that certain pollutants for which road traffic constitutes a major source are associated with short-term respiratory and cardiovascular effects. The evidence is strongest and most consistent for particulates.'

Professor Robert Davies and Dr J.C. Devalia: 'The equilibrium of the airways' natural barrier, the epithelial cell lining, is delicate ... even low levels of some vehicle derived pollutants may disturb that equilibrium, with resulting cell damage, inflammation, and increased susceptibility to allergic conditions including asthma and rhinitis.'

Professor Tony McMichael: 'it is clear that ambient urban levels of carbon monoxide exposure limit exercise tolerance in persons with angina pectoris, and reduce exercise performance in athletes ... people who work in traffic also have substantial exposure to CO (for example, police motorcyclists).'

Dr David Phillips: concluded that the evidence on cancer was not yet clear cut, but 'given the data from experiments ... and the evidence from occupational exposure to some components of petroleum fuels and engine emissions, it is a highly plausible hypothesis that environmental exposure to traffic pollution poses a carcinogenic risk to the general population.'

It seems reasonable to conclude that health issues are indeed real, and should be taken seriously.

The growth in volume of traffic

In Britain, we each spend, on average, just over an hour a day on travel, achieving an overall door-to-door speed of about 20 miles per hour, and travelling 21 miles a day. Forty years ago it was eight miles a day. Current forecasts imply that it may be approaching 50 miles a day by the year 2025, and still increasing.

It is not always realized how much of all transport is short-distance. A third of all personal trips are on foot. Even for car journeys 57% of them are less than five miles, and the average is eight miles. Similarly for freight traffic, 73% of all goods lifted in the UK are set down within the same region, and the average length of haul is less than 50 miles.

If we look at the make-up of traffic as a whole, 45% is in built-up areas, and 14% on motorways. For all classes of road, cars are by far the most numerous vehicles, and for the country as a whole over 80% of the vehicle-miles are travelled by cars, with 16% by vans and lorries and only 1% by bus and coach (which provide for nearly 20% of the vehicle journeys by road).

Thus private cars form the bulk of traffic. Within this, a third of car journeys are for work purposes (including education) and two-thirds for a wide range of other reasons—shopping, personal business, social, recreational and pleasure trips. Car ownership is widespread—two-thirds of households have one or more cars—but the usage is not evenly spread over the population. In particular, car ownership is very strongly related to income; over 60% of men have access to a car as the main driver, but less than 30% of women; and car use is on a very much lower level among the elderly.

So analysis of the current statistics leads us to focus on car use rather than lorries, on short distance travel for non-work purposes, particularly done by young and middle-aged men of the middle and higher income groups.

The largest part of traffic growth has been due to cars, not lorries. Indeed, car traffic, already the largest base, grew almost exactly twice as fast as goods vehicle traffic throughout the 1980s. For freight, there has been an increase in the tonnage of goods moved, broadly taken up by the use of larger vehicles; most of the extra freight traffic on the roads is due to an increase (around 1% a year) in the average length of haul, as origins and destinations get more spread out. By contrast, the average occupancy of cars has been decreasing, as well as an increase in the average journey length and in the total number of trips. There has been an increase in the proportion of journeys less than five miles, and in the proportion of non-work journeys.

In addition, the social characteristics of traffic growth are showing new features. The 'new elderly', brought up with cars, will tend to keep them when they retire, and car use among women is increasing very rapidly, partly for reasons of security. Children are being driven to school, rather than walking. As a result, there has been a decline in the traditional base of the bus market without, as yet, evidence of new markets developing from the increase in bus miles run, and fares levels, which followed deregulation.

The increase in traffic levels has taken place in a context of increasing pressures for development of rural and suburban areas, and changes in retailing and service provision all of which tend to encourage widely spread origins and destinations for which car use is increasingly necessary. Rising incomes enable the whole process to continue. Overall, the 'love affair with the car' has developed into a sort of dependence, in which psychological factors, influenced by education and advertising, play an important role. But the key driving force is seen to be the great convenience offered by personal transport in giving a control over time and space which has never previously been possible.

Transport policy acted to increase the growth in traffic

Although the scale of current transport problems is new, their existence is not new at all, and nor is their recognition. For many years there have been two coexisting streams of thought among British policy-makers and advisers on how to cope with the car and the problems it causes. One view has been to control car use in order to keep it within bounds defined by broader social objectives—both Tripp, in the 1930s, and Buchanan in the 1960s, argued that residential and other areas should be kept insulated from excessive car use (Tripp, 1942; GB Ministry of Transport, 1963). But there was always an ambiguity in the argument, encroached upon by aspects of the other view: that the growth in car use was inevitable and it was necessary to provide sufficient road infrastructure to accommodate it. It was this view that provided the dominant orthodoxy for transport planning in the 1960s and 1970s. Planners and local authorities who took a different approach—looking to public transport as a substitute for road construction, for example—were generally seen as going against the trend. Their initiatives tended to be partial, and short-lived.

The dominant element of transport policy was the construction of road capacity broadly intended—as far as possible—to provide for enough road space to cater for traffic increases which were in the main expected to occur due to economic growth and increased incomes. However, there was concern throughout that period that 'roads generate traffic', or, more precisely, extra road capacity induces additional traffic. Although the idea was consistently resisted, it would not go away, and is now accepted (GB SACTRA, 1994; GB Department of Transport 1994):

> SACTRA (the Standing Advisory Committee on Trunk Road Assessment) has concluded . . . that induced traffic is of greatest importance in the following circumstances:
> – where the network is operating or is expected to operate close to capacity;
> – where the elasticity of demand with respect to travel costs is high;
> – where the implementation of a scheme causes large changes in travel costs.
> The Department agrees with this conclusion.

The main focus in considering the implications of this, so far, has been the effect on the economic evaluation of the time savings from road improvements. (Induced traffic enjoys some benefits itself, but as congestion increases these benefits are outweighed by the greater and greater costs imposed on other vehicles, due to the non-linear relationship between the speed, and density, of traffic. As a result, induced traffic shortens the period of relief offered by a new road, and in congested conditions reduces its economic benefit.) However, from a broader point of view it may be that the environmental and health implications are more important, since the existence of induced traffic will almost always increase emissions to a greater level than they otherwise would have been.

The 'new realism' in transport thinking

In the search for solutions, every five years or so, the Department of Transport has produced forecasts of traffic growth. In 1989, revised national road traffic forecasts were produced, which had a profound effect on transport policy, because the projected increases of 83% to 142% traffic growth by 2025—which was consistent with past experience—were inconsistent with what could be supported by the road network.

The media reported these forecasts as a clever coup by the Department of Transport to win more money from the Treasury for road building. But then there was a quiet period, as local authorities worked out what their own road capacity requirements would be to meet their share of this expected growth. It became clear that in towns there simply was no way that road capacity could be expanded at rates which would match such growth. The consequence was a matter of arithmetic, not politics. On current trends, the numbers of vehicles per mile of road could *only* increase, and logically congestion could only get worse (in intensity, or duration, or geographical spread). The new realism was the recognition that, in towns, supply of road space would not—could not—be increased to match demand; therefore demand would have to be reduced to match supply.

This is the reason why over that period *demand management* quietly, but quickly, became part of the urban transport policy of every political party. Urban transport policy *in principle* now nearly everywhere proposes an environmentally-friendly package, but one that is justified in economic rather than environmental terms. The package usually consists of:

1. containment or reduction of the total volume of traffic;
2. improved and expanded public transport systems;
3. better provision for pedestrians and cyclists;
4. traffic restraint and traffic management, aimed at reduced flows and increased reliability rather than maximizing the throughput of vehicles;
5. the control of land use changes and new development, in such a way as to reduce journey length and car use wherever possible;
6. and sometimes the package expresses interest in charging road users directly for the congestion and environmental damage they cause, in order to reduce that damage, reduce traffic, and simultaneously provide the funds to pay for the other parts of the policy.

However, implementation in practice is still lagging far behind agreement on the principles. One problem is that these policies are rarely all implemented together, and the omission of some elements reduces or even negates the effects of others. For example, in the absence of good public transport, park-and-ride facilities can provide for an increase in the total volume of traffic, rather than the intended reduction.

Convergence of transport policies for health and economic efficiency

If it were only health that needed to be weighed against the manifest advantages of unrestricted vehicle use, it is difficult to believe that there would be much success in such a policy. However, there are other important elements in transport policy which—for reasons quite separate from health—are leading to the same conclusion, and this makes it possible to consider broader and more ambitious policy objectives than might have been possible even ten years ago. Recognition of the effects of traffic growth on health are in tune with policy arguments that have been derived from considerations of economic efficiency and environmental protection.

For these reasons, the health argument is likely to find an unusually favourable hearing: there is a window of opportunity with very positive possibilities for radical policy initiatives.

Acknowledgements

This chapter also draws on the author's contribution to the Ashden Trust Report (Goodwin, 1994).

References

Goodwin PB (1994) Vehicle pollution and health: policy implications. In Read C (ed) *How Vehicle Pollution Affects Our Health*. Ashden Trust, London

Great Britain Department of Transport (1994) *Trunk Roads and the Generation of Traffic: Response by the Department of Transport to the Standing Advisory Committee on Trunk Road Assessment*. HMSO, London

Great Britain Ministry of Transport (1963) *Traffic in Towns (The Buchanan Report)*. HMSO, London

Great Britain Standing Advisory Committee on Trunk Road Assessment (1994) *Trunk Roads and the Generation of Traffic*. HMSO, London

Green M (1994) Introduction. In Read C (ed) *How Vehicle Pollution Affects Our Health*. Ashden Trust, London

Read C (ed) (1994) *How Vehicle Pollution Affects Our Health*. Ashden Trust, London

Tripp A (1942) *Town Planning and Road Traffic*. Edward Arnold, London

25
Assessing the full cost of cars: can the market deliver?

Kenneth J. Button

*Centre for Research in European Economics and Finance,
Loughborough University, UK*

The motor car has always been a mixed blessing. Its introduction was not welcomed by competing modes of transport and it was seen at the outset as potentially dangerous to other road users. As its use has grown new hazards have emerged—in particular, those relating to atmospheric pollution (Button and Rothengatter, 1993). Motorized transport is a significant contributor to the emission of local, health damaging gases (such as carbon monoxide, sulphur dioxide and volatile organic compounds) and particulates. Cars emit considerable quantities of nitrogen oxide (NO_x) and other gases that have transboundary implications stretching beyond the immediate area of transport activity (e.g. in the form of acid rain). The car is almost exclusively powered by fossil fuels and, as a result, in many industrialized countries, motorized transport is the fastest growing source of carbon dioxide (CO_2) emissions which are viewed as one of the main contributors to the potential global warming phenomenon.

Further, cars are noisy, roads often create severe problems of community severance in our cities and derelict cars are visually offensive. The social account should also include the environmental and health implications associated with the construction of motor vehicles and of the infrastructure upon which they rely. This environmental degradation can have consequences for the health of both the current generation and future generations. Many of the effects are related to immediate physical illnesses while others affect the food chain and the general ecology of the planet on which later generations must live (GB Royal Commission on Environmental Pollution, 1994). The importance of setting policies regarding the future of car use within the context of ensuring sustainable development in its

Health at the Crossroads: Transport Policy and Urban Health.
Edited by Tony Fletcher and Anthony J. McMichael © 1997 John Wiley & Sons Ltd

fullest sense has now been recognized as a major long-term concern in most industrialized countries (e.g. GB Department of the Environment, 1994).

Set against this series of problems, however, should be seen the benefits of the increased mobility and access that the modern motor vehicle allows. It also represents an integral part of an industrial and social complex that in Western countries is associated with higher living standards and longer life expectancies than in the past. The key issue is, therefore, one of developing balanced transport and related policies which maximize the net contribution of the motor vehicle to society (Button, 1993). This is not a static issue but one which is becoming more pressing over time as the number of cars increases and their use expands.

Various approaches have been advocated in recent years to achieve this objective but, judging by the intensity of current debates, serious problems still remain. It is, indeed, now recognized that the environmental and health problems generated by motor traffic are more pronounced and complex than were recognized in the past (GB House of Commons Select Committee on Transport, 1994; GB Royal Commission on Environmental Pollution, 1994). Equally, traditional policies of accommodating motor traffic by providing infrastructure to meet its quasi-unrestricted demands have gradually given way to ideas of management and more rational pricing. Public opposition to extending motorways into sensitive rural areas and the physical difficulties of providing additional road capacity in urban centres have provided a practical edge to the intellectual arguments for the change. Fiscal prudence on the part of macroeconomic policy-makers has also played its role. The reality of translating this new thinking into practical measures has proved hard, and implementation has been difficult to accomplish.

As these changes in priority have taken place so the role of economics and, in particular, the relevance of markets have begun to take a more central place in debates. Economists have traditionally been interested in natural resource management and social welfare, a category to which environment and public health considerations belong, but have sometimes in the recent past been marginalized in debates about environmentally related issues. One reason for this has, perhaps, been the rather narrow definition sometimes placed on economics and to misperceptions about the role of markets.

The aims of this chapter are, first, to look at what markets can achieve in making the motor car a more socially efficient component of modern society and, second, to offer some discussion about what markets cannot do. In terms of layout, there is an initial discussion of the broad principles of markets and how they may be seen to relate, in particular, to the health hazards posed by motorized transport. This is followed by an examination of some of the ways in which market-based instruments (although seldom strictly market-based principles) have to date been applied in the transport field together with a brief discussion of other ways in which markets may help in developing environmentally sensitive transport policies.

Markets

It is important to appreciate what exactly markets can do. The underlying idea of markets is that, if people can trade goods and services for which they have relatively little use, in return for goods and services that they find more valuable, then they benefit. In conducting this trade, prices are revealed which indicate the opportunity costs of the decisions taken. By looking across these revealed prices in a range of different markets, individuals can elect to participate where they find it worth their while trading. This is very much the notion of economics which underlies modern Western society.

While markets can confer considerable benefits, their limitations have been long recognized and unfettered markets, in fact, have never been allowed to exist even under the most laissez-faire regimes. Indeed, even Adam Smith (1904) in his classic work, the *Wealth of Nations*, while extolling free markets, appreciated that the world falls far short of perfection and that markets seldom meet the exacting, ideal standards he would have wished. Nevertheless, we live in market economies and these economies, especially when contrasted to the centrally planned economies of the former communist states of Europe, not only provide a high material standard of living as measured in narrow economic terms of gross domestic product but also still have relatively good environments to be enjoyed by their citizens.

So what are the limitations of markets and how, in particular, do they relate to transport? To begin with, to be fully efficient, markets need to be ubiquitous and cover all goods and services. Of course, in reality, markets are not comprehensive and many resources are consumed outside of markets—the so-called 'externalities'. The underlying problem, which was highlighted by the Nobel Laureate, Ronald Coase (1960), is that there are no property rights associated with many natural resources such as the atmosphere and, hence, there is no market mechanism which allocates their use effectively. Since the market is not throwing up pricing signals indicating the opportunity costs involved in the exploitation of such resources, the outcome is excessive exploitation of these 'commons'. Put in a specific transport context, the users of cars are not directly aware of the costs they are imposing in terms of damage to health and the environment and, therefore, make excessive use of car transport.

The most obvious policy response in a market context is for property rights to be allocated so that use of these resources is constrained to the optimal level. This, however, poses practical problems of to whom the property rights should be allocated initially and how to ensure that they are subsequently traded efficiently in a market context. In the case of pollution with very long-term implications, such as CO_2 emissions, there is also the problem of how to treat the property rights of future generations as well as the current one. We return to some of these issues below.

Negative externalities are often seen to be at the heart of most environmental and public health problems but there are also other factors which create market imperfections. For a variety of technical reasons, for example, some markets may be unstable and this can lead to periods of over-supply. Further, markets which are characterized by monopolistic competition (that is, where many suppliers offer slightly different outputs) are also prone to excess capacity. If these markets use environmental resources as inputs then this, even in the absence of any externality effect, can lead to adverse environmental damage. Again seeking a transport example, one might think of an excessively competitive public transport market where large numbers of buses or taxis battle for traffic but each achieves low load factors. Each bus or taxi operator may take due cognizance of the environmental damage created by his operations but the sub-optimally large number of vehicles creates a situation where the overall damage is excessive.

Government interventions in markets can also sometimes worsen a situation where negative externalities already exist (Button, 1992). For example, in the transport context government provides and operates most roads but does not charge an economic price for their use. The problem is not so much one of whether total costs of providing the infrastructure are covered, but whether user payments at the margin adequately reflect the allocated marginal costs, including congestion costs. Inappropriate charging results in excessive use of much of the road network, especially in urban areas, which adds to the pollution and noise generated by the traffic flow. Other measures, such as direct subsidies in support of particular services for traffic management reasons, may lead to an excessive use of transport vis-a-vis other activities that can be equally damaging.

There are also situations where markets fail because of the transaction costs involved in their operation. Consider, as a very naive example in transport, the situation in which two vehicles moving in opposite directions confront one another on a road. They could in theory bargain and negotiate a price which would allow them to pass one another, but simple rules such as the legal requirement to drive on the left or to give way at cross-roads are much more efficient. Markets are, in effect, not costless mechanisms and in some cases it is preferable to forsake the benefits of trading to conserve transaction costs. While it is not a universal rule, these types of transaction costs tend to become proportionately more important the smaller the scale of the trade taking place and the larger the number of participants involved. This may, for instance, colour policy judgements when deciding how to tackle externalities generated by large, stationary sources, such as power stations, and that from numerous, mobile units such as motor vehicles.

Markets and market instruments

Quite clearly, if one considers the damage being done to the environment and, more specifically, to health, by the motor car, then at present the general view would seem to be that the market, for the types of reason set out above, is working imperfectly. One or two caveats should, though, be injected.

First, there are opportunity costs associated with all actions—there is no such thing as a 'free lunch'. This means that even in an optimal situation there will be some pollution and safety hazard associated with transport simply because the implications of removing this element of social cost are excessive in terms of what else is forgone. The issue is, therefore, one of whether markets currently create damage in excess of this level.

Second, in some instances it is difficult to know precisely what degree of amelioration is appropriate. This is not only a technical matter of imperfect scientific knowledge (e.g. as with gas emissions causing global warming) but also reflects poor information regarding social preferences. Indeed, in some cases social preferences may appear perverse, as when many millions of pounds are expended to reduce the extremely remote chance of another major underground fire started in the same manner as the King's Cross Station disaster that could, instead, have been used to improve safety features on, say, roads and almost certainly would save many more lives and reduce the number of serious injuries.

Market imperfections, however, can be reduced (Button, 1994). Ideally, one would 'internalize' the environmental implications of the motor car within the market by allocating property rights to environmental resources (European Conference of Ministers of Transport, 1994). In an environmental and public health context, it is important to appreciate what a full 'internalization' of the environmental consequences of the motor car would achieve. It would result not only in appropriate levels of abatement (for example, through different traffic patterns, changes in the volume of traffic and the use of alternative, 'cleaner' modes) but also in optimal reactions by those adversely affected (for example, in terms of location choices). In the longer term, the mechanism provides a stimulus to develop new technologies and lifestyles which economize on environmental intrusions.

Such allocations of property rights are, as indicated above, a theoretical solution, but one that is practically difficult to accomplish in all but exceptional circumstances. The underlying concept, however, is a useful one. It offers guidance as to how changes may be brought about in an efficient manner. It is always important to remember that change, achieved in an economically efficient manner, releases resources for uses elsewhere in the system. This is both socially desirable and can be used in compensation packages designed to make policies more politically attractive to the electorate. While it is difficult to use the market to allocate directly environmental resources, considerable advances can be made by using market instruments to achieve specified, albeit perhaps not optimal, levels of improvement (Organisation for Economic Co-operation and Development, 1994). Some examples follow.

Lead has long been recognized as impairing the normal intellectual development and learning abilities of children. In the USA the decision to phase out leaded fuel was made on the basis of a marketable permit system whereby refineries were allocated decreasingly small allocations of lead which they could then trade amongst themselves. This stimulated the maximum use of the most efficient refineries, which not only reduced the output of other pollutants, but also brought about the change at a low financial cost (Hahn, 1989).

In the case of lead the number of refineries involved was relatively small and enforcement of rules relatively easy, making this quasi-market approach tractable. It is unlikely, however, to be viable for many other pollutants. Market instruments in these latter cases may still be used, though, in the form of (Pigouvian) pollution charges or subsidies. Although there are clearly differing distributional implications, a given level of pollution abatement can be obtained by either charging a per-unit fee for the pollution a motor car generates or by paying its user a subsidy to reduce the problem. (Institutionally, the UK has accepted the OECD's 'polluter pays' principle and, thus, has practically ruled out the second of these options.)

The attraction of charges on pollution lies mainly in their incidence at the margin. Correctly applied, they force road users to adopt changes which ultimately have identical costs of abatement for the final unit of pollution removed (that is, at this point it is not cheaper to meet the desired target by car user X reducing pollution by one more unit with car user Y increasing pollution by one unit.)

These fiscal instruments can come in two broad forms. They may be universal in their applicability and aimed at a particular, global problem that transcends the transport sector. A carbon tax on all forms of fossil fuel to meet an international CO_2 target would fall into this category (for example, of the type the European Union has tried to develop). It would provide efficient signals across all users of fossil fuels to economize with the incidence being equalized at the margin. There is no prior assumption that the particular contribution of transport to this change is proportionately larger or smaller than other sectors—it depends on, amongst other things, society's perception of the importance of motorized transport and the availability of substitutes for the car.

Alternatively, there may be a specific, environmental pollution abatement target set for motorized transport. The specificity of such a policy perhaps reflects concerns about the distributional implications of measures such as general carbon taxes. Ongoing examples of such charges in this case include the premium paid for leaded fuel in most European countries and the systems of tax rebates given in some Scandinavian countries when old cars are handed in for recycling. They have also been used in a slightly different way in Germany to stimulate the uptake of higher environmental emissions standards prior to the statutory date.

These, and similar devices, represent market instruments rather than the strict internalization of the environment within the market. They are efficient means of achieving externally determined targets, possibly based on scientific advice, designed to meet public health and other criteria. Even these, however, may not always be appropriate policy tools (Rothengatter, 1994). In some cases where the potential damage is extremely severe and the transaction costs of deploying market instruments is high, the use of command-and-control measures such as bans and regulations may represent the logical policy option. The alternate-day banning of cars with odd and even number plates in Athens, and the banning of cars entirely when critical ozone level thresholds are crossed, is a practical illustration.

When it comes to wider environmental issues such as acid rain or global warming these types of physical action may also be necessary to ensure cross-country agreements can be reached. Such measures as the European Commission's regulations on the fitting of catalytic converters to cars come within this framework. Even here, however, markets are not without their uses since they can provide insights into the appropriate intensity of these regulatory policies.

The use of market insights

There is a further way in which markets can be useful in handling the full costs of the car. While direct markets for the environment are poorly developed, there are other markets where environmental and health considerations are implicitly traded. The prices of houses which are, to all intents and purposes, identical except for the traffic noise to which they are subjected often vary quite dramatically. There is also evidence that levels of some more immediately obvious atmospheric pollution can also affect house prices (Button, 1993). Information thrown up by these latter markets can often be usefully tapped to gain insights into the values society places on environmental attributes. These insights can then offer guidance as to the types of abatement levels policy-makers should be aiming for. They can also provide important inputs into the assessment of transport investment proposals although they are not yet used in this role in the UK (GB Department of Transport, 1989).

What these markets help to reveal is the value that people place on safety and health considerations (Smith, 1990). There is often the mistaken impression—not helped by some of the more popular literature on the subject—that by looking at the amounts that individuals spend on safety features of cars, for instance, one is seeking to place a value on a life. What is, in fact, being done is to analyse trade-offs to gain an idea of how much individuals and society are prepared to pay to reduce the risk of death or injury. Decisions of this type are made implicitly, and sometimes explicitly, all the time. Such market-based information helps to establish the benefits of bringing about particular changes in the environmental impacts of the car. These benefits can then be matched against the costs.

How reliable are the monetary figures produced by these economic studies of markets which implicitly trade environmental effects? They certainly tend to vary according to the type of environmental or health effect one is focusing on (Quinet, 1994; Bleijenberg et al., 1994). In some cases, especially where research has been quite extensive over the years, and where the problem can be relatively easily interpreted on a single scale, such as traffic noise nuisance, a relatively consistent picture is emerging. In other areas, for example relating to greenhouse gas emissions, it is more difficult to find appropriate markets to explore and the underlying measurement problems are greater. Unfortunately, there is often a tendency in debates to treat all these types of calculation as being equally accurate or reasonable. This is simply not the case, and there is still much work to be done looking at implicit trade-offs before all environmental cost calculations can be viewed in a comparable way. Nevertheless, important and useful information is being generated.

What are the ways forward?

A consideration, seldom discussed by economists, is whether there may be some better method of approaching the environmental and health aspects of transport policy other than through notions of markets. One could, of course, simply dictate standards or regulations without any regard to their economic implications. Indeed, this is sometimes done. The problem is that the economy is a system and adjustments in one segment have ripple effects, both through all other sectors and on the dynamic development of the overall system. Ultimately, perhaps our understanding of these delicate social linkages will become sufficient to make it possible to intervene and control the system. At present, this is hardly the case—as efforts to control relatively simply phenomena such as the rate of inflation demonstrate. We are, therefore, left with a situation that market type approaches, with all their weaknesses, offer possibly the best framework in which to view the environmental and health implications of modern motorized transport.

What we are seeing, however, is a slowly expanding appreciation of the ways in which particular policy instruments can be applied in the transport sector to improve the current situation. Not all have been successful, but in some cases careful and limited interventions have produced successful policy outcomes (Barde and Button, 1990). Some of these have involved non-market approaches, in the sense they have been regulatory measures, but they were initially thought through in a market context (that is, looking at costs and benefits).

Conclusions

The aim of this chapter has been to set the role of markets in the transport–health–environment debate into context. We live in a market economy and, despite their numerous imperfections, such economic systems have many demonstrable advantages over other forms of organizational structure. The crucial thing to remember about markets is that they are not an end in their own right—as Adam Smith acknowledged. They are a means of achieving particular ends and specific goals, and they are often very good at doing this. Further, even in circumstances where they do not work perfectly, they may prove better than alternatives. Human beings generally like being proactive and want to intervene, feeling perhaps that intervention inevitably brings better results than allowing nature to take its course. As in medicine and other fields, this has not always proved the case with environmental and economic matters.

One could view these conclusions as being excessively pessimistic, but this would not be entirely correct. A lot has been done to reduce many of the traditionally recognized public health problems posed by motor cars. They are now much safer than in the past. The use of leaded fuel is declining. Catalytic converters are reducing the problems of NO_x emissions. Vehicles are quieter. We now have a structure of longer-term petrol duty increases as a measure to contain CO_2 emissions. Some of the change has come about through the use of market instruments, although they have not been the main policy tool. Other issues, especially relating to some local health problems, are relatively new concerns that clearly require action either through command-and-control policies or the adoption of new fiscal measures. Their 'newness', coupled with our lack of a full understanding of the underlying causes and effects, naturally stirs public concern. The challenge is to mobilize market and other instruments to tackle them effectively. The issue is not really that markets are causing these problems but rather that markets, as currently operated, simply do not fully embrace them.

References

Barde J-P, Button KJ (eds) (1990) *Transport Policy and the Environment: six case studies.* Earthscan, London

Bleijenberg AN, van den Berg WJ, de Wit G (1994) *Social Costs of Traffic: A Literature Review.* Centrum voor Energiebesoparing en Schone Technologie, Delft

Button KJ (1992) *Market and Government Failures in Environmental Policy: The Case of Transport.* OECD, Paris

Button KJ (1993) *Transport, the Environment and Economic Policy.* Edward Elgar, Aldershot

Button KJ (1994) Alternative approaches towards containing transport externalities: an international comparison. *Transportation Research Part A-Policy and Practice, 28,* 289–305

Button KJ, Rothengatter W (1993) Global environmental degradation: the role of transport. In Banister D and Button KJ (eds), *Transport, the Environment and Sustainable Development,* Spon, London

Coase RH (1960) The problem of social cost. *Journal of Law and Economics, 3,* 1–44

European Conference of Ministers of Transport (1994) *Internalising the Social Costs of Transport.* ECMT/OECD, Paris

Great Britain Department of the Environment (1994) *Sustainable Development: The UK Strategy (Cm 2426).* HMSO, London

Great Britain Department of Transport (1989) *COBA 9 Manual.* Department of Transport, London

Great Britain House of Commons Select Committee on Transport (1994) *Transport-related Air Pollution in London (HC-506).* HMSO, London

Great Britain Royal Commission on Environmental Pollution (1994) *Eighteenth Report: Transport and the Environment (Cm 2674).* HMSO, London

Hahn RW (1989) Economic prescriptions for environmental problems: how the patient followed the doctor's orders. *Journal of Economic Perspectives, 3 (2)*, 95–114

Organisation for Economic Co-operation and Development (1994) *Managing the Environment: The Role of Economic Instruments*. OECD, Paris

Quinet E (1994) The social costs of transport: evaluation and links with internalisation policies. In European Conference of Ministers of Transport, *Internalising the Social Costs of Transport*. ECMT/OECD, Paris

Rothengatter W (1994) Obstacles to the use of economic instruments in transport policy. In European Conference of Ministers of Transport, *Internalising the Social Costs of Transport*. ECMT/OECD, Paris

Smith A (1904) *An Inquiry into the Nature and Causes of the Wealth of Nations* (ed Cannan E). Methuen, London

Smith VK (1990) Can we measure the economic value of environmental amenities? *Southern Economic Journal*, 56, 865–878

26
Sustainable transport policies: state of the art

Felix Walter, Stefan Suter and René Neuenschwander

ECOPLAN Economic and Environmental Studies, Bern, Switzerland

Health is certainly a key objective in a sustainable transport policy. We would call a development 'sustainable' if the impact—in our context the impact of the transport system—does not exceed the environment's capacity to regenerate and is therefore permanently tolerable. In a broader context, however, we should not forget that objectives like the conservation of resources and the needs of future generations and of people outside the established market economies belong to the concept of sustainability.

There are far more synergies than conflicts between a 'more healthy' and a 'more sustainable' development, especially in the fields of transport. Nevertheless, our civilization and the transport system in particular remain a long way from this long-term objective of the 1992 Earth Summit in Rio de Janeiro. However, what to change and where to begin remain hotly disputed.

The scope of this chapter is to give an overview of strategies and instruments that have been used so far in pursuit of a sustainable transport policy, especially at the urban level. In particular, it explores one aspect of how economists see the problem: transport generates what are called external costs, costs not borne by transport users but by society as a whole. Air pollution, for example, impairs visibility (smog), damages materials and plants and adversely affects human health. Other examples of external costs are the costs of traffic noise, uncovered costs of traffic accidents or time losses due to congestion. Although an exact calculation of external costs of transport is not possible, a conservative assessment can provide reliable lower limits for the external costs. An overview of the results of several European studies shows that the reasonable range of the external costs of transport in Europe is about 1.5 to 2.5% of gross domestic product (Figure 26.1).

As accidents, air pollution and noise all affect human health, it can easily be seen that health problems are important external costs. They are thus key

Health at the Crossroads: Transport Policy and Urban Health.
Edited by Tony Fletcher and Anthony J. McMichael © 1997 John Wiley & Sons Ltd

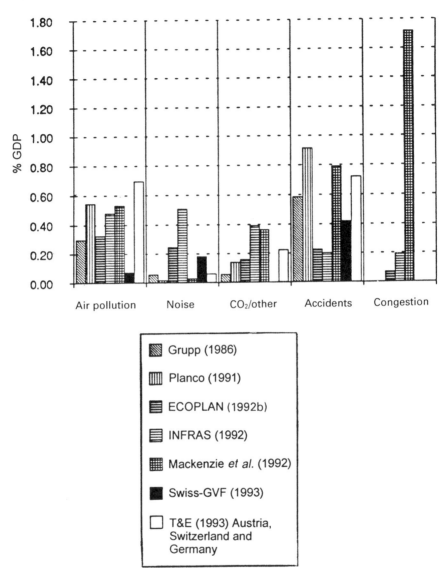

Figure 26.1 External costs of car traffic (% of GDP) as estimated in seven different studies

problems to be solved when talking about sustainable urban transport. Further, when we think about the impact of transport systems upon global warming and the depletion of resources, we should note that these health problems are part of a broader discussion.

Even if the focus of transport policy is often at the urban level, not all the problems can and should be solved at this level. Many problems are not limited to urban areas and a number of instruments can only be implemented at a national or international level. The following short overview of European strategies in transport policy is therefore not strictly limited to urban policy—nor to health problems. We distinguish three spatial levels of strategies: strategies at the European level; strategies at the national level; and strategies at the urban level.

Strategies at the European level

At the level of the European Union there are vigorous discussions about economic instruments. But in reality measures other than price strategies dominate the transport policy of the European Union.

Infrastructure policy

In the next ten years the EU plans to construct approximately 7500 miles of new motorways. This is the main answer to the expected growth of transport demand that accompanies the completion of the European internal market.

Emission standards

These standards for fuels and for motor vehicles have led to a marked reduction in emissions of air pollutants per mile driven and will continue to play an important role. But the growth of traffic more than offsets this technological progress. Hence, most of the harmful effects of transport have not diminished but have grown in the last decade, and transport's share of overall emissions of CO_2, volatile organic compounds and nitrogen oxides (NO_x) will still be rising over the next few years. This is the essential conclusion we must draw from the regulatory strategy of standard setting.

Economic instruments

First, in May 1992 the Commission of the European Union suggested the introduction of an energy/CO_2 tax as a contribution to stabilization of CO_2 emissions. The suggested level of the tax is only 4 ECU per 100 litres. After the summit of December 1994, a common solution is further away than ever before.

Second, and perhaps most important, are decisions to harmonize transport taxes and charges. In October 1992 the Council of the European Union adopted a directive fixing the minimum rate of excise duty on diesel and fuel. This minimum rate is quite low, but it is a first step to a harmonized introduction of higher fuel prices. In June 1993 the Council decided to set minimum rates for taxes and charges on heavy goods vehicles, from 1 January 1995. This same decision also authorized member states to introduce or to maintain tolls and user charges. This decision will lead to a general increase in the cost of road haulage. Five European countries have already decided to cooperate in introducing user charges.

Strategies at the national level

Besides various strategies in relation to infrastructure policy and emission regulation, the use of economic instruments has become increasingly prominent in European countries. Some countries have begun to integrate ecological aspects into taxes.

– In Scandinavian countries (Finland, Norway, Sweden), for instance, sales taxes are differentiated according to the emission standards of the cars.
– The same is true for recurrent annual charges which in several countries (Sweden, Austria, Germany, Finland, Greece) are differentiated according to engine size and other factors affecting fuel use.

Fuel taxes are the most important measure at national level to internalize the external costs of transport: again there are large differences between European countries. Figure 26.2 summarizes the fuel taxes in those countries for the beginning of the year 1994. It shows that:

– In all European countries, excise tax and VAT (value added tax) form the largest part of the taxation of fuel. Most of this revenue is used to finance the extension and the maintenance of the road network.
– Most countries have an extra charge on leaded petrol.
– Only Norway, the Netherlands, Sweden and Finland levy environmental or CO_2 taxes. The taxation of fuel has so far only very poorly reflected environmental concerns.
– What finally counts is the overall taxation level, not the name of the taxes. Looking at the large differences between 'ordinary' petroleum tax, the introduction of new low environmental taxes may not seem very relevant.

Strategies at the urban level

The negative effects of transport are most important in urban areas. That is why a special urban transport policy is needed to prevent the traffic collapse and to improve quality of life in cities. Strategies towards sustainable policies for urban transportation have been developed in many cities, and typically comprise a combination of measures such as those in favour of pedestrians and cyclists, the improvement of public transport and changes in urban planning. But the *sine qua non* is restriction of car use. Here economic instruments play an important role.

The OECD European Conference of Ministers of Transport (OECD/ECMT)

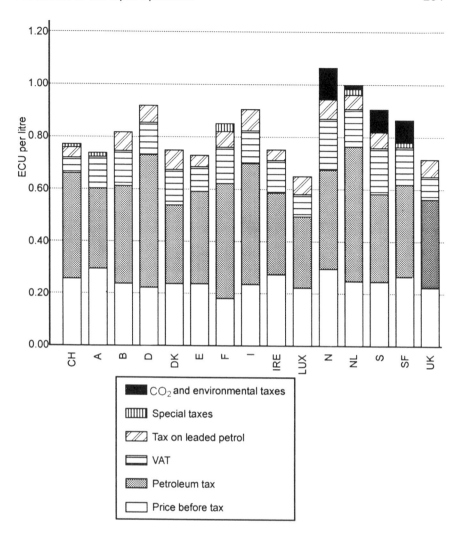

Figure 26.2   The taxation of fuel in European countries, 1994. CH, Switzerland; A, Austria; B, Belgium; D, Germany; DK, Denmark; E, Spain; F, France; I, Italy; IRE, Ireland; LUX, Luxembourg; N, Norway; NL, Netherlands; S, Sweden; F, Finland; UK, United Kingdom

project 'Urban Travel and Sustainable Development' showed that the cities examined have adopted a wide variety of policies (i.e. 449!) to change mobility patterns (Dasgupta, 1993). Figure 26.3 gives an overview of the most important policy measures implemented in the last two decades or planned for the future. We will briefly discuss some of the strategies.

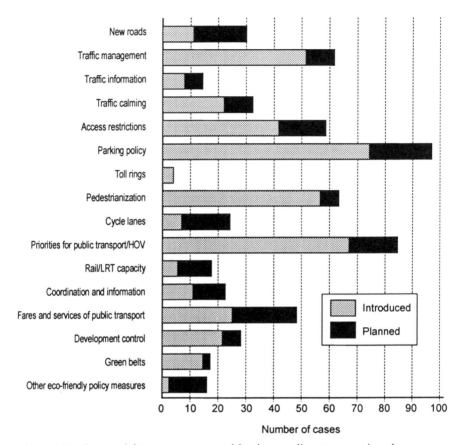

Figure 26.3   Past and future transport and land use policy measures in urban areas

Change in urban planning

For a long time spatial separation and the functional division of working and living has been a guiding principle of urban planning. This policy had major effects on land use in urban areas: a low urban density and a high need for mobility.

The new strategy in urban planning is aimed primarily at reducing the need to travel by selecting locations for living, working, shopping and recreation in such a way that the need for mobility (that is, travelling by car and driving longer distances) will decrease. This change of strategy in the direction of a more compact and mixed land use and of joint planning of transportation and land use can be considered the starting point for the more sustainable development of transport.

As an example, the principles and measures applied by the Dutch Government correspond to the new strategy in urban planning (Barendrecht, 1993):

1. High-density living.
2. New urban areas must have high-quality public transport within walking distance.
3. The location policy for business and facilities aims at locating activities that attract many employees and/or visitors as near to public transport as possible.
4. The quality of public transport and cycling links must be improved.
5. Cities must implement a stringent parking policy, discouraging long-term parking in particular.
6. The price of travelling via public transport must compete with that of car use.

The last three points reflect a further important change in urban planning in recent years: urban planning is no longer the 'art of satisfying transport demand'. It is accepted that transport policy measures are one strong condition for successful urban planning. Such policy measures are the subject of the two following sections.

Improving public transport

Because of its capacity and efficiency, public transport is well suited to ensuring large flows of traffic and preserving the environment. Therefore public transport is destined to play an expanding role in sustainable urban development. The question is, how can road users be induced to travel by public transport instead of using the car. In the past, the answer usually was 'let's make public transport more attractive'. In many cities the population agreed with a transport policy that gave priority to public transport.

The experience of the city of Zurich has shown the possibilities and the limits of such a policy. The following policy measures in favour of public transport were part of a plan to promote public transport (Ott, 1993):

1. A speed-up programme for public transport (separate bus tracks, maximum priority for public transport vehicles at traffic lights directly operated by trams and buses).
2. The introduction of a regional rail network interlinked with the national rail network ('S-Bahn') with more capacity and new connections and stations.
3. The introduction of a basic interval timetable and a tariff agreement.
4. The incorporation of the individual transport operators within the Zurich Transport Authority (ZVV).
5. A major marketing strategy.

There were clear positive results from this enormous effort: from 1985 to 1990, the number of travellers on public transport increased by 30%. The approximate 470 public transport trips per person and year on municipal transport services are noteworthy. The main negative result was that only a few former road-users switched to public transport: the opening of the regional metro system did not result in less car traffic (ECOPLAN, 1991). One reason for this disappointing outcome is the so-called 'fundamental law of traffic congestion', the fact that any reduction of congestion due to road users switching to public transport tends to increase attractiveness of car use. This again raises the car traffic volume and leads to congestion. Zurich has come to the inescapable conclusion that promoting ecological transport modes is not sufficient; it is essential to limit the attractiveness of private car travel. A further negative result of the policy measures in favour of public transport are the ZVV's enormous budgetary deficits (INFRAS, 1992).

Restrictions on car use

Access limitations. In many European cities, access to central zones is restricted (Button, 1992). This can be done by banning cars entirely from certain areas (for example, pedestrian zones), by limiting the access to a certain zone to holders of a permit (for example, Milan, Bologna) or by number plate controls (for example, the odd/even number plates allowed on alternative days in Athens since 1992).

From an economic point of view, access limitations may be inefficient. They impose rigid barriers to people's behaviour and cannot take into account the different preferences of road users. This would not be the case if the permits were tradable.

Experience with access restrictions has shown the following advantages and disadvantages (Rothengatter, 1993):

1. Limitations of car use in city centres are widely accepted within the population (Internationaler Verband für öffentliches Verkehrswesen und Socialdata, 1992).
2. Once introduced, they lead to a marked and immediate reduction of traffic flow at low investment costs.
3. Access limitation encourages people to find ways of circumventing the rules: in Athens, for instance, falsified car number plates were fitted to vehicles to facilitate all-week driving.
4. Traffic flow in areas around the restricted zone increased and this posed problems to public transport.

Road pricing. Road pricing is the most important economic instrument to internalize external costs of urban transportation.

1. The main reason for the introduction of urban toll rings in the Norwegian cities Oslo, Bergen and Trondheim was to finance urban road networks and to meet the demand of increasing traffic (Solheim, 1992). In Oslo and Trondheim a portion of the collected funds is used for public transport infrastructure and amenities for pedestrians and cyclists. The Trondheim system is completely automatic with electronic payment. In Oslo, the introduction of the toll ring led to a considerable reduction of traffic volume in the short term, but has had only minor effects on the long-term trends. The modal split did not change in favour of public transport.

2. The introduction of an electronic toll ring system in the Stockholm region is part of a plan to solve the environmental and congestion problems.
3. A new road pricing technology to reduce congestion is to be tested in Cambridge: the costs of using congested roads will be deducted from a tax card (similar to telephone cards). It is estimated that the introduction of the congestion metering system would cut traffic emissions by approximately 50% (Larkinson, 1992).

Lessons learned from European cities such as Oslo, Bergen or Trondheim are that road pricing schemes offer the best opportunities to:

1. collect money to finance road building and maintenance;
2. reduce traffic volume and therefore congestion;
3. influence the modal split away from car traffic; and
4. internalize the external costs.

Parking policy. Parking policy should be a major element of a green urban transport policy. Because every car trip begins and finishes on a parking lot, parking policy is a suitable instrument to influence mobility patterns. Parking policy measures are: parking time restrictions, reductions in the number of surface parking lots in city centres, extension of park-and-ride facilities and—most important—higher parking fees.

Parking fees allow temporally and spatially differentiated increases in the cost of car use and can therefore be a flexible part of an urban internalization strategy. From an economic point of view (ECOPLAN, 1992a), parking fees should not only charge for the costs of land use and maintenance of the parking lot, but should also contribute to the internalization of external costs.

The discussion on parking policy is often hardly rational but highly emotional. Retailers and their organizations complain that higher parking fees and a reduced supply of parking facilities in central urban areas would induce car users to orient themselves away from the city centre towards the urban fringe shopping centre. However, German studies have shown that city centres with a relatively low supply of car parking and high modal split in favour of environmentally friendly transport modes (public transport, walking, cycling) are actually more successful than those with more parking facilities (Apel, 1990). Despite the usual opposition of retailers, there has been a significant change in public awareness. The political acceptance of parking fees has grown in recent years.

Conclusion

The discussion of the different transport policy measures has shown:

1. that there are several effective instruments and strategies to attain a more sustainable urban transport policy; and
2. that some cities have already implemented such policy measures.

The successes and failures (according to the OECD Group on Urban Affairs) of urban policies can be assessed as shown in Table 26.1.

The assessment makes clear that 'the approach of the infrastructure engineers' has failed. Central to this approach is the idea of unlimited growth. The answer to the question 'How can we get people to move, to feel free and liberated?' usually was: 'Let us build motorways, bypasses and parking lots' (Berger, 1992). The objective of transport policy was mainly to satisfy growing demand by providing new transport infrastructure and public transport services. The public sector first of all acted as investor. Hence the political acceptance of transport policy was high because this policy was seemingly lucrative for all those involved. But it is now understood that neither road investments nor the improvement of public transport have solved the major problems of urban transport.

Nor did 'the approach of the technicians' succeed in solving the problems of urban transport. The faith in the development of emission reduction technologies as the only way out of the unpleasant situation proved to be wrong. However, the

Table 26.1   Subjective assessment of successes and failures of urban policies: actual experiences (upper symbols) and potentials (symbols in brackets) (Webster, 1993)

Actions taken	Conges- tion	Air pollution	Noise	Visual effects	Public transport	Road safety	Global warming
Road investment and traffic management	+ (– – –)	– –	– –	–	–	+	– – –
Road pricing (tolls) and parking policy	+ + (+ + +)	+ (+ +)	+ (+)	+ (+ +)	+ + (+ +)	+ + (+ +)	+ (+ +)
Improvement of public transport	(– – –)	(– –)			+ + +	+	–
Land use planning	+ (– –)	+ (– –)		–	+	+ (+)
Pedestrian and cyclist policy, traffic calming	–	+ (+)	+ (+)	+ + (+)		+ + (+ + +)	
Emission control	+ (+ +)	+ + (+ +)	(+ +)				+ (+ + +)

Key: The first line shows the *experiences* actually made, i.e. the success of the various actions taken with regard to the different problems of urban transport:

+some measure of success	– made the problem slightly worse
+ +successful	– – made the problem worse
+ + +highly successful	– – – made the problem much worse

In the second line, it is assessed whether the instrument and strategies have the *potential* to contribute more to a solution of the problems or whether their potential has been overrated:

(+) slight potential for improvement	(–) did not quite live up to expectations
(+ +) high potential for improvement	(– –) did not live up to expectations
(+ + +) very high potential for improvement	(– – –) did not at all live up to expectations

experts from OECD/ECMT are still optimistic with regard to the potential of further developments in emission control (see the last line of Table 26.1). What about 'the approach of the economists' that suggests a wider and more consistent use of market forces through the use of economic instruments (parking fees, road pricing) as the existence of external costs indicates that the price signals in the transport sector are wrong (OECD, 1993)? The potential of a transport policy which sets financial incentives to change mobility behaviour and to increase the efficiency of the use of existing transport infrastructure is viewed particularly favourably (see second line in Table 26.1). That is, in a future urban transport policy in which the road users pay for both internal and external costs, transport will be on a dynamic path towards sustainability.

Furthermore, Table 26.1 shows that a green urban transport policy must consist of a policy mix. As a rule, one sole instrument does not optimally cover all of the fields of a sustainable or 'green' urban transportation system. Cities with high shares of non- or little-polluting means of transport like Amsterdam, Stockholm, Zurich, Bologna, Basle and Gröningen have used several instruments and strategies to achieve this distribution. Thus, it seems that only an interdisciplinary approach will be appropriate for tackling the serious problems of urban transport.

Despite this well-known fact, in most European cities the dilemma of achieving a green urban transport policy remains:

1. On the one hand, it is not possible to change the modal split in favour of less polluting transport modes only by promoting public transport, low or zero emission vehicles, cycling and walking. Such a policy is too expensive and too little effective to attain a green urban transportation system.
2. On the other hand, the political will for necessary restrictive policy measures to reduce private car use is often not strong enough.

This chapter has also shown that the implementation of the necessary policy measures is not a problem of scientific knowledge, but one of political acceptance. Hence, an important step towards a sustainable urban mobility is to strengthen the supportive viewpoints and to overcome the opposing viewpoints among the different interest groups within society.

References

Apel D (1990) Verkehrssysteme, parkraumkonzept und innenstadtentwicklung. In Apel D, Lehmbrock M *Stadtverträgliche Vekehrsplanung—Chancen zur Steuerung des Autoverkehrs durch Parkraumkonzepte und bewirtschaftung.* Berlin

Barendrecht M (1993) *Planning in the Netherlands.* (Unpublished paper presented at the International Conference 'Travel in the City—Making it Sustainable'; 7–9 June 1993, Dusseldorf)

Berger HU (1992) Welcome Address. In Frey RL, Langloh PM (eds) *Use of Economic Instruments in Urban Travel Management.* Universität Basel, Basel

Button K (1992) Alternatives to road pricing. In Frey RL, Langloh PM (eds) *Use of Economic Instruments in Urban Travel Management.* Universität Basel, Basel

Dasgupta M (1993) *Urban Problems and Urban Policies: OECD/ECMT Study of 132 Cities.* (Unpublished paper presented at the International Conference 'Travel in the City—Making it Sustainable'; 7–9 June 1993, Dusseldorf)

ECOPLAN (1991) Szenarien zu s-bahn und siedlung. In *Auftrag der Direktion für Verkehr, Energie und Wasser des Kantons Bern,* Bern

ECOPLAN (1992a) External costs of urban transport in Berne and parking fees as a part of an internalization strategy. In Frey RL, Langloh PM (eds) *Use of Economic Instruments in Urban Travel Management.* Universität Basel, Basel

ECOPLAN (1992b) Externe Kosten im Agglomerationsverkehr, Fallbeispiel Region Bern. Studie im Rahmen des Nationalen Forschungsprogramms 25 'Stadt und Verkehr', study no. 15B, Bern

Grupp H (1986) Die sozialen Kosten des Verkehrs, Gundriss zu ihrer Berechnung. *Verkehr und Technik,* Heft 9 und 10. S. 359366; 403407

INFRAS (1992) *Internalisieren der Externen Kosten des Verkehrs, Fallbeispiel Agglomeration Zürich.* INFRAS, Zurich.

Internationaler Verband für Öffentliches Verkehrswesen und Socialdata (1992) *Einschätzungen zur Mobilität in Europa.* UITP, Brüssel und München

Larkinson J (1992) Research into road pricing: the UK Department of Transport's Programme. In Frey RL, Langloh PM (eds) *Use of Economic Instruments in Urban Travel Management.* Universität Basel, Basel

MacKenzie JJ, Dower RC, Chen DDT (1992) *The Going Rate: What it Really Costs to Drive.* World Resources Institute

OECD (1993) *Taxation and the Environment.* Complementary Policies, Paris

Ott R (1993) *Making Public Transport More Attractive.* (Unpublished paper presented at the International Conference 'Travel in the City—Making it Sustainable'; 7–9 June 1993, Dusseldorf)

Planco Consulting (1991) Externe Kosten des Verkehrs: Schiene, Strasse und Binnenschiffahrt. From the Deutsche Bundesbahn, Essen

Rothengatter W (1993) *Obstacles to the Use of Economic Instruments in Transport Policy.* OECD/ECMT, Paris

Solheim T (1992) Introducing urban tolls: the Norwegian experiences. In Frey RL, Langloh PM (eds) *Use of Economic Instruments in Urban Travel Management.* Universität Basel, Basel

Swiss-GVF (1993) *Grundlagen zur Kostenwahrheit im Verkehr. Vorschläge für eine Gesamtverkehrsrechnung unter Einbezug von externen Kosten und Nutzen.* GVF-Bericht 3/93. Bern

T&E (The European Federation for Transport and Environment/author P Kageson) (1993) *Getting the Prices Right. A European Scheme for Making Transport Pay its True Costs.* T&E Report 93/7. Brussels

Webster FV (1993) *Successes and Failures in Urban Policies.* (Unpublished paper presented at the International Conference 'Travel in the City—Making it Sustainable'; 7–9 June 1993, Dusseldorf)

27
Overview—future directions in policy and research

John Whitelegg

Ecologica Ltd, Lancaster, UK

The case for an alternative vision of the future of transport has never been stronger. The last two years have seen a significant consolidation of a large number of analyses and interpretations of transport policy, transport impacts and sustainable development, all of which point inexorably in the direction of fundamental change. Current policies and expenditure priorities are not delivering environmental, economic and social progress. We are locked into a situation where increases in the demand for transport erode the effectiveness and efficiency of travel and transport for everyone and accelerate the tendency towards non-sustainability.

Transport policy is now at a critical juncture. The publication of the Royal Commission report (GB Royal Commission on Environmental Pollution, 1994) and the Standing Advisory Committee on Trunk Road Assessment (SACTRA) report (GB Department of Transport, 1994) have had a dramatic effect in legitimizing and amplifying what has been a long-standing criticism of the 'predict and provide' philosophy of successive governments. This clarification of the poverty and naiveté of the last 30 years of transport planning has coincided with the realization that traffic does damage human health and that transport problems are public health problems. If we add to this powerful cocktail of insight some serious concerns about value for money and lack of evidence that roads do benefit local economic development and create jobs then we have all the preconditions for a major reassessment of policies and priorities and a shift to a new set of priorities and a new paradigm. To help sort out our objectives and policy options, it is important to focus on the concept of sustainability in transport.

Health at the Crossroads: Transport Policy and Urban Health.
Edited by Tony Fletcher and Anthony J. McMichael © 1997 John Wiley & Sons Ltd

What is sustainable transport?

A great deal has been written about sustainable transport and how it can be achieved (Whitelegg, 1993; Kageson, 1994; ECOPLAN, 1994). It is clear from this discussion and from the documentation of practical successes that there are a number of characteristics that clearly define sustainable transport. Three are described below.

Policies that work to achieve objectives and targets

Sustainable development is a practical process that leads somewhere. Every sector of the economy and every aspect of human activity has a contribution to make towards the primary goals of sustainability. These include reducing energy consumption, reducing raw material consumption, reducing the production of waste, reducing emissions especially CO_2, and protecting biodiversity through the protection of ecology and habitat. Targets already exist for CO_2, and transport represents a particularly difficult sector for CO_2 reduction. On current trajectories, it is highly unlikely that transport can deliver anything like the scale of reduction necessary to achieve a stabilization of CO_2 emissions at 1990 levels by the year 2000.

Sectoral targets for CO_2 emissions have not been set in the UK, and transport policies have not been adjusted so that investments and priorities can play their role in achieving international treaty obligations and commitments. This amounts to a clear decision not to implement sustainability policies.

Targets and objectives are equally important at the local level. CO_2 reduction strategies and strategies to reduce health damaging emissions can be implemented at the local level and are being implemented in Portland (Oregon) and discussed in Melbourne (Australia). Urban areas and corridors can work to clear targets, for example, 35% fewer passenger kilometres (pkm), 20% fewer city centre parking places, 50% fewer lorries in an urban area, 50% reduction in road tonne kilometres (tkm) on an inter-urban route. The lack of such targets encourages sloppy thinking and woolly concepts of sustainability.

The protection of human health

Human health has risen to very near the top of transport policy agendas and sustainability discussions. There is a particular concern for the health of children and a realization that a concern for future generations (the intergenerational equity issue in sustainability) is meaningless if we damage the health of the current generation of children. There is ample evidence that children's health is being damaged through exposure to traffic (Wjst *et al.*, 1993) and that all sections of the population are at risk when living in close proximity to heavily trafficked streets (Whitelegg *et al.*, 1993).

A sustainable transport policy would set out to minimize the exposure of vulnerable groups to the damaging influences of traffic noise, vehicle exhaust emissions and the stress caused by the constant fear of road traffic accidents and community severance. Equally important is the loss of quiet countryside and recreational activities such as cycling away from the noise, smell and visual intrusion of new roads. The loss of countryside and the loss of 'tranquil areas' has been thoroughly documented by CPRE (Sinclair, 1993).

Transport policies can have a health-nurturing effect through the promotion of community activities, physical exercise (e.g. cycling) and reduced susceptibility to a number of diseases. Healthy cities are unlikely to be associated with dense traffic flows, air pollution and noise disruption.

The development of economic activity

Sustainable transport policies are not in any way inimical to economic activity. They do not seek to reduce the costs of transport in order to encourage longer distance movements of freight and passengers, but they do seek to provide businesses with high quality access conditions and a wide range of choices for the movement of goods and people. In combination with increasing the costs of transport, such policies will provide more encouragement to local firms to seek out market opportunities and better commuting conditions for workers. Sustainable transport policies will benefit a large number of local communities through a net increase in jobs. At best, the non-sustainable alternatives can only offer jobs at a few locations, and then only in association with large amounts of lorry movement and pollution. Sustainable development is not a process of job destruction or de-industrialization, but it does require a major rethink of attitudes towards traditional views of economic growth and the demand for transport. More importantly, there is considerable evidence (reviewed later) that sustainable transport and sustainable development can create jobs more successfully and use scarce resources more effectively than non-sustainability based on cheap transport and new transport infrastructure.

How do we know that we are running on a non-sustainable trajectory?

This question is much easier to answer now we have the report of the Royal Commission on Environmental Pollution (GB Royal Commission on Environmental Pollution, 1994). This report describes in some detail the problems associated with current levels of transport investment and infrastructure, and the impossibility of continuing with existing policies. Both freight and passenger transport have declined in efficiency in the past 30 years. We drove 22% more miles in 1990/91 compared to miles driven in 1985/86, but still do roughly the same sort of thing, such as go to work, school, shop and leisure facilities. This is an important indicator of inefficiency. In freight transport we move the same goods over increasingly long distances, giving rise to the complexities of distribution and sourcing so vividly revealed by Böge (1994) in the German yoghurt study.

More effort for the same work done

Böge (1994) maps the flow of materials into a yoghurt and chocolate pudding production plant in southern Germany, and quantifies all the lorry movement associated with the supply chain. Most of these raw materials can be sourced much closer to the factory than is currently the case. The reasons they are sourced at very long distances have a great deal to do with the cheapness of transport and the cheapness of components when bought in large quantities from a high volume source. When this is coupled with additional advantages to be obtained from seeking out distant sources of cheap labour, the attraction of thousands of lorry-miles can be seen to be perfectly rational within the parameters of the prevailing economic system and its cost structures.

Return of the smog

The eradication of the 'pea souper' following the 1952 London smog and new clean air regulations is often quoted as one of the success stories of environmental and public health intervention. The 1990s have seen the return of poor air quality and an increase in respiratory illness (particularly asthma) and fatalities. The December 1991 smog in London was responsible for approximately 200 excess deaths and 1994 saw frequent poor air quality warnings. The main culprit is motor vehicle exhaust emissions and there is a proven link between air pollution from this source and poor health. Walters (1994) has concluded:

- recent evidence has convincingly shown that death rates from heart and lung disease are up to 37% higher in cities with high levels of fine particulates;
- people exposed to high traffic levels experience more respiratory symptoms and worse lung function than people who live in areas with less traffic; and
- three traffic-related pollutants: particulates, NO_x and ozone are all associated with a fall in lung function and an increase in respiratory symptoms in healthy people as well as those with asthma.

These conclusions are amplified in a large number of studies in the USA, particularly the work of Dockery (1996).

Increasing levels of congestion

In spite of elevated levels of expenditure on additional road capacity over the last ten years, congestion problems have increased in severity. The vast majority of local authorities have voiced a concern about congestion levels and related pollution issues in urban areas, noting in passing that average speeds in urban areas are now less than they were 20 years ago. The construction of bypasses and inner ring roads has not solved congestion problems. Several urban areas in Lancashire, including Preston, Burnley and Blackburn, have both bypasses and inner relief/ring roads and serious congestion problems. Congestion is no worse in towns like Lancaster that have avoided inner relief roads and do not have bypasses other than the M6. Pfleiderer and Dieterich (1994) have noted the impact of new road capacity on creating new traffic and the GB Standing Advisory Committee on Trunk Road Assessment (SACTRA, 1994) has arrived at the same conclusion in a report to the government.

Congestion problems indicate the ability of traffic to fill available space and the necessity for a sustainable approach based on demand management, parking reduction and pricing policies to increase the cost of transport.

Suffer the little children

Children suffer many of the effects of our high levels of car dependency. They are deprived of independent mobility, injured and killed as they attempt to use roads and pavements, deprived of learning experiences and exposed to lung damaging pollutants. Researchers in both Sweden (Björklid, 1992) and the UK (Whitelegg, 1994) have drawn attention to the very serious consequences of such a concerted attack on the welfare of children.

Pig in a poke

Current levels of expenditure on transport in the UK are approximately £5 billion per annum. Rarely can so much non-military expenditure have been allocated by so few with so little analysis of value for money and with so little to show for it. It is very rare indeed for any ex-post validation or audit of expenditure to take place. If roads are justified on the grounds that they relieve congestion or create jobs, then these outcomes should be monitored and results published. I suggest that performance tables for new roads would make more interesting reading than similar tables for hospitals and school exam results.

There are a large number of alternatives available for reallocating this expenditure (e.g. Transport 2000, 1993) and the alternatives that have been suggested are unlikely to be as bad value for money as current priorities. There is an urgent need for research to identify value for money in alternative budget strategies.

What evidence is there that sustainable transport ideas are being implemented?

Dramatic progress is being made in Germany and the Netherlands in advancing car-free city concepts and car-free residential areas. The first European car-free city conference took place in Amsterdam in March 1994, and established a European car-free city club with 30 participating cities (the UK participants are Glasgow, Leeds, Aberdeen, Nottingham, Doncaster, Edinburgh and Birmingham).

The city of Bremen is currently implementing a car-free residential area development in the suburb of Hollerland, which has enormous relevance for UK cities and the practical implementation of sustainable transport policies. Bremen's experiment is based on a legally binding contract between residents and the city council not to keep or use a car in the new development.

Michael Glotz-Richter, the planner responsible for the Hollerland project, sees the whole idea as much more than a transport policy matter. Car-free residential areas are about urban design, quality of life, public space, community activity, health and liberating scarce resources devoted to catering for the car and reallocating them to energy efficient homes, kindergarten facilities and attractive public space. This holistic view has won the support of politicians and those who want to seek out a better quality of life for themselves. In effect, they are redefining quality of life to exclude the car, and charting a new course in the relationship between people, cities and technology (Glotz-Richter, 1994).

Car-free in the context of a residential area like Hollerland covering 2.6 hectares and supplying 250 homes releases a quarter of the total area for other uses. Thirty parking spaces will be provided instead of the 200 normally required in such a development, and these will be used for car-sharing and car-pooling schemes. The scheme is not one that simply shifts car parking to the edge, but is fundamentally different in its design objectives—which are to exchange car benefits for the greater benefits of clean air, green space, safety for children and the elderly, and a distinctive and high quality living environment. The car cannot deliver these benefits, and it destroys the environment and social conditions of many hundreds of people in its daily use.

The car-free residential area gives the residents of Bremen a choice between dirty polluted living environments, and an environment where the children can breathe clean air and play safely on the streets.

The city council has had to overcome a large number of obstacles to get as far as it has done. One of these obstacles was a parking ordinance from the Third Reich laying down generous parking/garaging arrangements for new residential developments. Parking norms are a major source of encouragement to higher levels of dependence on motorization and the time is long overdue in Britain and Germany for much reduced provision of car parking spaces of all kinds in urban areas.

The Hollerland project has revealed just how much hard cash goes to prop up car dependence. Reducing parking provision in Hollerland has saved DM 3 million. This means that rents and house prices can be reduced and building quality improved particularly from an environmental point of view. Car-free residential areas can therefore reduce energy consumption and global warming from transport source and from domestic premises because of more energy efficient homes. This is a remarkable achievement summarized by Glotz-Richter (1994) as 'the money is not lying in the road'.

Car-free residential areas depend for their success on the overall quality of public transport infrastructure and facilities for pedestrians and cyclists. This is guaranteed in the case of Hollerland with high quality connections into a city wide bike system and the tram system. The development will be completed by

1996, and will be watched very carefully indeed for the experience that will be invaluable for the next wave of car-free areas.

Three other projects taking their cue from Hollerland are already at various stages of development. In Amsterdam, the Westerpark Quarter is an inner city site formerly used by gas, water and electricity utilities and will now become the first car-free residential area in the Netherlands, supplying 600 housing units. In Berlin, Lichterfelde-Sued is a 72 hectare site formerly used for military purposes, and is proposed for a car-free residential area supplying 2000 units. Also in Berlin, Eldenauer Strasse, a former slaughter yard, is proposed for a car-free development.

In discussions of sustainability, freight transport is often overlooked. This is surprising given the rapid growth of road freight and the enormous unpopularity of lorries in an urban environment. There are a large number of practical solutions available for moving freight in ways that are more environmentally acceptable and certainly reduce noise and pollution and improve the quality of the living environment. One of the best examples of a coordinated strategy is the Netherlands. A non-governmental Dutch plan (Werkgroep 2duizend, 1993) has outlined a plan for urban distribution centres to reduce lorry movements in cities, operational strategies to reduce empty running, arrangements for picking up return loads, and substantial investments in multimodal transport and transfer points between road/rail/water transport. The substantial environmental benefits of the 'new course scenario' are summarized in Table 27.1.

Dutch cities have a great deal to offer to the transport and urban planner in search of solid evidence that new policies can be generated and implemented. Delft and Groningen both have a 50% modal share for cycling and walking, and have moved a long way in the direction of reducing auto-dependency. Cycling has considerable potential for improving the health of the population (British Medical Association, 1992) and in Groningen has been the subject of 20 million ECU expenditure since 1986 to achieve high levels of use. Leiden has an ambitious plan, not yet implemented, to reduce the number of lorries in the urban area by 80%.

A recent report from the European Federation for Transport and the

Table 27.1. Environmental effects of 'new course scenario' compared with a business-as-usual scenario (basic scenario 2015; 1990 = 100)

Environmental effect	Basic scenario	New course scenario	Sustainability target
Energy use	147	54	50
CO_2 emissions	148	57	50
NO_x emissions	70	14	18

Source: Werkgroep 2duizend (1993).

Environment (ECOPLAN, 1994) reviews European 'best practice' under a number of different headings. These include:

1. land use planning;
2. walking and cycling;
3. traffic management;
4. public transport;
5. parking; and
6. road pricing.

Each heading is associated with a description of specific examples where these policies are being implemented or monitored.

Land use planning

The Dutch experience is described where new developments are allocated to specific sites according to their traffic generating characteristics. Large traffic generators are steered in the direction of nodes of high public transport accessibility. Similar policies are in place in Bern (Switzerland) and in Vienna (Austria).

Walking and cycling

Munster (Germany), Groningen and Amsterdam (Netherlands) and Tonsberg (Norway) are described as positive examples of progress with cycling's share of transport in response to specific policies favouring that mode.

Traffic management

This category includes access limitation, traffic calming and traffic information systems. Gothenburg (Sweden) is quoted as a positive example of successful reduction of noise and pollution as a result of introducing a traffic 'cell' system. Bologna and Milan (Italy) have limited access to the central zone for motorized traffic. This has produced a 30% reduction. Lubeck and Aachen (Germany) have banned cars in the city centres.

ECOPLAN, surprisingly, does not mention the experience of the state of North Rhine Westphalia in Germany, which has introduced over 10 000 traffic-calmed areas including 30 kmph restricted areas with important benefits for air pollution levels and road traffic accidents. The traffic-calmed areas are mainly in Düsseldorf, Cologne, Essen, Bochum and Dortmund.

Public transport

Zurich is described as a positive example: 'from 1985 to 1990 the number of travellers increased by 30%. The approximately 470 public-transport trips per inhabitant and year on municipal transport are unique on this planet'. Unfortunately, very few car drivers abandoned their cars and switched to public transport. This has also been the experience of the Manchester tram system, and there are serious problems with a sustainable transport strategy based on the assumption that progress can be made by switching car drivers to public transport.

Germany has a large number of very successful public transport operations receiving substantial new investment in rail, bus, tram and ticketing systems. The design of effective public transport requires considerable coordination between modes, simple ticketing, and monthly/annual card systems and traffic management policies that give public transport the edge over cars. There are no technical problems in any of these areas, but there is a need for planning, coordination and investment. The preconditions for this have been removed in Britain by rail privatization and deregulation.

Parking

The provision of generous amounts of car parking space at work and in city centres works to increase the advantages of car use and against the interests of sustainable transport. The provision of parking spaces by employers including universities and local authorities is a serious obstacle to modal switching. There are a number of examples of transport policies based on reducing car parking places in city centres and improving the alternatives, including the alternative of park-and-ride. These include Amsterdam, Nuremberg, Munich, Bologna, Stockholm and Gothenburg.

Road pricing

'Road pricing' refers to measures taken to have road users pay in proportion to use. This is currently the subject of heated debate, and it is still far from clear how, if at all, it would produce sustainable transport. Various forms are already in place in Oslo, Bergen and Trondheim (Norway), Stockholm (Sweden), Singapore and Hong Kong, and one is under discussion for Cambridge (England). It is clear that road pricing as a means of fully internalizing the external cost of transport would work if applied to all journeys over all roads. It is highly unlikely that it will be applied with this amount of rigour and commitment to the 'polluter pays principle' and so it will remain problematic and possibly negative as a contribution to sustainability.

The European Sustainable Cities Good Practice Guide

In May 1994, the expert group on the urban environment of the European Commission produced its first annual report detailing examples of good practice

Table 27.2 a. Examples on the theme integrating urban environment and land use planning

	Country	
Emsher Park	D	Renewal of old industrial areas
Reggio Emilia	I	Integration of environmental analysis in support of the Local Land Use Plan
Strasbourg	F	Integrated environment project
Evora	P	Recovery of the historical run-down city centre
Lyon	F	Operational tools for a recovery of public spaces
Val Maubuee	F	Strengthening of ecological function of public spaces

b. Examples on the theme integrating environment and urban mobility and accessibility

Copenhagen	DK	General travel management policy
Zurich	CH	General travel management policy
Groningen	NL	General travel management policy
Oslo	N	Toll ring
Lyon	F	Parking policy
Karlsruhe	D	Intermodality tramway/train
Nancy	F	Bi-mode trolleybus network
Saint Brieuc	F	Public taxi to meet demand
Perugia	I	Policy in favour of pedestrians
Freiburg	D	Environmental cards on public transport networks

D, Germany; I, Italy; F, France; P, Portugal; DK, Denmark
CH, Switzerland; NL, Netherlands; N, Norway.
Source: European Commission (1994).

in Europe. Sixteen cities or regions are described (Table 27.2) in sufficient detail to permit rapid transfer of good ideas and good practice to other cities and regions.

There is no shortage of innovative planning and sustainable transport in action in Europe, but there is a lack of clear political commitment and vision to move quickly to correct the mistakes of the car-dependency era in European and North American history. There is still no one example of a thoroughly integrated, sustainable transport system in place embracing the whole spectrum of land use planning, walking and cycling, fiscal policies, severe traffic restraint and public transport initiatives. There is, however, enough in place to show that there is a surfeit of good policy alternatives and good ideas about how to get to where we want to be from where we are now—and how to do this within current budgets and by careful attention to local geography and local community aspirations.

Conclusion

Current, non-sustainable transport policies represent a large-scale experiment with people's lives. It is very costly, it is thought to have large benefits, but we know it has significant disbenefits, including health damage, and cannot be sustained into the future. The experiment is car-dependency. The time has now arrived to vary the diet and to experiment with other kinds of mobility, accessibility, urban form and living environments. The experiments that are now needed are in the direction of reducing this dependency and reallocating expenditures.

It has taken us 70 years to arrive at our present condition of car-dependency, so it would be reasonable to plan a 20–30 year programme of alternatives based on car-free cities, car-free residential areas, transfers of freight from road to rail and waterway/inland shipping, land use planning to increase the density and accessibility of all the things we travel for within one or two miles of where we live. None of this should be prescriptive. Unlike the present charade of a free market these alternatives will, for the first time, make choices available. If people do choose to live and work in dirty, heavily trafficked environments, then that is not a problem as long as they have the choice of clean, low noise, low pollution, safe environments. Public health specialists and environmental health officers have a role to play in making choices available and moving public policy in the direction of healthier people and healthier places. There is nothing to lose and everything to gain.

References

Björklid P (1992) Children's traffic environment and road safety education from the perspective of environmental and developmental psychology. (Unpublished paper presented at the International Conference on Road Safety in Europe, Berlin, 30 September–2 October 1992)

Böge S (1994) The well travelled yoghurt pot: lessons for new freight transport policies and regional production. *World Transport Policy and Practice*, 1, 7–11

British Medical Association (1992) *Cycling: Towards Health and Safety*. BMA, London

Dockery DW (1996) Acute respiratory effects of particulate air pollution. In *Abstracts from the Urban Air Pollution and Public Health Conference*, Environmental Change Research Centre (University College London), 23 September 1994 (in press)

ECOPLAN (1994) *Green Urban Transport: a Survey*. Preliminary report, January 1994. Ecoplan, Brussels

European Commission (1994) *European Sustainable Cities: Good Practice Guide*. Office for Official Publications of the European Communities, Luxembourg

Glotz-Richter M (1994) Living without a car: the Bremen-Hollerland experiment. *World Transport Policy and Practice*, 1, 45–47

Great Britain Department of Transport (1994) *Trunk Roads and the Generation of Traffic: Response by the Department of Transport to the Standing Advisory Committee on Trunk Road Assessment.* HMSO, London

Great Britain Royal Commission on Environmental Pollution (1994) *Eighteenth Report: Transport and the Environment.* HMSO, London

Great Britain Standing Advisory Committee on Trunk Road Assessment (SACTRA) (1994) *Trunk Roads and the Generation of Traffic,* HMSO, London

Kageson P (1994) *The concept of sustainable transport.* Personal communication

Pfleiderer R, Dieterich M (1994) New roads generate new traffic. *World Transport Policy and Practice, 1,* 29–31

Sinclair G (1993) *The Regional Lost Land: Land use change in England's Regions and Counties,* 1945–1990. Council for the Protection of Rural England, London

Transport 2000 (1993) *Transport 21: An Alternative Transport Budget.* Transport 2000, London

Walters S (1994) What are the respiratory health effects of vehicle pollution? In Read C (ed) *How Vehicle Pollution Affects Our Health.* Ashden Trust, London

Werkgroep 2duizend (1993) *A New Course in Freight Transport.* Foundation Werkgroep 2duizend, Amersfoort (Netherlands)

Whitelegg J (1993) *Transport for a Sustainable Future: the Case for Europe.* Belhaven Press, London

Whitelegg J (1994) Where the street ends: transport planning and children. (Unpublished paper presented to the Accessible City Conference, Toledo, 19–21 October 1994)

Whitelegg J, Gatrell A, Naumann P (1993) *Traffic and Health.* Lancaster University, Lancaster

Wjst M, Reitmeir P, Dold S *et al.* (1993) Road traffic and adverse effects on respiratory health in children. *British Medical Journal, 307,* 596–600

28
Future directions in policy and research: a public health perspective

Jens Steensberg

Embedslægeinstitutionen Frederiksborg AMT, Hillerød, Denmark

Twenty-five years ago a Danish author, the late Per Lange, wrote a small essay entitled: 'At the shore of traffic' (Lange, 1969). He quoted the English poet W.E. Henley who, in the early days of motoring, wrote in breathless praise of this new means of transport:

> The heart of Man
> Tears at Man's destiny
> Ever; and ever
> Makes what it may
> Of his wretched occasions,
> His infinitesimal
> Portion in Time.
> Hence the Mercedes!

As an invalid Henley probably felt that the automobile in a strange way replaced his congenital defects and made him whole. As we are all in a sense invalids, motorism may have been of importance to enhance the vital sense of human beings. It may have granted a sort of higher vigour which could in older times only be gained on horseback. The motorists are the knights of today. This may sound surprising but was confirmed some years ago by William Rootes, the British car manufacturer:

> Since the shields and lances of the Middle Ages no human invention has satisfied the manly ego like the automobile (Lange, 1969).

Evidently Mr Rootes had not anticipated that one day the world would be overpopulated by those knights, fighting so united under the holy banner of egoism that they may eventually be choked by their own weapons—like the prehistoric sabre-toothed tiger on its own teeth.

At the time that Per Lange wrote this essay, the British Royal Commission on

Health at the Crossroads: Transport Policy and Urban Health.
Edited by Tony Fletcher and Anthony J. McMichael © 1997 John Wiley & Sons Ltd

Environmental Pollution in its First Report (GB Royal Commission on Environmental Pollution, 1971) warned that it would be dangerously complacent to ignore the potential implications of the increasing number of motor vehicles. In its most recent report from 1994 it is stated that the unrelenting growth of transport has become possibly the greatest environmental threat facing the UK, and one of the greatest obstacles to achieving sustainable development (GB Royal Commission on Environmental Pollution, 1994). If one adds the pain, grief and loss of life and limb caused by road accidents, along with the range of adverse non-traumatic health impacts, it is clear that these concerns are most timely.

This chapter summarizes some of the main points of view presented in the preceding chapters—seen in a public health perspective. Some additional comments on decision-making and the implementation of public policies are also presented. They illustrate the difficulties we meet on our way to obtaining healthy urban transport policies.

A public health view of transport

What is public health?

Public health is not a concrete intellectual discipline but a field of social activity. It combines sciences, skills and beliefs that are directed to the maintenance and improvement of the health of a whole community. It is concerned with the prevention of disease, the prolongation of life and the promotion of the quality of life of human populations, and aims at reducing the burden of ill health and disability. Public health permeates through all the social, environmental and other activities of populations.

The prevailing social values determine the perception of health problems—so to some extent public health is a political activity. But, essentially, public health is an ethical enterprise committed to the notion that all persons are entitled to protection against the hazards of this world and to the minimization of disease, disability and premature death (Beauchamp, 1976).

Public health services must provide information, be able to diagnose problems, and have either the ability to initiate action by mobilizing appropriate resources or the ability to influence those responsible for executive action to undertake corrective or preventive activities. Public health practitioners identify major causes of illness and disease, devise methods of prevention, treatment or care, and thus identify priorities. However, many of their proposed solutions are difficult to implement and often attack the current citadels of power. Their results do not occur immediately and are not as dramatic as those of curative medicine. It is only if the public health practitioner can influence or deploy the resources of those in other sectors of society that truly effective activities can be developed (Holland and Fitzsimons, 1991).

The spiritual heirs of the British sanitary movement are faced with a challenge at least as great as that which faced people like Edwin Chadwick. In the opinion of Ashton (1991) the work of the public health pioneers has, over many decades, been defined and codified, frozen in relation to another era and another way of looking at the world. Its practice now seems to have become reactive and bureaucratic, rather than proactive and innovative. John Ashton (1991) in his provocative paper mentioned the 'new public health', the understanding that health is fundamentally an ecological matter which depends on an optimal balance between populations and their environments. As we approach the millennium, in his view, the two fundamental challenges to human society are 'eco-sanity' and social justice.

Transport and public health

'Sustainability' is a fashionable word. It is both used and misused. Used correctly, it is a strategy for socio-economic development that meets the needs of the present generation, without compromising the ability of future generations to meet theirs. It demands that development be pursued within the constraints of the Earth's resource base and the biosphere's capacity, which some existing strategies cannot fulfil. Sustainability requires new approaches and practical measures in many sectors of society and reorientation at the highest political level (WHO, 1990). The chairman of the World Commission on Environment and Development, the Norwegian prime minister, Gro Harlem Brundtland—herself a medical doctor trained in public health—has stressed the interdependence of health and sustainable development.

Transport is a public health issue just as much as clean water and clean air. The health-damaging effects of transport are experienced by everyone, but mostly by those in disadvantaged groups who are more likely to live in areas of high traffic density. The poor are breathing the air that the rich pollute. 'We need to develop imaginative and well-financed transport policies that will put the car firmly in its place as one among many options rather than the only one. Otherwise we will miss a vital opportunity to create a more equitable, humane and healthy society'. These were the concluding words of a recent article in the *British Medical Journal* (Godlee, 1992).

For public health impact to be an important criterion in transport policy formulation across many sectors of government, health scientists must impress upon the departments of transport, environment, manufacturing, education and others the often fundamental impact of their policies upon public health. As Tony McMichael said (McMichael, this volume, p. 10) it is essential to have good studies on the health impacts; that all participants learn better how to evaluate and deal with the uncertainties that surround all of science; that formal risk assessment is used to clarify and quantify the nature and magnitude of the public health impact; and, finally, that the results of these assessments are conveyed simply and clearly to all participants.

Accidents

Accidents constitute the third most common cause of death in the WHO European Region, after cancer and cardiovascular diseases. Although traffic fatalities have decreased in most (western) European countries over the last decade or two, motor vehicle accidents still account for approximately 40% of accidental deaths. For every death in a road accident, about 15 people are severely injured and 30 slightly injured. These injuries require complex and costly treatment technology, and medical and social services to care for the disabled (WHO, 1990). By preventing car accidents, safety precautions already in place may save more years of life than medical procedures for cancer and heart disease. If supported across the world, they will continue to be among the most successful public health initiatives ever taken (European Environment Extra, 1994).

National characteristics and problems are apparent when focusing on accident structure and special aspects of traffic safety. In all countries passenger car fatalities account for the highest percentage of killed road users, but considerable differences emerge in an international comparison. Thus, Great Britain, among western European countries, records the highest percentage of pedestrian fatalities. Reliable analyses are, however, hampered by the under-reporting of accidents (Brühning, this volume, pp. 118–20).

The risk of fatal injury in an automobile accident provides an excellent example of the 'prevention paradox': for the individual, highways are very safe and getting safer; yet, at the community level, the level of safety could probably be doubled if everyone wore seatbelts and air bags were installed in every car. This way of looking at the problem suggests that many modern risks are group rather than individual problems; we address problems at the collective level that we ignore or tend to neglect at the individual level (Beauchamp, 1988). The preventive paradox, described by Geoffrey Rose, is at the heart of prevention in modern society: 'a preventive measure which brings much benefit to the population offers little to each participating individual' (Rose, 1991).

Air pollution

During the first decades of industrialization in Europe inhabitants of cities were frequently offended by smells, gases and smoke emitted from factories and workshops. It was extremely difficult to trace directly any illness to these outpourings of industry and it was partly for this reason that effective legislation to control air pollution was slow in coming.

In England, John Simon, the Victorian medical officer, in 1878 insisted that it was surely not necessary to prove that air pollution causes specific disease (Wohl, 1983):

> to be free from bodily discomfort is a condition of health . . . When a man is living in an
> atmosphere which keeps him constantly below par . . . that is an injury to health

(though not a production of what at present could be called a definite disease) . . .
Every population includes a certain proportion who have sensitive bronchi; and such
sensitive people are frequently much troubled with those vapours as an effect on health . . .

The modern road vehicle is safer and quieter, consumes less fuel and pollutes less than its predecessor of even a few years ago, but the growing density of traffic and the infrastructure necessary to support it are profoundly affecting both urban and rural areas. Despite better design and more stringent controls, vehicle emissions are responsible for a substantial proportion of air pollution such as carbon monoxide, nitrous oxides, lead, formaldehyde, benzene, pyrene and soot. Even well maintained diesel engines emit particulates that may harm the respiratory tract and potentially carcinogenic hydrocarbons, and in many European cities traffic emissions are the main cause of photochemical smog (WHO, 1990).

It is interesting that as late as 1979 the UK Ministry of Transport felt able to state that there was no evidence that air pollution by motor vehicles had any adverse effect on health. It is now quite clear that transport emissions have a wide range of adverse short-term and long-term effects upon human health. If one takes an inclusive view of the many health impacts one can readily confirm the contemporary impression held by people who inhabit large traffic-congested cities. Their view—and that of McMichael (this volume, pp. 10–11)—is that this is not a healthy way to conduct our life.

Other aspects

If it were possible to draw up a list of the various problems facing society, noise would rank among the most insidious: vast numbers of people are exposed to noise at work, while travelling and at rest; the severity of ill-effects has been underplayed and overlooked; the nature of noise as an environmental stressor may well have a synergistic effect with other stressors and other forms of pollution; and the unique nature of noise as a pollutant presents us with complex technical, social, political and legal issues (Bugliarello *et al.*, 1976).

The source of noise outside the workplace which disturbs the largest number of people for the longest period is transport. Between 10 and 20% of the population in Western industrialized countries live in areas exposed to outdoor noise levels in excess of 65 dB(A). This level has in many countries been considered the upper limit of 'tolerance' or 'acceptability' (OECD, 1979).

We should not forget the disruption of social relations and neighbourhoods resulting from the domination of automobiles in the city landscape. The urban environment in many cities of the world, with maybe the Netherlands and Scandinavian countries as notable exceptions, has become hostile to walking and cycling. Mayer Hillman reminds us (this volume, p. 179) that cycling or walking can be used as part of the routine daily travel by most people from childhood through to old age. This form of physical exercise is conducive to positive health.

Decision-making

Knowledge

Scientific facts have a relative character and the results of biological research frequently remind us of our ignorance. In empirical sciences, like epidemiology, causal associations cannot be proven in an absolute sense. Although empirical science is often insufficient to satisfy the intellect it may, however, be sufficient to direct preventive action, and the effect of prevention may give the final proof of its justification. While admitting the imprecision of the biological sciences it should be remembered that the apparently exact technical sciences also rest upon uncertainties and judgements (Steensberg, 1989).

Scientific evidence is not the determining factor in regulatory action. It seems to be realized insufficiently by the public and politicians that decisions on prevention must be taken on the basis of inadequate knowledge. However, the degree of proof needed should increase with the severity of consequences following a wrong decision. An over-critical attitude to existing knowledge and unrealistic demands of proof may support the forces in society that are not willing to accept change, i.e. preventive action. The prevention of environmentally-caused disease cannot always await our understanding of the mechanism of causation. We should pay more attention to abatement strategies, irrespective of the causal factor. We should focus not only on human behaviour but also on the social, political, economic and physical environments that largely determine behaviour. Long-term concerns for the protection of our ecosystems, even with the ultimate aim of safeguarding man, do not yet weigh sufficiently heavily against other governmental goals, such as employment, economic stability or energy supply.

What goes on inside the 'black box' of decision-making is not a rational, logical process in which information and research determine policy outcomes. It is a highly political process in which power and entrenched interests are the main driving forces. Values play an important part in policy-making. Conservative governments are more likely to favour policies that put the emphasis on individuals and changes in lifestyle. Socialist governments are more likely to favour state action, both within health services and other sectors. Researchers must go beyond research to sell their ideas to policy-makers. It is not enough to publish scientific papers in learned journals. Ideas have to be packaged and presented clearly and attractively to make an impact (Ham, 1990).

David Gee (this volume, pp. 31–8) pointed to the fact that the experience of victims and common-sense observations often predate confirmation by experts, sometimes by several decades. Common-sense observations can turn out to be more accurate about health hazards than pronouncements by 'authorities' such as that made on vehicle pollution by the UK Ministry of Transport in 1979. Waiting for 'convincing' human evidence may be costly, in terms of deaths, ill health and treatment, but the benefit of the scientific doubt is still given to substances (or pollution), and not to the health of the people.

It must be understood that clear and definitive scientific evidence is often elusive. Ambient air pollution illustrates well the problems posed to epidemiological research by a predominantly 'ecological' (community-shared) exposure. The estimation of health risks typically depends on studies conducted at the population or group level either between geographic locations or across time, because it is very difficult to make discriminating measures of air pollution exposure at the individual level (McMichael, this volume, pp. 9–23). There are still many open questions in air pollution epidemiology. To address these, innovative research approaches will have to be used. They should effectively combine traditional study designs, achieve better exposure assessment and use larger and more diverse study populations (Katsouyanni, this volume, pp. 51–60).

The limited knowledge on the adverse health effect of air pollutants and the uncertainty involved in the development of air quality standards and guidelines makes it difficult to use them for quantitative risk assessment. Yet they provide a useful tool to monitor air quality and can help decision-makers to plan and monitor air pollution control strategies (Romieu, this volume, pp. 87–99).

The reduction in road accidents and injuries since the 1960s in most western European countries is a success story. Almost all accidents are a consequence of human error and we must continue to encourage safer driving behaviour, especially in moderating speeds and reducing drink-driving. We need to continue the efforts to improve safety further if the downward trend is not to reverse at some time in the future. In Denmark that point is approaching. It is therefore important that the efforts continue in all areas of safety research and policy, since the achievements are based on an integrated and multidisciplinary approach (Bly, this volume, pp. 125–38).

Participants

Scientists basically behave like other human beings in their interpretation of evidence. They are imperfect, influenced by their temperament, personal preferences and particular socio-cultural status. The 'objective' truth of the expert is only one of the many elements in the decision process. The wishes and goals of the population often differ from those of the experts. In the end we must accept that laymen—and women—have to balance the alternatives and decide on the priorities (Steensberg, 1989).

Our public administrations have a built-in tendency to decreasing effectiveness as they expand. Internal hierarchies and outward secrecy may impede an integrated and coordinated implementation of their tasks. Outside pressure for action is necessary to break bureaucratic inertia. Problems that politically have a 'crisis' character are more likely to be tackled wholeheartedly by an agency.

Politicians, in principle, should act as our generalists representing the comprehensive view, although the complexity of problems leads them to some degree of specialization. Yet, their pragmatic, short-term approach to policy-making, which is influenced by the prospects of re-election, tends to leave out even medium-term perspectives. The long-sighted views that are frequently found in party programmes and government declarations are misleading because of the great distance between ideological and practical policy.

Ministers have great difficulties in exercising actual political control over public policy, which in practice tends to be taken over by the administration. The late British Labour Minister of Housing, Richard Crossman, had to realize the tremendous effort it required not to be taken over by the Civil Service (Crossman, 1979). A couple of months after his appointment he made this observation on the administration in his diary:

> They are extremely good at working the procedures of the Civil Service. What they lack is a constructive apprehension of the problems with which they deal and any kind of imagination. Also they are resistant in the extreme to the outside advice which I think it is my job to bring in. So the battle between me and the Ministry will go on as I try to get these admirable officials, conscientious and thorough people, somehow widened, and a little blood pumped into their veins by people from the outside who know the realities which they handle in such an abstract and aloof way.

More than a year after taking office he speculated:

> How far down does my influence stretch? Perhaps to an Assistant Secretary level but certainly not below . . . this means that my policies are transmitted by the senior civil servants to their subordinates merely by word of mouth and very often in an unsympathetic form.

The short cycles of public attention to specific issues like 'environment' that are magnified by the mass media act as strong stimuli to legislation. The changing focus of attention may be important to allow for readjustments in the attitudes of our societies that could otherwise become too static. The episodic way in which the newsmedia take up causes, sensationalism and overreaction may, however, lead legislators towards overambitious rule-making. The media have increasingly concentrated attention around single cases which the politicians are forced to place on the agenda to the detriment of long-term concerns. Yet, in our democratic political systems the media are needed to inform the public and stimulate the authorities to act (Steensberg, 1989).

Organized interest groups are largely recognized as legitimate components of the political system. In, for example, the United States and Scandinavia, corporate systems with strong ties between interest organizations, legislative bodies and public administrations are seen. Groups representing consumers or environmental concerns are in a weak political position, and industrial viewpoints tend to be given more weight than do health and ecological concerns. Epstein (1979) illustrated the complex set of strategies that industry has evolved in support of the *status quo*. The essence of these strategies is to minimize the reality of risks due to a particular product or activity, to maximize the social benefits, and to exaggerate the costs and difficulty of regulation. The elements of these strategies are sometimes presented frankly as industry positions, but they often come from industry spokesmen and academic consultants as 'professional' viewpoints, with no hint of who employs the professionals.

The binding international cooperation within the European Union has in many ways limited the freedom of national administrations to act in the interest of the public's health. EU negotiations are primarily based on the trade and economic effects of a lack of harmonization among member countries although the arguments used in discussions might leave the impression that environmental and health aspects were the main concern. The decision process is complicated and very slow as consensus must be reached. Scientific disputes may act as a cover for controversies of a very different nature. So-called 'package deals' containing quite dissimilar proposed directives are sometimes used to reach political agreement; they have the character of horse trading and health problems tend to be ignored. The resulting compromises may be phrased in complicated regulatory texts that are difficult to adopt and implement at the national level. Conflicts of authority between the different directorates of the huge European Commission bureaucracy do not encourage an emphasis on health considerations. From a public health perspective it is problematic when a health problem is predominantly handled as a technical barrier to trade (Steensberg, 1989).

Intersectoral coordination

Effective prevention of environmental health problems that are the responsibility of several public administrations is difficult to coordinate. All seem in favour of coordination if it can be on their own conditions. The gradual development of mutual trust between agencies is a precondition if intersectoral harmonization is to be more than a gesture. The speed of decision-making is slowed down when several authorities are involved even if well documented and serious acute health problems should be prevented. The reactions of a responsible agency may be particularly slow when the preventive measures are technically complicated and economically demanding, and if, at the same time, there is no heavy pressure from other authorities or societal forces. In general, inter-agency coordination is facilitated if all the relevant authorities are under external stress (Steensberg, 1989).

In a penetrating examination of intersectoral coordination in environmental management, Schaefer (1981) concluded that certain conditions have to be met if environmental coordination is to be more than a gesture. It is necessary to build an effective political base of opinion and power and then to design adequate systems, assign authority, provide resources and translate plans into action. The development of the systems must be monitored, so that they can be adapted as required. In most countries, sectoral bureaucracies have to be brought under a considerable degree of control and given clear, consistent and persistent policy direction, if coordination schemes are not to founder.

The European Charter on Environment and Health identifies urgent issues to which governments and other public authorities should pay particular attention. It mentions urban development, planning and renewal, and the environment and health impact of transport, especially road transport. In the commentary to the Charter (WHO, 1990) it is stated that mechanisms for intersectoral cooperation must be established for policies (such as those related to transport) for strategic and physical planning and for individual developments. In some cases intersectoral collaboration may have to be mandatory; in others it may be effectively achieved by establishing less formal mechanisms. The short-term tensions between environmental health and economic objectives should be openly acknowledged, and there should be intersectoral links with clearly delegated responsibility and public accountability to make sure that these relations are effective.

Gregory Goldstein (this volume, pp. 169–76) has elaborated on the necessary intersectoral work. The health sector must undertake new roles based upon information, and policy and advocacy. He also outlined a communications strategy that allows results to be presented to decision-makers so that their significance for future action becomes evident.

The WHO *Healthy Cities* project has health on the social and political agenda of hundreds of cities, towns and villages all over the world (Hancock, 1993). For the most part we have city governments with departments whose roots are in the 19th century (public health, public works, housing, urban planning, parks etc.). They are trying to come to grips with a set of 21st century issues such as health, sustainability, equity and safety. These new concerns cut across the 19th century departments. Addressing them will need a new style of management. Maybe the 'healthy city movement' could stimulate a new way of organizing and managing our cities—just as the 'health of towns' movement contributed to change in the way cities were managed and governed in the 19th century. Eventually, cities may become 'places to grow people in'.

Policy implementation

The implementation game

The now famous Lalonde Report, 'A new perspective on the health of Canadians' (Lalonde, 1974) and the subsequent policy decisions, in the opinion of Carol Buck (1986), failed to deal adequately with the environment. Buck considered the barriers to achieving an environment that will create health. Possibly the most entrenched barrier is a philosophical one—the belief that an element of misery is part of the human condition. Inertia means that the sheer effort of introducing basic reform is an intrinsic deterrent to action. Another barrier to reform is the fragmented structure of the political and bureaucratic apparatus. The last-mentioned, and powerful, barrier is that of vested interests. To employers, landlords, investors and taxpayers in general, the cost of reform is a strong deterrent to action. Our hearts may be warm, but they are cooled by an examination of our purse.

Most governmental decisions leave considerable leeway in their implementation. Decisions can be reversed or ignored. The opportunity for slippage between decison and action is quite large. The American social scientist Eugene Bardach (1978) conceived of the implementation process as the 'playing of games'. It is a process of assembling the elements required to produce a particular programmatic outcome. It is the playing out of a number of loosely interrelated games whereby these elements are withheld from—or are delivered to—the programme assembly process on particular terms.

Citizens generally assume that, once we pass a law and decide to spend money, the purpose of the law and expenditure shall be achieved. They expect that the intended effects of the policy will be felt by society. These assumptions are not always warranted, but the implementation process does not come as readily to citizens' attention as does the enactment of legislation (Steensberg, 1989).

One of the most important barriers to prevention is delay in the implementation of already codified public policies. Constituencies representing health interests that may have been active in the legislative process tend to switch their interest to other matters once the law has been passed; it is useful if they continue to remind the administration of the original intentions of the legislators.

The implementation process is structured by statutory regulations. The clearer the legislative instructions are that guide the implementation, and the less ambiguous the legal language, the more likely it is that the outcome will be consistent with the intention. Pressure from interested parties may have resulted in idealistic regulations. A realistic picture of the side-effects of such rules may not appear until the implementation phase, resulting in exemptions and dilution of stated goals. The outcome may be a disregard for the long-term health goals in favour of short-sighted economic gains. Therefore, weaker parties such as the general public should be openly informed on the compromises made during the implementation phase.

A number of non-regulatory factors are particularly important for the outcome of environmental health decision-making. The problem of scientific uncertainty, the socio-economic conditions of society and the available technology form a general background that influences the administrative, political and judicial systems and the public. The administration and its political sovereigns not only are stimulated by external national and international forces but also by factors that are internal to the system. If we wish to understand and influence the politics of disease prevention we should pay attention to the characteristics of the implementation process and especially the many non-regulatory factors. A deeper appreciation of environmental health decision-making improves our chances of being able to prevent disease.

Sustainable transport policy

The Danish Ministry of Transport in 1993 published a white paper 'Transport 2005' presenting the Government's views on a sustainable transport policy (Trafikministeriet, 1993). The Danish Government wants to pursue four superior strategies to reach its goals:

1. Influencing the extent, and distribution on means of traffic, of transport work.
2. Improving alternatives to automobile transport.
3. Limiting pollution problems.
4. Strengthening transport planning and research.

The objectives for a sustainable transport policy in the UK suggested by the GB Royal Commission on Environmental Pollution (1994) follow the same general ideas. Targets are proposed for moving towards the objectives, supplemented by specific recommendations about measures that are believed to be needed to achieve the targets. The conclusions of this report are valuable as a background for further action by the British Government and could also give inspiration to decision-makers in other European countries.

'Road transport is not paying its way' says Sir John Houghton, Chair of the Royal Commission. In the opinion of Felix Walter *et al.* (this volume, pp. 287–98) the implementation of the necessary policy measures is not a problem of 'scientific' knowledge but of political acceptance. A green urban transport policy must consist of an 'interdisciplinary and dynamic policy mix', as they put it.

The dominant view among transport policy-makers and advisers of the 1960s and 1970s was that the growth in car use was inevitable and it was necessary to provide sufficient road infrastructure to accommodate it. Yet, it turned out that the provision of road capacity itself caused an acceleration in the growth in traffic (Goodwin, this volume, p. 274). The 'new realism' in the UK since around 1990 is the recognition that, in towns, the supply of road space could not be increased to match demand—which must, therefore, be reduced to match supply. Environmentally-friendly urban transport policies are now frequently presented, but implementation in practice is still lagging far behind agreement on principles. Carmen Hass-Klau (this volume p. 203) argues that Britain and the Continent are drifting apart in this field. She regrets that major elements of a 'car oriented' transport policy have to be pursued in Britain, because alternatives are missing and land use trends have already been set.

Whereas the traditional approach of the 'infrastructure engineers' or 'technicians' have failed or have had limited success, Felix Walter *et al.* (this volume, pp. 294–5) consider that the economic approach may be useful, i.e. through taxes, road pricing and parking fees. Transport costs resulting from environmental effects have so far mostly fallen on the community rather than on the users or the builders of the transport system. Seriously misleading price signals have resulted, leading to decisions in all areas of transport which have harmed the community

(GB Royal Commission on Environmental Pollution, 1994).

Seen in a market economic perspective, the key issue is one of developing balanced transport and related policies which maximize the net contribution of the motor vehicle to society. Kenneth Button acknowledges (this volume, pp. 277–86) that there is something wrong with the economic structures. Markets cannot be accused of having caused the present transport problems but rather markets, as currently operated, do not fully embrace them.

Following discussions at the Forum, a few words on economics, ecology and public health can be added to this text. In fact, the rationality of economics underlies a good deal of the philosophy of public health. Dedicated environmentalists have, however, characterized economics as increasingly being 'madness with a system in it, logical conclusions with forgotten or camouflaged premises'. 'Economics is the true foe of ecology' one of our contemporary Danish poets has said (Bjørnvig, 1978).

The American political scientist Dan Beauchamp has stated (1981) that in a complex society it is most unlikely that market mechanisms will adequately safeguard the interests of the entire class of individuals at risk. Markets cannot provide common or group protections or benefits, only public authorities can do so. He felt that it would be a public health goal to 'socialize' safety. This can be done by introducing safeguards against the predictable and recurrent failures of the marketplace and the political system which is dominated by producer interests.

The present system of transport is the consequence of policy choices over a century or more. Their cumulative effect has been to transform the ways in which land is settled, the ways in which people travel to work, and the ways in which families live. This present transport system is not sustainable. It imposes environmental costs which are so great as to compromise the choices, and the freedom, of future generations (GB Royal Commission on Environmental Pollution, 1994).

As public health workers we naturally pay most attention to the immediate health effects of accidents, air pollution and noise but we should not forget the broader issues of global warming and depleting resources. It may even be wise to pay attention to messages from philosophers, poets and artists stating that nature has rights in itself. It is not only here for the benefit of man.

The philosopher, musician and medical doctor, Albert Schweitzer, held a view of nature, a 'reverence for life', that is a source of inspiration also to public health workers. After having been trained as a medical doctor—he was not sufficiently dogmatic in his religious views to be sent out as a missionary—he knew what his task was in Central Africa in spite of the enormous difficulties he met. When asked whether he was a pessimist or an optimist he replied:

> my cognition makes me a pessimist but my determination and hopes make me an optimist. (Schweitzer, 1931)

Let us face the urban future as optimists!

References

Ashton J (1991) Sanitarian becomes ecologist: the new environmental health. *British Medical Journal*, 302, 189–190

Bardach E (1978) *The Implementation Game: What Happens After a Bill Becomes a Law.* MIT Press, Cambridge (MA)

Beauchamp DE (1976) Public health as social justice. *Inquiry, 13*, 3–14

Beauchamp DE (1981) *Rights, Justice and the Zero-risk Society: a Public Health Perspective on Risk.* (Unpublished paper presented at the annual meeting of the American Public Health Association, Los Angeles, 4 November 1981)

Beauchamp DE (1988) *The Health of the Republic: Epidemics, Medicine and Moralism as Challenges to Democracy.* Temple University Press, Philadelphia

Bjørnvig T (1978) Ogs for naturens skyld (Also for the sake of nature). *Ecological Essays.* Gyldendal, Copenhagen

Buck C (1986) Beyond Lalonde: creating health. *Journal of Public Health Policy, 7*, 444–457

Bugliarello G, Alexandre A, Barnes J (1976) *The Impact of Noise Pollution: a Socio-technological Introduction.* Pergamon Press, New York

Crossman R (1979) *The Crossman Diaries: Selections from the Diaries of a Cabinet Minister, 1964–1970.* Cape, London

Epstein SS (1979) *The Politics of Cancer.* Anchor Press/Doubleday, New York

European Environment Extra (1994) Finding the cure for Europe's hidden epidemic. No. 2

Godlee F (1992) Transport: a public health issue. *British Medical Journal, 304*, 45–50

Great Britain Royal Commission on Environmental Pollution (1971) *First Report.* HMSO, London

Great Britain Royal Commission on Environmental Pollution (1994) *Eighteenth Report: Transport and the Environment.* HMSO, London

Ham C (1990) Analysis of health policy—principles and practice. *Scandinavian Journal of Social Medicine, supplementum, 46*, 62–66

Hancock T (1993) The evolution, impact and significance of the healthy cities/healthy communities movement. *Journal of Public Health Policy, 14*, 5–18

Holland WW, Fitzsimons B (1991) Public health—its critical requirements. In Holland WW, Detels R, Knox G (eds) *Oxford Textbook of Public Health volume 3*, (pp. 605–611). Oxford University Press, Oxford

Lalonde M (1974) *A New Perspective on the Health of Canadians.* Government of Canada, Ottawa

Lange P (1969) Ved Traffikens Bred. *Dyrenes Maskerade.* Denmark

Organisation for Economic Cooperation and Development (1979) *The State of the Environment in OECD Member Countries.* OECD, Paris

Rose G (1991) *The Strategy of Preventive Medicine.* Oxford University Press, Oxford

Schaefer M (1981) *Intersectoral Coordination and Health in Environmental Management: an Examination of National Experience.* Public Health Papers 74. World Health Organization, Geneva

Schweitzer A (1931) *Aus mein Leben und Denken.* Felix Meiner Verlag, Leipzig

Steensberg J (1989) *Environmental Health Decision Making: the Politics of Disease Prevention.* Almqvist & Wiksell International, Copenhagen

Trafikministeriet (1993) *Trafik 2005: Problemstillinger, mål og Strategier.* Trafikministeriet, Copenhagen

WHO (1990) *Environment and Health. The European Charter and Commentary.* WHO Regional Publications No. 35, Copenhagen

Wohl AS (1983) *Endangered Lives: Public Health in Victorian Britain.* Dent, London

Index

Note: page numbers in *italics* refer to figures and tables

Index compiled by Jill Halliday